Exam Preparatory Manual for Undergraduates

DENTAL MATERIALS

Exam Preparatory Manual for Undergraduates

DENTAL MATERIALS

Editor

Lovely M MDS

Professor

Department of Prosthodontics

Sree Mookambika Institute of Dental Sciences

Kulasekharam, Tamil Nadu, India

Foreword

K Chandrasekharan Nair

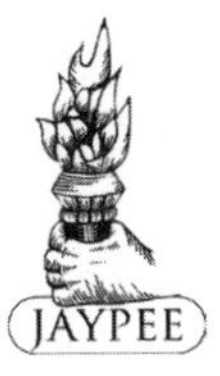

The Health Sciences Publisher

New Delhi | London | Philadelphia | Panama

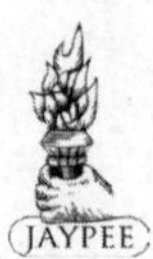

Jaypee Brothers Medical Publishers (P) Ltd.

Headquarters
Jaypee Brothers Medical Publishers (P) Ltd.
4838/24, Ansari Road, Daryaganj
New Delhi 110 002, India
Phone: +91-11-43574357
Fax: +91-11-43574314
E-mail: jaypee@jaypeebrothers.com

Overseas Offices

J.P. Medical Ltd.
83, Victoria Street, London
SW1H 0HW (UK)
Phone: +44-20 3170 8910
Fax: +44(0)20 3008 6180
E-mail: info@jpmedpub.com

Jaypee-Highlights Medical Publishers Inc.
City of Knowledge, Bld. 235, 2nd Floor, Clayton
Panama City, Panama
Phone: +1 507-301-0496
Fax: +1 507-301-0499
E-mail: cservice@jphmedical.com

Jaypee Medical Inc.
325, Chestnut Street
Suite 412
Philadelphia, PA 19106, USA
Phone: +1 267-519-9789
E-mail: support@jpmedus.com

Jaypee Brothers Medical Publishers (P) Ltd.
17/1-B, Babar Road, Block-B, Shaymali
Mohammadpur, Dhaka-1207
Bangladesh
Mobile: +08801912003485
E-mail: jaypeedhaka@gmail.com

Jaypee Brothers Medical Publishers (P) Ltd.
Bhotahity, Kathmandu, Nepal
Phone: +977-9741283608
E-mail: kathmandu@jaypeebrothers.com

Website: www.jaypeebrothers.com
Website: www.jaypeedigital.com

Inquiries for bulk sales may be solicited at: jaypee@jaypeebrothers.com

Exam Preparatory Manual for Undergraduates: Dental Materials

First Edition: **2016**

ISBN: 978-93-86056-80-1

Printed at Rajkamal Electric Press, Plot No. 2, Phase-IV, Kundli, Haryana.

Dedicated to

The Almighty God

My Professor

Dr K Chandrasekharan Nair

My Dear Husband

Dr Biji Thomas George

Contributors

Adeela Rafique BDS MSc
Assistant Professor
Department of Operative Dentistry
FMH College of Medicine and Dentistry
Lahore, Pakistan

Anil Kishen BDS MDS PhD
Associate Professor
Discipline of Endodontics
Faculty of Dentistry
University of Toronto
Ontario, Canada

Lekshmi Arun BDS MDS
Reader
Department of Conservative Dentistry
Sri Sai College of Dental Surgery
Vikarabad, Telangana, India

Lovely M MDS
Professor
Department of Prosthodontics
Sree Mookambika Institute of Dental Sciences
Kulasekharam, Tamil Nadu, India

Rajesh S Nair BDS MDS
Professor and Head
Department of Conservative Dentistry
Sree Mookambika Institute of Dental Sciences
Kulasekharam, Tamil Nadu, India

Savitha P Rao MSc
Assistant Professor
Department of Prosthodontics
Vokkaligara Sangha (VS) Dental
College and Hospital
Bengaluru, Karnataka, India

Shilpa Shetty MDS
International College of Oral
Implantologist (ICOI) Diplomate
Editor-in-Chief
The Journal of Indian Prosthodontic Society
Professor
Department of Prosthodontics
Vokkaligara Sangha (VS) Dental
College and Hospital
Bengaluru, Karnataka, India

V Prasanth BDS MDS
Faculty Member
Department of Prosthodontics
Government Dental College
Thiruvananthapuram, Kerala, India

Foreword

The science of dental materials began in the laboratory of GV Black at Northwestern University in 1900 with the first controlled experiments on dental amalgam.

The science progressed when excellent textbooks became available, for example, *The Science of Dental Materials* (1936) by EW Skinner. In the earlier times, dental material science focused exclusively on gypsum, waxes, metals and resins. By the early 1970s, dental materials acquired the status of biomaterials.

Ever since, the science has become more sophisticated. The specialty of dentistry has progressed with the turn of events that have occurred in the field of dental materials.

The recent times have witnessed the emergence of dental implants and incorporation of advanced technology of computer-aided system/computer-aided manufacturing (CAD/CAM). Dentists now require predictable results on bonding, esthetics and longevity of the restorations. Partly this is due to the enhanced patient demand for natural looking teeth which presumably would improve the self-esteem.

The study of dental materials has become an integral part of dentistry and the students should be well-versed with the nuances of modern developments. The transition from micro-levels to nano-levels and from generations of bonding to component-based total etching/self-etching systems would normally complicate the students' perception. But Dr Lovely M has candidly addressed the subject with a student's point of view.

I have no doubt that this book would enlighten generations of young dentists.

K Chandrasekharan Nair MDS
Professor
Department of Prosthodontics
Amrith Educational and Cultural Society (AECS)
Maaruti College of Dental Sciences
Bengaluru, Karnataka, India

Preface

This is the fourth in the sequence of study guides, the others being *Review of Complete Dentures, Review of Fixed Partial Dentures* and *Review of Removable Partial Dentures*.

Originally intended for the sole benefit of BDS students, the scope of this book is now expanded to include students and the dental fraternity in general, after receiving extremely positive feedback for the earlier books.

The objective of the book is to assist the students in understanding the principles involved in answering questions in essays and short notes format in the University Examinations in Dental Materials.

In normal circumstances, each question needs to be read at least twice to make sure the intended answer is correct and further time is lost in formulating the answer to suit the question.

In comparison to standard textbooks, the book is deliberately made succinct and precise, yet informative and exhaustive, thereby ensuring its suitability for last minute examination, preparation and review.

A careful perusal of the contents of the book will, therefore, enable the candidate to quickly grasp the question and to format an appropriate answer without loss of valuable time. Thus, the candidate secures himself or herself sufficient time to write and revise the answers in the short period allotted.

In response to the persistent demands received from many students, the book also includes the multiple choice questions (MCQs). Thus, in addition to aiding BDS candidates, it will be of great assistance to the students during their preparations for the entrance examinations and the first part examination of their MDS course too.

A topic on *Recent Advances in Dental Materials* has also been included for the benefit of students as well as for the interest of dentists in general.

I sincerely hope that our endeavor will be rewarded by the acceptance of the book by the dental fraternity.

Lovely M

Acknowledgments

I am extremely grateful to Professor K Chandrasekharan Nair, Professor, Department of Prosthodontics, Amrith Educational and Cultural Society (AECS), Maaruti College of Dental Sciences, Bengaluru, Karnataka, India, for encouragement and support despite his busy schedule.

I am thankful to my department colleagues, Dr SC Ahila, Dr NS Manikantan and Dr VM Shaju for all the help, and Dr James J Rex, Dr Vini K Varkey, and Dr Veena Baby for drawing the graphs and pictures. I especially wish to thank Dr Sandeep Krishna of SK Hospital, Thiruvananthapuram, Kerala, India, for helping me collect the question papers. I also thank Mr Rajesh Kumar D for all the computer typing and picture editing.

I also thank Dr Rema V Nair (MD, DGO), Director, Sree Mookambika Institute of Dental Sciences, Kulasekharam, Tamil Nadu, India, for providing the library facilities and help for the completion of this book.

Dr Anil Kishen, who contributed *Recent Advances in Dental Materials* along with Dr Adeela Rafique, is a renowned researcher and teacher in Dental Materials at the National University of Singapore and has numerous publications in this field; Dr Rajesh S Nair, who contributed *Multiple Choice Questions (MCQs) in Dental Materials in Restorative Dentistry*; Dr Lekshmi Arun, who contributed *Essays and Short Notes in Dental Materials in Restorative Dentistry*; Dr V Prasanth, who contributed *MCQs in Dental Materials in Prosthodontics*; and Dr Shilpa Shetty and Ms Savitha P Rao contributed *Recent Advances in Prosthodontic-related Dental Materials*. Two years of hard work put in by all the contributors have finally led to its completion in the present form.

I deeply thank all the contributors for their patience, effort and prompt work.

Last but not least, I thank my son Joshua George Thomas for tolerating the many hours of computer work patiently and letting me complete this endeavor. The book could not have been possible without the support and editing done by my husband Dr Biji Thomas George.

Contents

ESSAYS

SHORT NOTES

MULTIPLE CHOICE QUESTIONS

ANSWERS TO MULTIPLE CHOICE QUESTIONS

INVITED REVIEW ARTICLES

Essays

1. Define proportional limit, yield strength and ultimate tensile strength. Draw and label a stress-strain diagram.

PROPORTIONAL LIMIT

Proportional limit is defined as the greatest stress that a material will sustain without a deviation from the linear proportionality of stress to strain.

A material does not deform if the stress applied to a material is below the proportional limit value. Also, after the applied stress is removed, the material regains its original dimension.

YIELD STRENGTH/YIELD STRESS

The yield strengths is defined as the stress at which a material exhibits a specified limiting deviation from proportionality of stress to strain.

It is the stress at which the material starts to function in a plastlc manner in which a limited permanent strain has occurred in the material.

The amount of permanent strain may be indicated as 0.1%, 0.2%, or 0.5% of permanent strain. The amount of percent strain may be referred to as the percent offset.

On the stress-strain curve, the yield strength is represented by the value *y*. The parallel line bisecting the stress-strain curve is yield strength.

ULTIMATE TENSILE STRENGTH

The ultimate tensile strength is defined as the maximum stress that a material can withstand before failure in tension occurs.

After a maximum stress is applied to a material, it begins to elongate, and the stress calculated from the force and the original cross-sectional area before the final fracture occurs is the ultimate tensile strength.

The stress at the end of the curve is less than at some intermediate point on the curve.

An alloy that has been stressed to near the ultimate tensile strength will be permanently deformed.

Tensile Properties of Brittle Materials

Brittle materials are made into dumbbell-shaped specimens of known cross section and held in special grips to permit axial tensile loading with a minimum of localized stress concentration.

The other methods of testing brittle materials are by diametral compression test for tension, the Brazilian test, or the indirect tensile test.

The tensile stress is directly proportional to the load applied in compression.

$$\text{Tensile stress} = \frac{\text{Load}}{(\text{Diameter} \times \text{thickness})}$$

At stresses above the proportional limit (point PL), the actual stress curve (dashed line) terminates at the higher UTS (ultimate tensile strength) value, or at the point of fracture.

Cross-section of the wire decreases as it lengthens under tensile stress.

The ultimate tensile strength is based on the initial area (lower UTS value).

The decrease in cross-sectional area of the wire and the actual or true stress-strain curve is indicated by the upper solid line.

STRESS-STRAIN CURVES

The stress-strain relationship of dental materials can be measured by calculating the load and deformation.

The testing of many materials requires loads of 220 N (500 lb) or more and the measurement of deformations of 0.02 mm or less at uniform rates.

Method of Measurement

- The load is measured electronically with a strain-gauge transducer and recorded on the horizontal axis of the strip-chart recorder
- The deformation is measured when an extensometer is clamped over a given length of the sample and the deformation is recorded on the vertical axis of the recorder
- The measurements can be converted to a plot of stress versus strain by simple calculations
- The area of specimen remains constant during the test. This curve is called an engineering stress-strain curve
- Stress-strain curves for two hypothetical materials of different composition are shown as stress-strain curve **(Fig. 1)**
- The stress in MN/nv is plotted vertically and the strain is plotted horizontally
- Hence, it is seen that for each material as the stress is increased, the strain is increased and as the stress is doubled, the amount of strain is also doubled.

Properties of Stress-strain Curves

The stress-strain curves represent materials with various combinations of physical properties. The stiffness, strength, ductility and toughness can be evaluated. This can be done in the same stress-strain graph **(Fig. 2)**.

The material obeys Hooke's law; the elastic stress will be proportional to elastic strain.

For such a material, the stress-strain diagram starts from the origin (O) as a straight line. Along this linear path, the material behaves elastically and it springs back to its initial shape and size at the instant the force is removed.

After a certain stress value, the line becomes nonlinear and stress is no longer proportional to strain.

The stress value at P, the point above which the curve begins from a straight line, is known as the *proportional limit*.

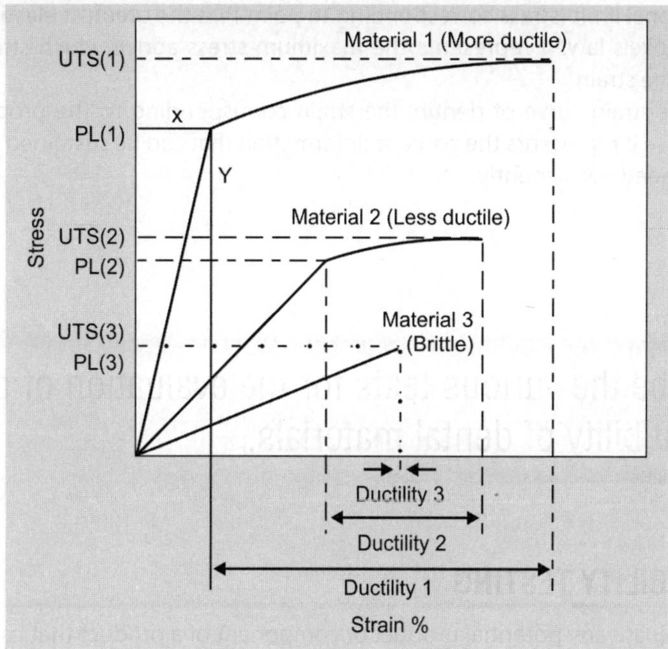

Fig. 1: Stress-strain plots of materials that exhibit different mechanical properties
Abbreviations: UTS, ultimate tensile strength; PL, proportional limit

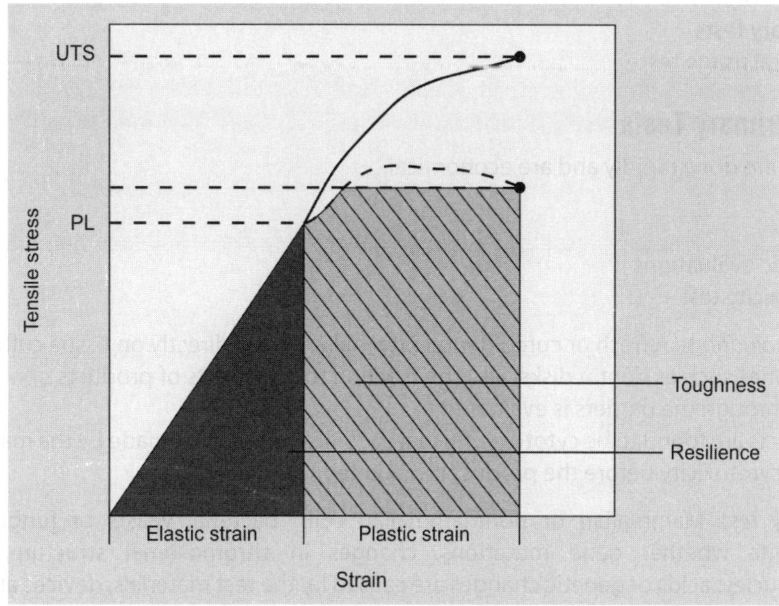

Fig. 2: Proportional Limit
Abbreviations: UTS, ultimate tensile strength; PL, proportional limit

The proportional limit (stress corresponding to point P) is the greatest elastic stress possible according to Hooke's law. It represents the maximum stress above which stress is no longer proportional to the strain.

For the stress-strain curve of dentin, the strain corresponding to the proportional limit is important because it represents the percent deformation that can be sustained in dentin before it becomes damaged permanently.

2. Describe the various tests for the evaluation of biocompatibility of dental materials.

BIOCOMPATIBILITY TESTING

It is done to eliminate any potential product or component of a product that can cause harm or damage to oral or maxillofacial tissues.

CLASSIFICATION OF BIOCOMPATIBILITY TESTS

- Primary tests
- Secondary tests
- Preclinical usage tests.

Group I: Primary Tests

These tests are done rapidly and are economical.

Types

- Cytotoxic evaluations
- Genotoxicity test.

Cytotoxic evaluations: A fresh or cured dental material is placed directly on tissue culture cells or on membranes such as dentin disks, and the reaction to the effects of products or components that leach through the barriers is evaluated.

If products are found to be cytotoxic, further modifications can be made by the manufacturer to prevent cytotoxicity before the product is marketed.

Genotoxicity test: Mammalian or nonmammalian cells, bacteria, yeasts or fungi are used to determine whether gene mutations, changes in chromosomal structure, or other deoxyribonucleic acids or genetic changes are caused by the test materials, devices and extracts from materials.

Group II: Secondary Tests

At this level, the product is evaluated for its potential to create systemic toxicity, inhalation toxicity, skin irritation, and sensitization and implantation responses.

Systemic Toxicity Tests

In the systemic toxicity tests such as the oral median lethal dose (LD50) test, the test sample is administered daily to rats for 14 days either by oral dosage or by dietary inclusion. If 50% of the animals survive, the product has passed the test.

Efforts are being made to develop other systemic toxicity tests that require far fewer animals.

Dermal Toxicity Tests

The dermal toxicity test is important because of the great number of chemical substances that are capable of producing an inflammatory response in most susceptible people after the first exposure. Once a toxic material, product, or component is identified, it can be replaced, diluted, neutralized and chelated to reduce the risk for toxicity.

Irritation is defined as an inflammation brought about without the intervention of an antibody or immune system.

Sensitization is an inflammatory response requiring the participation of an antibody system specific for the material allergen in question.

To simulate dermal toxicity, the test material is held in contact with the shaved skin of albino rats/guinea pig for periods ranging from 24 (one exposure) to 90 days (with repeated exposures). The animal must receive an occlusive covering to prevent mechanical loss of the contacting agent, even by evaporation.

An *allergen* is defined as a substance that is not primarily irritating on the first exposure but produces reactions more rapidly in subsequent exposure to similar concentrations.

Method of testing:

- The test material is introduced intradermally and, after 24 hours, the resulting dermal reaction is assessed
- For the main test, the highest concentration of the test material that causes no more than slight erythema and edema is selected
- After an interval of 7 days, the test material of the same concentration is placed on gauze patches and applied to cover the previously injected sites
- Fourteen days later, the test material is applied to the shaved flank of the animals. After removal of the dressings at 24, 48 and 72 hours, the skin reactions at the sites are evaluated and graded.

Inhalation Toxicity Tests

- These are performed on rats, rabbits or guinea pigs in an exposure chamber with aerosol preparations by releasing the spray material around the head and upper trunk of the animals. The animals are subjected to 30 seconds of continuous spray at 30-minute intervals
- After 10 consecutive exposures, the animals are observed over a 4-day period
- If any animal dies within 2–3 minutes, the agent is considered very toxic.

Implantation Tests

- The use of in vivo implantation techniques helps to review the physical characteristics of the product, such as form, density, hardness and surface finish that can influence the character of the tissue response
- The animal species is selected according to the size of the implant test specimen and the duration of the test in relation to the life span of the animal
- For short-term tests (12 weeks) in subcutaneous tissue or muscle, animals such as mice, rats, hamsters, guinea pigs and rabbits are commonly used
- For long-term tests (2–12 weeks) in muscle or bone, animals such as rabbits, dogs, sheep, goats and subhuman primates are used. For subcutaneous and muscle implantation, the test implant material is packed into various types of plastic tubes (variations of polyethylene or teflon)
- For bone implantation, the lateral cortex of a femur or a tibia or both are exposed and holes are drilled using low-speed, intermittent cutting under profuse irrigation with physiologic saline solution to prevent overheating of the bone
- Cylinders of the test implant material are inserted into the drilled holes by finger pressure
- The diameter of the implant and the implant bed in the bone must match well
- Histopathologic evaluation for the formation of new bone without intervening connective tissue is done.

Group III: Preclinical Usage Tests

The US Food and Drug Administration (FDA) can approve a product after passing the primary and secondary tests

Dental materials have a long 7-year period to prove efficacy after the product has reached the open market with FDA approval.

The product is required to have the ADA Seal of Acceptance after all the biologic, laboratory and clinical evaluations.

Implant materials require more long-term data.

Pulp and Dentin Usage Test

- This test is designed to assess the biocompatibility of dental materials placed in dentin adjacent to the dental pulp
- Nonrodent mammals with recently erupted, intact permanent teeth are selected and Class V cavity preparations are done with 1 mm or less of tubular dentin between the floor of the cavity preparation and the pulp. Some cavities are retained for control specimens
- As a negative control, zinc oxide-eugenol (ZOE) is used
- For a positive control, Class V cavity preparations are done and are luted under pressure
- The animals are then sacrificed after 7 days, 28 ± 3 days and 70 ± 5 days, routine histopathologic processing of the specimens are done and are graded for degree of inflammatory response, reparative dentin formation in the pulp and microleakage.

Biocompatible materials cause minimum or no pulpal response.

Pulp Capping and Pulpotomy Usage Tests

- A calcium hydroxide (CH) product is used as a negative control. The animals are sacrificed after 7 ± 2 days and 70 ± 5 days
- Biocompatible materials form a bridge directly against the capping material, with minimal destruction of pulp tissue at the time the pulp capping agent was applied.

Endodontic Usage Tests

- For this test, the same types of animals are used, but the pulp is completely or almost completely removed from the pulp chamber and root canals, and replaced by the obturating test material and control material ZOE alone or ZOE combined with a sealer
- The animals are sacrificed after 28 ± 3 days and 13 ± 1 weeks
- The teeth are removed together with their surrounding apical periodontal (soft and hard) tissues in a single block, and degree of inflammation is evaluated in the periapical tissues.

Amalgam Controversy the Latest Update

The use of mercury in dental fillings is considered safe and effective in all countries practicing modern dentistry except Norway and Sweden, that have introduced legislation to prohibit or restrict use of amalgam fillings.

World Health Organization (WHO) has suggested phasing down of Amalgam use over a period of time.

3. Classify dental impression materials. What is the composition of an ideal irreversible hydrocolloid impression material? How is it manipulated? What are the failures associated and merits with the use of this material?

CLASSIFICATION OF IMPRESSION MATERIALS

- Elastic
- Inelastic/Rigid impression materials.

Elastic Impression Materials

- Hydrocolloids
- Elastomeric impression materials.

Hydrocolloids

- Agar (reversible)
- Alginate (irreversible).

Elastomeric Impression Material

- Addition silicone
- Condensation silicone
- Polyether
- Polysulfide.

Rigid Impression Materials

- Impression plaster
- Impression waxes
- Zinc oxide eugenol
- Impression compound
- American Dental Association (ADA) classification
- Classification of impression materials.

Nonelastics

- Impression compound
- Impression plaster
- Waxes
- Zinc oxide-eugenol.

Aqueous Elastomers

- Reversible hydrocolloids (agar)
- Irreversible hydrocolloids (alginate).

Nonaqueous Elastomers

- Polysulfides
- Condensation polymerizing silicones
- Addition polymerizing silicones [poly(vinyl siloxanes)]
- Polyethers.

ALGINATE

- ANSI/ADA Specification No. 18.

Composition

Substance	%	Function
Potassium alginate	(18%)	Reacts with calcium ions
Calcium sulfate dihydrate	(14%)	Reacts with potassium alginate to form insoluble calcium alginate gel

Contd...

Contd...

Potassium sulfate/Potassium zinc fluoride	(10%)	Gypsum hardener
Tri-sodium phosphate	(2%)	Retarder (Increases the working time)
Diatomaceous earth	(56%)	Filler
Organic glycols	Traces	For dustless alginates
Wintergreen, peppermint	Traces	For flavor
Pigments	Traces	Color
Ammonium salts and chlorhexidine	2%	Disinfectant

Components and their Functions

Filler

Diatomaceous earth increases the strength and stiffness of the alginate gel, produces a smooth texture and ensures a firm gel surface that is not tacky. It also aids in forming the sol by dispersing the alginate powder particles in the water.

Zinc oxide acts as a filler and influences the physical properties and setting time of the gel.

The amount of filler present controls the flexibility of the set impression material from what is called soft-set to hard-set. The injection type is more fluid after mixing and more flexible after setting.

Retarder

The concentration of sodium phosphate differs depending on regular and fast-set alginates. There are tray and injection types available.

Retarders are sodium or potassium phosphate, potassium oxalate, or potassium carbonate, trisodium phosphate, sodium tripolyphosphate and tetrasodium pyrophosphate. The latter two are now the most commonly used.

If approximately 15 g of the powder is mixed with 40 mL of water, gelation will occur in about 3 to 4 minutes at room temperature.

Reactor

Any type of calcium sulfate can be used as the reactor. The dihydrate form is generally used, but sometimes the hemihydrate form is used as it produces an increased shelf life of the powder and gives better dimensional stability of the gel.

Gypsum Hardener

Potassium titanium fluoride is added as an accelerator for the setting of the stone to ensure that a hard, dense stone cast surface is produced against the impression.

Shelf Life

Materials should be stored in a cool environment.

Gelation Process

Reaction

- Alginic acid is prepared from a plant and is a linear polymer of anhydro-β-D-mannuronic acid of high molecular weight
- The potassium, sodium and ammonium salts of alginic acid when reacted by a calcium salt produce an elastic gel
- When potassium alginate salt reacts with calcium sulfate dihydrate, calcium alginate gel and Potassium sulfate is formed
- The soluble alginate and the calcium sulfate dihydrate are both included in the powder and as the powder is mixed it reacts with sodium phosphate to form insoluble calcium phosphate
- Calcium sulfate reacts rapidly to produce the insoluble calcium alginate from the potassium or sodium alginate in an aqueous solution
- A third water-soluble salt, trisodium phosphate, prolongs the working time
- Calcium sulfate will react with the other salt in preference to the soluble alginate till the trisodium phosphate is exhausted.

$$2NaPO_4 + 3CaSO_4 \rightarrow Ca\,(PO_4)_2 + 3Na_2SO_4$$

When the supply of trisodium phosphate is exhausted, the calcium ions begin to react with the potassium alginate to produce calcium alginate as follows:

$$K_2\,n\ \text{Alginate} + n\ CaSO_4 \rightarrow n\ K_2SO_4 + \text{Ca Alginate}$$

Gel Structure

In a sodium or potassium alginate, the cation is attached at a carboxyl group to form an ester or a salt.

When the insoluble salt formed by the reaction of the sodium alginate in solution reacts with the calcium salt, the calcium ions replace the sodium ions in two adjacent molecules to produce a cross-linking between the two molecules.

As the reaction progresses, a cross-linked molecular complex or polymer network forms. This network resembles a brush-heap structure of the gel.

The final structure is a brush heap of a calcium alginate fibril network enclosing unreacted sodium alginate sol, excess water, filler particles and reaction byproducts, such as sodium sulfate and calcium phosphate.

Availability

- Preweighed for an individual impression
- Bulk form in a can
- The two-component system consists of two pastes; one contains the alginate sol and the other contains the calcium reactor.

MANIPULATION

Proportioning and Mixing

Water/Powder Ratio

- 15 g in 40 mL of water

- A powder and water scoop is provided for accurate proportioning by volume
- Changes in the water/powder ratio will alter the consistency, setting times of the mixed material and the strength and quality of the impression.

Mixing Time

- For regular alginate, it is 1 minute
- For fast-set alginates, it is 45 seconds.

Working Time

- The fast-set materials have working times of 1.25 to 2 minutes
- Mixing time of 45 seconds for the fast-set types
- The working time of the regular-set materials may be from 3 minutes to 4.5 minutes
- Mixing time should not exceed 60 seconds.

Setting Time

- Setting times range from 1 to 5 minutes
- The ANSI/ADA specification requires no less than 1 minute or more than 2 minutes for the fast-set materials and no less than 2 minutes or more than 4.5 minutes for the regular-set materials.

Factors Affecting Setting Time

Setting time can be increased by:

- Reducing the temperature of the water, not advisable to use water cooler than 18°C or warmer than 24°C for mixing
- Altering the water-powder ratio will reduce the strength and accuracy of the alginate
- Slow setting alginate can be used.

Controlling Gelation Time

- The gelation time is measured from the beginning of mixing until gelation occurs. It is the time from the start of mixing until the material is no longer tacky or sticky when it is touched
- The optimal gelation time is between 3 and 4 minutes at room temperature (20°C)
- For fast setting (1–2 minutes) and normal setting alginate (2.5–4 minutes)
- Gelation time is best regulated by the amount of retarder added during manufacturing
- The higher the temperature, the shorter is the gelation time.

MERITS AND DEMERITS OF IRREVERSIBLE IMPRESSION MATERIAL

Strength

- Maximum gel strength is required to prevent fracture and to ensure elastic recovery of the impression on its removal from the mouth
- Strength is altered if too much or too little water is used in mixing. Insufficient spatulation results in failure of the ingredients to dissolve sufficiently. Over-mixing breaks up the calcium alginate gel network as it is forming and reduces its strength.

Viscoelasticity

The tear strength is increased when the impression is removed with a snap. The speed of removal must be a compromise between a rapid movement and the comfort of the patient.

Accuracy

- Most alginate impression materials are not capable of reproducing the finer details as that of other elastomeric impression materials
- The roughness of the impression surface is sufficient to cause distortion at the margins of prepared teeth
- Surfactants can be used to produce a smooth surface, but addition of a layer of solution over the surface of the impression also obscures the accuracy.

Dimensional Stability

Once the impression is removed from the mouth and exposed to the air at room temperature, shrinkage or evaporation results in **syneresis** and, if the impression is immersed in water, swelling will occur due to **imbibition**.

Compatibility with Gypsum

All forms of gypsum are compatible with hydrocolloid impression as gypsum hardener (titanium fluoride) or accelerator is used in the material.

Disinfection

- The irreversible hydrocolloids may be disinfected by 10-minute immersion in, or spraying with, an antimicrobial agent such as sodium hypochlorite and glutaraldehyde
- After disinfecting, the impression is wrapped in a disinfectant-soaked paper towel, placed in a sealed plastic bag for 10 minutes and later the model is poured.

FAILURES WITH REVERSIBLE AND IRREVERSIBLE HYDROCOLLOID IMPRESSION MATERIALS

Effects of Mishandling

Grainy Material

- Improper mixing
- Prolonged mixing
- Undue gelation
- Water-powder ratio too low.

Separation of Tray

- Adhesive not applied
- Lack of mechanical interlocking.

Tearing

- Inadequate bulk
- Premature removal from mouth
- Moisture contamination
- Premature removal from when tray seated in mouth
- Prolonged mixing.

External Bubbles

- Air incorporated during mixing.

Irregularly Shaped

- Material too cool or grainy
- Moisture or debris on tissue voids.

Rough or Chalky

- Inadequate cleansing of impression
- Inadequate cleaning of stone model
- Excess water or potassium sulfate solution left in impression
- Premature removal of impression
- Improper manipulation of stone
- Premature removal of model
- Leaving model in impression pouring too long.

Distortion

- Impression not poured immediately
- Movement of tray during gelation
- Premature removal from mouth
- Movement of tray during gelation
- Improper removal from mouth.

ADDITIONAL APPLICATIONS OF HYDROCOLLOIDS

Laminate Technique

This is the combined agar-alginate technique. The tray hydrocolloid is replaced with a mix of chilled alginate that bonds to the syringe agar.

Disadvantages

- The bond between the agar and the alginate is not always strong
- The higher viscosity alginate displaces the agar during seating
- The dimensional inaccuracy of the alginate limits the use to single units.

Duplicating Materials

To duplicate dental casts or models, hydrocolloid-type duplicating materials are used. They have the same composition as the impression materials, but their water content is higher.

Recent Developments

Dustless Alginates

The material is coated with a glycol.

Ionized Alginates

Two-paste alginates have developed which incorporate a silicone component which have superior tear resistance compared to unmodified alginate.

Color Changing Fast Setting Alginate (Kerr)

Advantages

3-step color change, 120 hours dimensional stability, optimal tear strength and low deformation:
- Working time—1.50 min
- Setting time—2.30 min.

AgiNot FS AlgiNot FS™ (Alternative to Alginate)

Advantages

- Cost-effective, good accuracy and performance
- AlgiNot is also available as fast set
- The improved thixotropic consistency reduces slumping and displacement from the impression tray
- No hand mixing (cartridge or Volume™ automix dispensing)
- A single impression can yield multiple stone pours
- Impressions remain stable and can be disinfected
- Work time (Cartridge): 1 min/Set time (Cartridge): 2 min
- Work time (Volume): 1.15 min/Set time (Volume): 2.15 min.

4. What are colloids? Discuss the composition, manipulation and properties of agar.

COLLOIDS

The word 'colloid' is derived from 'kola', meaning glue.

A colloid is a heterogenous mixture of two phases, where the two phases are not readily differentiated (the colloidal state represents a highly dispersed phase of fine particles within another phase, somewhere between a solution and a suspension).

AGAR

Agar is an organic hydrophilic colloid (polysaccharide) extracted from certain types of seaweed. It is a sulphuric ester of a linear polymer of galactose.

Filler controls the strength, viscosity and rigidity of the impression material.

Composition

- Agar (8–15%)
- Water (80%)
- Borax (Increases the strength or density of the micelle)
- Potassium sulfate (accelerator)
- Diatomaceous earth, clay, silica, wax, rubber and similar inert powders (filler)
- Thymol (bactericide)
- Glycerine (plasticizer)
- Pigments and flavours (traces).

MANIPULATION OF AGAR IMPRESSION MATERIALS

Gelation Process

- Gelation is the conversion from sol to gel. It is a solidification process. The physical change from the sol to gel is due to temperature change. To return to sol state, the gel must be heated to a liquefaction temperature (70°–100°C)
- It transforms into a gel between 37° and 50°C.

Factors Affecting Gelation

- The molecular weight
- The purity of the agar
- Ratio of agar to other ingredients.

Availability

- The material is supplied in sealed containers to prevent evaporation of water
- It is brought to a fluid state by heating the tube in boiling water in a processing unit for 10 to 45 minutes
- After boiling, the material can be stored at 65°C for up to 8 hours
- It is important that the entire tube of material is softened.

Steps in Manipulation

- Advanced preparation of the material
- Preparation immediately before making the impression
- The making of the impression.

Preparation of the Material

- The hydrocolloid is usually supplied in two forms—syringe and tray materials
- The only difference between the syringe and tray material is the color and a greater fluidity of the syringe material
- The first step is to convert the material from gel to the sol state by placing the material in liquefaction bath at 100°C for a minimum of 10 minutes
- After it has been liquefied, the material is stored in the sol condition until it is needed for injection into the cavity preparation or for filling the tray.

Preparation Immediately before Making the Impression

Conditioning or tempering:

- A tube of hydrocolloid sol is removed from the storage bath
- The tray is filled
- A gauze pad is placed over the top of the tray material
- The tray is placed in the tempering section for 3–10 minutes at 45°C.

Points to follow during preparation of the material:

- The loaded tray should not be kept in the bath for more than 10 minutes
- Gauze is placed on the material loaded on tray before placing it in the storage bath to prevent imbibition
- The gauze is removed and the contaminated surface layer of material is peeled off along with the gauze
- This fresh surface adheres easily to the syringed material that was injected over the prepared teeth
- The syringe material is taken from the storage bath and applied to the prepared tooth surface
- When the material is extruded from the syringe, the temperature lowers further.

Impression Making

- The tray is positioned and seated with light pressure and held in place passively
- Gelation is achieved by circulating cool water, approximately 18° to 21°C through the tray for 3 to 5 minutes
- Waiting an extra minute greatly increases the strength and tear resistance
- The impression is removed with a sudden jerk.

Wet Field Technique

It is a type of impression technique in which the areas before impression are flooded with warm water and the syringe material is introduced quickly to cover the occlusal and incisal areas. The tray material is then seated over the syringe material.

Agar-alginate Combination Impressions

In this procedure, a syringe type of agar in a cartridge is heated in boiling water for 6 minutes and stored in a 65°C water bath 10 minutes before use.

Method of impression

- The regular set type is mixed with 10% more water and placed in a tray
- The agar is injected around the preparation and the mixed alginate is seated on top of the agar
- The alginate sets in about 3 minutes and the agar gels within this time as a result of being cooled by the alginate
- During the setting of the alginate and gelling of the agar, a bond forms between them
- The impression may be removed in about 4 minutes.

PROPERTIES

Viscoelastic Properties

The elastic recovery of the hydrocolloid is never complete and it does not return entirely to its original dimension after deformation.

Permanent Deformation is Avoided when

- The material has adequately gelled
- The impression has been removed rapidly
- The undercuts present in the cavity preparation are minimal.

Distortion during Gelation

- Occurs during the transformation from a sol to a gel
- As the sol is a poor thermal conductor, rapid cooling may cause a concentration of stress near the tray where the gelation first takes place
- Water at approximately 20°C is more suitable for cooling.

Reproducibility

Multiple cast cannot be poured.

Double-die technique

- One impression is made and cut apart into individual dies of the prepared teeth
- The second impression is made in a triple tray so that both arches and the occlusal relationship are recorded
- Both maxillary and mandibular impressions are poured at the same time and attached to a simple hinge articulator.

Gelation Temperature

After boiling for 8 minutes, the material should be fluid enough to be extruded from the container.

After tempering, the sol should be homogenous and should set to a gel between 37° and 45°C when cooled, as required by ANSI/ADA Specification No. 11.

Permanent Deformation

Permanent deformation should be less than 1.5% after the material is compressed 10% for 30 seconds. This permanent deformation is slightly lower than that of alginate impression materials.

Flexibility

The ANSI/ADA Specification requirement for flexibility allows a range of 4% to 15%.

Strength

- The compressive strength of a typical agar impression material is 8000 g/cm^2
- ANSI/ADA Specification minimum is 2500 g/cm^2
- The tear strength of agar impression materials is about 700 g/cm.

Compatibility with Gypsum

- Not all agar impression materials are equally compatible with all gypsum products
- The impression should be washed free from saliva and any trace of blood, which retard the setting of gypsum
- The washed impression is blown with an air syringe.

Dimensional Stability

- When stored in air, agar gels lose water and contract
- Replacing the agar in water resulted in absorption and swelling
- Agar impressions are best stored in 100% relative humidity and should be poured in one hour.

5. What are the ideal requisites of an impression material? Mention the composition, properties, advantages and disadvantages of addition silicone rubber base impression material.

IDEAL REQUISITES OF IMPRESSION MATERIALS

1. Should have pleasant odor, taste and color.
2. Should not be toxic and should be biocompatible with oral tissues.
3. Should have adequate shelf life.
4. Should be economical.
5. Should be easy to use with the minimum of equipment.
6. Should have adequate setting time, satisfactory consistency and texture.
7. Should readily wet oral tissues.
8. Should have elastic properties with no permanent deformation after strain.
9. Should possess adequate strength to resist tear on removal from the mouth.
10. Should have adequate dimensional stability.
11. Should accurately reproduce cast or die.
12. Should be compatible with cast and die materials.
13. Disinfection should be easy, without loss of accuracy.

ADDITION SILICONE

Synonyms

- Vinyl polysiloxane
- Polyvinylsiloxane.

Composition

Base and catalyst pastes contain a form of vinyl silicone.

Base Paste

Contents

- Polymethyl hydrogen siloxane
- Siloxane prepolymers
- Hybrid silicone
- Filler
- Coloring agents.

Catalyst Paste

Contents

- Divinyl polydimethyl siloxane and other siloxane prepolymers
- Chloroplatinic acid (the accelerator or catalyst)
- Filler
- Retarder (present in the paste that contains the platinum catalyst)
- Coloring agents
- Palladium or platinum (scavenger)

Availability

It is available in different consistencies:

- Low
- Medium
- Heavy
- Very heavy.

Chemistry

- The addition reaction polymer is terminated with vinyl groups and is cross-linked with hydride groups activated by a platinum salt catalyst
- There are no reaction by-products as long as the correct proportions of vinyl silicone and hydride silicone are maintained and there are no impurities.

PHYSICAL PROPERTIES

Working and Setting Times

- Compared to condensation silicones and polysulfides, the addition silicones are more sensitive to ambient temperature

- Working and setting times can be extended by the addition of a retarder and by cooling the mixing slab
- The two types of setting materials available are fast-setting material and regular-setting vinyl polysiloxanes.

Elasticity

- Distortion is not present on removal from undercuts as they exhibit the lowest strain-in-compression values (permanent distortion)
- The heavy-body putty material builds up elastic response while in the working stage and then distortion occurs when the material elastically rebounds
- The stiffness is proportional to the consistency of the material, putties are stiff, but light-bodied materials are flexible.

Rheology

- It is the most pseudoplastic impression material
- Because of its pseudoplastic nature, single step material can be used both as syringe and tray material
- Single-phase material, when syringed, flows readily and yet holds its shape when placed in an impression tray.

Tear Energy

The resistance to tearing is adequate, similar to that of the condensation silicones. If not handled correctly, these materials will tear rather than stretch like the polysulfides.

Dimensional Stability

- Vinyl polysiloxane impression materials are the most dimensionally stable of all the elastomers
- No volatile reaction by-products are formed if mixed accurately
- The clinically set material cures completely, hence no dimensional change occurs
- The primary dimensional change occurs from thermal shrinkage as the material cools from mouth temperature to room temperature
- Because of its excellent dimensional stability and superior elasticity multiple casts can be made with the same degree of accuracy.

Biocompatibility

- These are highly biocompatible
- During the removal of the impression, if thin margins of impression material get lodged in the sulcus, this can cause severe gingival inflammation.

Shelf Life

- The vinyl polysiloxanes have a 2-year shelf life.
- The shelf life can be prolonged by storing the material in a cool, dry environment.

ADVANTAGES OF ADDITION SILICONE

- The addition type of reaction does not produce a byproduct and, hence, addition silicone is the most dimensionally stable impression material
- Multiple cast can be made with the same accuracy.

DISADVANTAGES

- It is basically a hydrophobic material. To make the material hydrophilic, a surfactant has to be added to the paste
- Sulfur contamination from natural latex gloves inhibits the setting of the addition silicone impression materials.

6. Classify elastomeric impression materials. Write in detail about polysulfide rubber.

CLASSIFICATION OF ELASTOMERIC IMPRESSION MATERIAL

Depending on the Type of Chemical Reaction

- Polysulfide
- Condensation polymerizing silicone
- Addition polymerizing silicone
- Polyether.

Depending on Consistency

- Low
- Medium
- Heavy
- Very heavy putty.

Categories based on viscosity

- *Type 0*: very high viscosity: (putty)
- *Type 1*: high viscosity: (heavy body)
- *Type 2*: medium viscosity: (medium body)
- *Type 3*: low viscosity: (light body)

Impression materials are also classified as
- Hydrophilic (contact angle is from 80° to 105°).
- Hydrophobic (contact angle is from 40° to 70°).[1]

POLYSULFIDE IMPRESSION MATERIAL

Chemistry

- The basic ingredient of the polymer paste is a polyfunctional mercaptan or polysulfide polymer
- Polyfunctional mercaptan is a linear polymer which provides pendant mercaptan groups as chain cross-linking sites
- This polymer cross-links with lead dioxide by condensation reaction of the lead dioxide with the SH groups of the polysulfide polymer.

Reaction Occurs in Two Steps

- Chain-lengthening polymerization from the reaction with the terminal—SH groups
- Cross-linking from the reaction with the pendant—SH groups. (Form three-dimensional network).

The condensation reaction byproduct is water. Loss of water from the set material can affect the dimensional stability of the impression.

Composition

Base Paste

- Polysulfide pre-polymer—80% (reactant)
- Filler (e.g. lithopone and titanium dioxide) to provide the required strength—5%
- Calcium sulfate—thickener and reinforcer—15%

Catalyst Paste

- *Reactor*: Lead dioxide that produces the dark-brown color—78%
- *Plasticizer*: Dibutyl phthalate 17% thinner
- *Sulfur: Reactant—4%*
- *Retarders*: Oleic or stearic acid, control the rate of setting.

Each paste is supplied in a tube and equal lengths of each paste are dispensed to give the correct ratio of polymer to cross-linking agent.

Manipulation

- Equal lengths of each paste are dispensed onto a mixing pad or glass slab
- The catalyst paste is first collected on a stainless steel spatula and then distributed over the base
- It is mixed until the mixed paste is of uniform color with no streaks of the base or catalyst paste
- Adhesives used with polysulfide rubber impression materials include butyl rubber or styrene acrylonitrile dissolved in chloroform or a ketone.

Handling Technique

- Tray material is mixed first and loaded on to the tray
- A second person begins mixing and filling the syringe
- The material is injected from the filled syringe within and around the prepared teeth
- The filled tray is then carried to place and seated over the syringe material
- The two materials should cure together.

Factors Affecting Working and Setting Times (Tested by Oscillating Rheometer)

- An increase in temperature accelerates the curing rate and, thus, decreases both setting and working times
- Cooling is done by storing the materials at a low room temperature or by mixing on a chilled, dry glass slab
- Retarders increase the setting time
- Adding a drop of water decreases the setting time
- Altering the base—accelerator ratio is not a recommended method as it alters the physical properties as the accelerator paste contains a retarder as well as a reactor.

Physical Properties

Elasticity

- Elastic properties improve with curing time
- Recovery of elastic deformation is less rapid for the polysulfides and hence they exhibit the most permanent deformation following strain in compression compared with the other materials
- Polysulfides also sustain more distortion when the strain rate is slow.

Rheology

- Polysulfide is the least stiff of the elastomeric impression materials
- The flexibility allows the set material to release from undercut areas and be removed from the mouth with a minimum of stress
- The unset material displaces any unwanted fluid present while seating the impression and the excess material extruded from the tray does not flow easily, causing discomfort to the patient.

Tear Energy

Polysulfides have the highest resistance to tearing. Thin sections of polysulfide impression material are less likely to tear than other silicone impression materials.

Dimensional Stability

The stone cast should be poured up immediately because the impression is the most accurate immediately after removal from the mouth.

Factors causing dimensional change

- During setting, contraction occurs due to loss of byproduct water, which causes shrinkage
- They also absorb fluids if exposed to water, disinfectant, or a high-humidity environment over time
- After setting, there is incomplete recovery of deformation
- Polysulfide rubber materials have more dimensional change than polyether and addition polymerizing silicone and should be poured immediately.

Biocompatibility

- Polysulfide has the lowest cytotoxicity among impression materials
- They are radiopaque.

Shelf Life

- Tubes are tightly closed when not in use and stored in a cool environment
- ADA specification No. 19 requires that after storage of the base and accelerator for 7 days at 60 ± 2°C, the material must still meet the test for permanent deformation.

Pros and Cons of Polysulfide Impression Materials

Permanent Deformation

Strain

- The strain in compression under a stress of 1000 gm/cm^2 is a measure of the flexibility of the material
- The polyethers containing thinner are more flexible than the regular material
- The silicones are stiffer than the polysulfides of comparable consistency and the addition silicones are slightly stiffer than the condensation silicones.

Flow

- The flow is measured on a cylindrical specimen 1 hour old and the percent of deformation is determined 15 minutes after a load of 100 gm is applied
- Flow properties are recorded as per requirements of ANSI/ADA Specification No. 19.

Hardness

- The shore A hardness increases from low to high consistency
- Hardness was measured at 1.5 minutes after removal from the mouth and after 2 hours
- The polysulfides and the low, medium and high viscosity addition silicones do not change hardness significantly with time
- The hardness of condensation silicones, addition silicone putties and the polyethers increase with time.

Tear strength

A few polysulfides have high tear strengths of 7000 gm/cm but the majority have lower values in the 2500–3000 gm/cm range.

Detail reproduction

Except for the very high viscosity products, they all should reproduce a V-shaped groove, of 0.020 mm wide line in the elastomer and the elastomer should be compatible with gypsum products.

Creep compliance

- The initial creep compliance shows polysulfide to be the most flexible and the polyether the least
- Polysulfides have the poorest recovery from deformation, followed by the condensation silicone and then the addition silicone and polyether
- Polysulfides have the greatest viscoelastic quality and require more time to recover, followed by the condensation silicone, the polyether and the addition silicone.

Wettability of rubber impression materials

The hydrophilic addition silicones and the polyethers were wetted the best and the condensation silicones and hydrophobic addition silicones the least.

Disinfection of Rubber Impressions: 2% glutaraldehyde

Recent Advances in Rubber Impression Materials

- A visible light-cured polyether urethane dimethacrylate rubber impression material has been developed
- It is available in low and heavy consistencies that are supplied in a light-tight plastic syringe and tube
- These materials have very long working time but short setting time when exposed to blue light and physical properties equal to addition silicones. These materials have the highest resistance to tearing (6,000–7,500 g/cm) compared to any other rubber impression material.

Modifications

Instead of lead dioxide reactor, organic hydroperoxide can be used (e.g. butyl hydroperoxide), but these compounds have poor dimensional stability.

REFERENCE

1. Chu CS, Smales RJ, Wei SHY. Requirements of an impression material for fixed prostheses. Gen Dent;1997;45:548-55.

7. What are elastomers? Mention the composition of condensation silicone rubbers. Enumerate the common merits and demerits encountered with the use of non-aqueous elastomeric impression materials.

DEFINITION: (ADA) SPECIFICATION No. 19

- Elastomer refers to the non-aqueous elastomeric impression materials
- Elastomers are a group of rubber-like elastic impression materials
- An elastomeric material consists of large molecules or polymers that are joined by a small amount of cross-linking. Stretching causes the polymer chains to uncoil only to a specific amount that is recoverable, when the stress is removed.

CONDENSATION SILICONE IMPRESSION MATERIAL

Availability

Condensation silicone paste materials and putty are available in various colors as pastel pinks, blues, greens and purples.

Composition

Base Paste

- Contains low molecular weight silicone called dimethyl siloxane, which has reactive terminal hydroxyl groups
- Fillers as copper carbonate or silica having particle sizes from 2 μ to 8 μ in concentrations from 35% to 75% for low to putty consistencies.

Accelerator

The accelerator may be a liquid that consists of stannous octoate suspension and alkyl silicate, or it may be supplied as a paste by the addition of a thickening agent.

Reaction

- The polymer consists of an α-co-hydroxy-terminated polydimethyl siloxane
- The polymer reacts with trifunctional and tetrafunctional alkyl silicates, commonly tetraethyl orthosilicate, in the presence of stannous octoate ($Sn[C_7H_1SCOO]_2$)
- These reactions take place at room temperatures and, hence, these materials are called room temperature vulcanization (RTV) silicones
- The accelerator has short shelf life because the stannous octoate may oxidize and the ortho-ethyl silicate is not stable in the presence of the tin ester

- Ethyl alcohol is a by-product of the condensation setting reaction
- Ethyl alcohol evaporates resulting in a contraction of set silicone rubber.

Working and Setting Times

- The initial and final setting times are determined using a penetrometer with a needle and weight selected to suit these materials
- The Vicat penetrometer, with a 3 mm diameter needle and a total weight of 300 gm, has been commonly used
- A metal ring, 8 mm high and 16 mm in diameter, is filled with freshly mixed material and placed on the penetrometer base. The needle is applied to the surface of the rubber for 10 seconds and a reading is taken. This is repeated every 30 seconds
- The initial set is that time at which the needle no longer completely penetrates the specimen to the bottom of the ring
- The final set is the time of the first of three identical nonmaximum penetration readings
- When the material has set, the penetration of the needle will be the same at each application.

RELATIVE MERITS AND DEMERITS OF ELASTOMERIC IMPRESSION MATERIALS

Handling Characteristics

Polysulfide

- The setting process of the polysulfide alters with temperature and humidity. A high temperature, high humidity gives shorter working and setting times
- The working time and setting time are 6 and 13 minutes respectively
- The **condensation-cured silicones** vary in setting time due to nonuniform mixing procedure
- The **polyether and addition-cured silicone** impression materials more consistent
- In addition-cured silicone putties, wearing latex gloves during manipulation can alter setting time.

Mechanical Properties

Stiffness

The relative stiffness of the set materials can be ranked as follows:
Polysulfide (PS) < condensation cured silicones (CCS) < addition cured silicones (ACS) <polyether (PE). (Excluding the putties and comparing similar viscosity materials).

Permanent Deformation

All of the elastomeric impression materials are viscoelastic in behavior and, hence, need to be removed from the mouth by a sharp tug

Permanent deformation graded as follows:
PS > PE > CCS > ACS

Polysulfides are most prone to permanent deformation while the addition silicones are the least prone to permanent deformation.

Tear Strength

- The polysulfides have the highest tear strength, followed by the polyethers and finally the silicones
- The tear strength should be sufficient to prevent failure, but not so high as to result in deformation.

Reproduction of Surface Detail

All of the elastomeric impression materials are able to reproduce the details of the surface very accurately when a low viscosity material is used. The reproduction is so good that the stone dies are unable to reproduce it.

Factors affecting surface reproduction

Poor technique: Nonhomogeneous mix results in improper setting in areas of impression.

Hydrophobic in nature: If the surface of the tooth has become contaminated with saliva, the impression material is unable to wet it—this can give rise to loss of surface detail. The contact angles for water on the set materials have been measured as 49.3°, 82.1° and 98.2° for polyether, polysulfide and an addition-cured silicone respectively. Polyethers have maximum wettability compared to others.

A surfactant has been added to these materials to alter the hydrophobicity.

Dimensional Stability and Accuracy

Polymerization shrinkage

Polyether and addition cured silicones have the lowest polymerization shrinkage, followed by the polysulfides. The condensation-cured silicones have the highest degree of contraction due to polymerization shrinkage.

PE<ACS < PS < CCS

Thermal contraction

The polyethers have the highest thermal contraction (320 ppm/°C), followed by the polysulfide (270 ppm/°C) and then the silicones (200 ppm/°C). These can be ranked as follows: CCS< ACS < PS < PE

The higher the filler loading, the smaller is the contraction.

Dimensional change on setting

The condensation silicones have the largest dimensional change, about –0.6% due to evaporation of volatile byproducts and the rearrangement of the bonds resulting from polymerization.

The addition silicones have the smallest change, about –0.15%, polyethers at about –0.2% and the lead dioxide and copper hydroxide-accelerated polysulfides at about –0.4%.

Storage stability

- The polysulfides contract on storage. Thus, the model will always be slightly larger than the tooth
- The polyethers are very stable on storage. If placed in a high humidity environment, they will absorb water and expand, resulting in a model smaller than the original tooth
- The condensation-cured silicones show contraction with time due to the loss of the alcohol byproduct

- The addition-cured silicones are extremely stable once set and show no dimensional change on storage.

Compatibility with Model Materials

- Polysulfides cannot be electroplated with copper to produce reinforced dies, as the polysulfide reacts with the electrolyte
- Polyether impression materials absorb water and cause distortion during the plating process
- The condensation- and addition-silicones can be plated with either copper or silver.

Acceptability

- The polysulfides have an unpleasant odor due to the mercapto groups
- The polysulfides are also difficult to clean off clothing if spilled
- The polyether and silicone impression materials are highly acceptable and very clean to handle.

Cost

The elastomers are more expensive than the hydrocolloids and the rigid impression materials, of which the addition-cured silicones cost more.

DISINFECTION OF IMPRESSION MATERIALS

The Effects of Disinfectants on the Accuracy of Impression Materials

Polysulfides

This impression material can be disinfected by immersion for up to 30 minutes.

Polyethers

Polyether impression materials swell after 10 minutes when immersed in a variety of disinfectants. Hence, spray disinfectants are used for <10 minutes, such as chlorine compounds.

Condensation-cured Silicones

All the disinfection procedures are acceptable but the period of immersion should not exceed 30 minutes.

Addition-cured Silicones

- Immersion for 30 minutes in a glutaraldehyde is ideal for addition, polysulfide and condensation silicones
- Chlorine compound spray disinfectant is used for irreversible hydrocolloid and polyether impression materials.

8. Classify elastomeric impression materials. Describe the chemistry, composition, setting reaction and properties of polyether rubber base impression material.

CLASSIFICATION OF IMPRESSION MATERIALS

Depending on Type of Chemical Reaction

- Polysulfide
- Condensation polymerizing silicone
- Addition polymerizing silicone
- Polyether.

Depending on Consistency

- Low
- Medium
- Heavy
- Very heavy putty consistencies.

POLYETHER IMPRESSION MATERIAL

(Introduced in Germany in the late 1960s).

Chemistry

It is a polyether-based polymer that is cured by the reaction between aziridine rings which are at the end of branched polyether molecules.

The main chain is a copolymer of ethylene oxide and tetrahydrofuran cross-linking, in which setting is brought about by an aromatic sulphonate ester

This produces cross-linking by cationic polymerization via the imine end groups

This material was the first elastomer to be developed primarily to function as an impression material.

Composition

Base paste

- Contains the polyether polymer
- *Filler*: a colloidal silica
- *Plasticizer*: Glycol ether or phthalate.

Accelerator paste

- Contains the alkyl aromatic sulfonate
- *Filler*: Colloidal silica
- *Plasticizer*: Glycol ether or phthalate.

Properties

Working and Setting Times

The curing rate of the polyethers is less sensitive to temperature change than that of the addition silicones.

Factors affecting setting time

- Modification in base-accelerator ratio
- Use of the thinner. The thinner reduces the stiffness of the set material without increasing the permanent deformation.

Elasticity

- The polyethers are the stiffest of the impression materials, excluding the high-viscosity putties
- Compression set testing indicates that the polyethers are slightly less elastic than the vinyl polysiloxanes.

Rheology

The pseudoplastic characteristics permit the original single-viscosity materials to be used as both syringe and tray materials.

Tear Energy

Tear resistance is better than that of the condensation silicone impression materials and most of the addition silicone impression materials, but is more prone to tearing than polysulfide. Polyether is the most radiolucent impression material; hence, it cannot be detected in the radiographs.

Dimensional Stability

- The dimensional change of the polyether impression materials is small, as they have no reaction byproduct
- The recovery is nearly complete. Thus, the polyether impressions can be poured even after several days and the resulting casts will have the same accuracy
- The polyethers exhibit the least amount of distortion from the loads imposed on the set material
- Polyether absorbs water or fluids and the simultaneous leaching of the water-soluble plasticizer is observed if it is not kept in a dry, cool environment to maintain its accuracy.

Strain in Compression, in Increasing Order

- Addition silicone< condensation silicone< polyether< polysulfide
- Recovery of elastic deformation following strain is less rapid for the polysulfides than for the other three kinds of materials.

Stiffness in Increasing Order

Polysulfide< condensation silicone< addition silicone< polyether.

Biocompatibility

- Contact dermatitis from the polyether has been reported
- Recent studies indicate no cytotoxic effects associated with the imine catalyst
- If pieces of the impression material are left in the sulcus, there can be minor to severe irritation.

Availability

- Monophase or single-viscosity material
- Regular
- Light body
- Putty.

Disinfection

- Two percent glutaraldehyde is ideal
- Impression material itself may contain a disinfectant, which may be present in some dental stones.

Handling of the Stone Cast

- Wettability of dental stone with polyether impression is much easier than silicone materials
- The stiffness of polyether makes it difficult to remove the stone cast from the impression.

Shelf Life of Polyethers

Storing in a cool, dry environment prolongs the shelf life.

Recent advances in impression techniques apart from the material manipulation techniques

- Optical impressions
- CAD-CAM system (Acquisition only)
- Scan and mill system CEREC

9. Classify impression materials. Write about the composition, chemistry, manipulation and physical properties of Zinc oxide-Eugenol impression paste. Discuss the factors controlling its setting time.

CLASSIFICATION OF IMPRESSION MATERIALS

- Elastic
- Inelastic/Rigid impression materials.

ELASTIC IMPRESSION MATERIALS

- Hydrocolloids
- Elastomeric impression materials.

Hydrocolloids

- Agar (reversible)
- Alginate (irreversible).

Elastomeric Impression Materials

- Addition silicone
- Condensation silicone
- Polyether
- Polysulfide.

INELASTIC/RIGID IMPRESSION MATERIALS

- Impression plaster
- Impression waxes
- Zinc oxide eugenol
- Impression compound.

ZINC OXIDE-EUGENOL PASTE (ADA-16)

Composition

Base Paste

- Zinc oxide (80%)
- Plasticizer (15%)
- Zinc acetate
- A trace of water.

Catalyst Paste

- Oil of cloves or eugenol (15%)
- Gum rosin and oils (65%)
- Filler (talc or kaolin) (16%)
- MgCl, accelerator and moisture (4%).

Functions of Components

Zinc Oxide

Base material.

Plasticizer

Fixed vegetable or mineral oil to offset the action of the eugenol as an irritant.

Eugenol

- Eugenol/Oil of cloves which contains 70–85% eugenol
- Forms a chelate with zinc oxide.

Fillers

- Kaolin and talc, diatomaceous earth
- For strength.

Hydrogenated Rosin

- Quickens the setting and makes the impression paste more cohesive, so that it can be softened in hot water for easy removal from the cast
- Other gums, resins, or waxes, for example, carnauba wax, kauri gum, or coumarine resins, can be substituted for gum rosin.

Canada Balsam

Canada balsam and Peru balsam are often used to increase flow and improve mixing properties.

Accelerators

Zinc acetate, calcium chloride, primary alcohols and glacial acetic acid can be used in either one or both pastes.

Magnesium Chloride

Hastens the slow-setting reaction of zinc oxide and eugenol mixture. The metallic salts of acetic, hydrochloric and nitric acid also act as accelerators.

Chemistry

- Zinc oxide hydrolysis and a subsequent reaction between zinc hydroxide and eugenol to form a chelate

  The reactions are represented by the following:

  $ZnO + H_2O \rightarrow Zn(OH)_2$

  Base acid salt reaction:

  $Zn(OH)_2 + 2HE \rightarrow ZnE_2$ (Zinc eugenolate) $+ 2H_2O$

Setting Reaction

- Two molecules of eugenol react with one molecule of zinc oxide to form a chelate, zinc eugenolate
- The methoxyl group and the phenolic hydroxyl group form two five-membered chelate rings with zinc
- If the zinc oxide powder is completely dehydrated before it is mixed with eugenol, the resulting paste will not harden. The presence of water is essential for the setting reaction
- Zinc oxide with 2% water will give mixtures that require 24 hours to harden, whereas the

presence of 5% water in the zinc oxide reduces the setting time to about 15 minutes
- Set impression consists of an amorphous zinc eugenolate matrix, which binds the unreacted zinc oxide together.

Manipulation

- The two pastes are provided in contrasting colors
- Equal proportions of base and catalyst paste are mixed together on a slab or mixing pad with a flexible spatula
- Mixing is continued for approximately 1 minute until a uniform color is observed.

Setting Time

The working time includes the time for mixing, filling the tray and seating the impression in the mouth. (Between 3 and 6 minutes)

The final setting time is defined as the time at which the material is hard enough to resist penetration under a load. [10 minutes for Type I pastes (hard) and 15 minutes for Type II pastes (soft)].

Control of the Setting Time

- Adding a small amount of an accelerator, such as zinc acetate, or a drop of water to the eugenol paste before blending the two pastes can shorten the setting time. Water is not generally added
- Cooling the spatula and mixing slab may help increase the setting time, provided the temperature is not lower than the dew point
- Adding certain inert oils and waxes during mixing, such as olive oil, mineral oil and petrolatum, can prolong setting time. This can reduce the rigidity of the set material and result in an Inhomogeneous mix
- Altering the ratio of the two pastes can result in retardation or acceleration, depending on which paste contains the accelerator
- The longer the mixing time (within limits), the shorter is the setting time.

Physical Properties

Accuracy

- These impression materials are sufficiently fluid to record the fine detail in the mouth
- There is little or no dimensional change associated with the setting process
- The set material is not elastic, so it will not record undercuts
- The set material appears to be stable on storage
- Impression pastes are compatible with dental stone cast materials. The paste can be removed from the stone by softening it in water at 60°C.

Flow

Those materials that show a decrease in flow at various time intervals also have a shorter setting time and a shorter time interval between the initial and final sets.

Rigidity and Strength

Impression paste can be compounded to increase resistance to flow at mouth temperature such that it is comparable or superior to that of compound.

Dimensional Stability

A negligible shrinkage (<0.1%) may occur during hardening.

Uses

Used as final impression material for edentulous arches:
- As surgical dressing
- As a bite registration paste.

Modification

Eugenol Free

- Carboxylic acid is used instead of Eugenol
- Carboxylic acid reacts with zinc hydroxide by the hydrolysis of zinc oxide to form a salt as follows:

$$Zn(OH)_2 + 2RCOOH — (RCOO)2Zn + 2H_2O$$

Luralite Impression Paste

Is easy to mix, pleasant tasting free-flowing zinc oxide eugenol paste, which will not distort soft tissue.

The impression can be reinserted to test, and is dimensionally stable and extremely accurate.

10. Classify gypsum products used in dentistry. How do plaster of Paris and dental stone differ from each other? How do you control setting times and setting expansion of various products?

CLASSIFICATION OF GYPSUM PRODUCTS

Type 1. Impression plaster
Type 2. Dental plaster

Type 3. Dental stone
Type 4. Stone, high-strength, low-expansion
Type 5. Stone, high-strength, high-expansion.

DIFFERENCES BETWEEN DENTAL PLASTER AND DENTAL STONE

(International Standard ISO 6873:1998)

Manufacturing

Dental Plaster

Gypsum (β-hemihydrate)

- Also called as 'alabaster'
- Plaster is a gypsum that is ground to a fine powder and the material is heated at 120°C in an open pan. This results in partial dehydration of the gypsum to yield the hemihydrate.

Heating of gypsum

Overheating the gypsum results in completely dehydrated $CaSO_4$, of which there are three types (crystalline modifications):
- $CaSO_4$(I) high-temperature form
- *$CaSO_4$*(II) insoluble anhydrite (mineral)
- *$CaSO_4$*(III) soluble anhydrite.

Dental Stone

Hydrocal (α-hemihydrate)

Obtained by heating under steam pressure in an autoclave. The hemihydrate produced can recrystallize to yield a more regular crystal form.

Crystacal/densite stone

Hemihydrate crystals of a very regular nature can be obtained by adding gypsum to the boiling *$CaCl_2$* solution.

Color

Dental Plaster

Cheap and white in color.

Dental Stone

- More expensive and are available in various colors
- Most common are green and yellow.

Particle Size and Shape

Dental Plaster

- Calcined hemihydrate particles are larger; and are irregular and porous.

Dental Stone

- The particles of the autoclaved material are smaller, regular and nonporous.

Water-Powder Ratio

Dental Plaster

- Calcined hemihydrate (plaster) 50–60 mL/100 g
- Porous particles as in dental plaster absorb lot of water
- The porosity of set plaster is greater than the porosity of set stone.

Dental Stone

- Autoclaved hemihydrate (dental stone) 22–35 mL/100 g.

Mechanical Properties of the Set Material

Dental Plaster

- Less dense than dental stone.

Dental Stone

- Harder and stronger than plaster.

Applications

Dental Plaster

- When strength is not of primary importance, plaster is used for mounting casts and some orthodontic study casts.

Dental Stone

The material of choice for

- Master cast used in construction of dentures
- Dies for crowns, bridge and inlay work
- Binders for casting investments.

SETTING TIMES AND SETTING EXPANSION

The setting is accompanied by

- Evolution of heat (exothermic reaction)
- Development of strength (interpenetration of crystallites)
- Setting expansion.

Steps in Setting

- Calcium sulfate hemihydrate dissolves in water to give Ca_2 and SO_4 2 ions. The solubility of hemihydrate is about 0.8%

- Induction period is the time between mixing and the formation of the saturated solution, in which the mix flows
- At the end of the induction period, the glossy surface is lost and crystal growth begins
- The dissolved calcium sulfate hemihydrate reacts with the water and forms calcium sulfate dihydrate
- The solubility of calcium sulfate dihydrate is very low and a supersaturated solution is formed
- This supersaturated solution is unstable and calcium sulfate dihydrate crystals precipitate out as stable crystals
- Nucleation is provided by impurities such as unreacted gypsum
- Spherulites are rosettes of long, needle-like crystals growing from isolated sites of nucleation
- As the stable calcium sulfate dihydrate precipitates out of the solution, more calcium sulfate hemihydrate is dissolved and this continues until all the hemihydrate has dissolved.

Initial Set

- The setting time is measured by the ability of the setting plaster or stone to withstand a stress. The initial set takes place when the lighter needle *fails to indent* the surface of the setting plaster when lowered gently to the surface
- During the initial set, trimming can be carried out.

Final Set

- At the final set, the material has become hard and brittle and cannot be cut with a knife
- The device consists of a mass of 300 g applied to a flat needle of diameter 1 mm. The material is set when the needle fails to indent the surface by more than 2 mm.

Working and Setting Times

- *Impression plaster*: The working time is 2–3 minutes
- *Gypsum-bonded investment*: Working time approaches 8 minutes
- *Impression plaster*: The setting time is 2–3 minutes
- *Gypsum-bonded investment*: The setting time can vary from 20 minutes–45 minutes
- *Dental plaster*: The setting time is 5–10 minutes
- *Dental stone*: Setting time can be up to 20 minutes.

Factors Observed during the Setting Reaction

- Initially the mix of hemihydrate and water can be poured
- The material becomes rigid, but not hard ('initial set')—at this stage, the material can be carved but not molded
- Final set follows when the material becomes hard and strong
- The linear expansion is in the range 0.3–0.4% for most plasters and 0.05–0.3% for dental stones. This expansion is caused by the outward thrust of the growing crystals of dihydrate
- The expanded set material contains crystals of dihydrate and pores. The volume of crystals of the set material is less than the initial volume of the hemihydrate. (less by 7%)
- If mixed plaster is placed under water at the initial set stage, a greater expansion on setting occurs. This is hygroscopic expansion.

Factors Affecting Setting Time

Spatulation

Increase in spatulation time will decrease setting time.

Temperature

The higher the temperature, the faster is the setting time.

Humidity

Moisture from atmosphere lengthens the setting time.

Colloidal Systems

Blood, saliva etc. act as retarders.

Accelerators

- Potassium sulfate
- Sodium chloride
- Sodium sulfate
- Calcium sulfate dihydrate.

Potassium Sulfate

- Potassium sulfate (K_2SO_4) reacts with the water and hemihydrate to produce 'syngenite' ($K_2(CaSO_4)_2 H_2O$) which crystallises rapidly and forms more crystal growth
- This reduces the overall expansion and accelerates the setting reaction
- When present as a 2% solution in water, it will reduce the setting time from approximately 10 minutes to 4 minutes.

Sodium Chloride

Sodium chloride provides additional sites for crystal formation. The higher density of crystals limits the growth of the crystals and, hence, reduces their ability to push each other apart, causing a reduction in expansion.

Calcium Sulfate Dihydrate

The addition of a small amount of calcium sulfate dihydrate will provide additional sites for nucleation and will reduce both the working and the setting times.

Sodium Sulfate

- Sodium chloride and sodium sulfate can be used as accelerators in low concentrations but act as retarders in high concentrations
- In low concentrations, they aid in the dissolution of the plaster powder, but interfere with the nucleation of gypsum in high concentrations.

Retarders

Borax

- The addition of borax ($Na_2B_4O_7\ 10H_2O$) counteracts the increased rate of setting due to the inclusion accelerators. Borax retards the setting process
  For example, hydrated sodium borate.
- When the plaster, or stone, powder is mixed with an appropriate aqueous solution of borax (0.9% w/v), the powder particles become coated with a thin layer of $Ca_2B_6O_{11}5H_2O$ (*'colemanite'*) which is very insoluble and delays the dissolution of powder (increased induction period).

Potassium Citrate

- Potassium citrate acts as a retarder and is sometimes added in addition to borax
- Accelerator to retarder ratio in correct proportion can produce the correct degree of expansion and the correct working and setting times
- The low setting expansion of stone and densite makes it ideal for dies and models.

SETTING EXPANSION

- On setting, the crystals impinge on one another as they grow and try to push each other apart with large empty spaces form between the crystals resulting in an apparent expansion on setting though the volume decreases
- The setting expansion is measured using a 'v'-shaped trough of length 100 mm
- The trough is fitted with one fixed and one movable end wall, the latter contacting a measuring gauge (dial gauge)
- To measure the setting expansion, the trough is greased and lined with a polythene sheet and filled with plaster (or stone) of a particular water/powder mix
- The movable end wall is adjusted to initially contact the trough and the dial gauge set to zero
- At the end of the induction period, the plaster or stone begins to expand and this expansion can be measured from the movement of the end wall.

Hygroscopic Setting Expansion

- Exposure of setting plaster, or stone, to excess water *before* the initial set results in an increased expansion
- The increased expansion is due to reduced surface tension effects which tend to cause coalition of the spherulites when a limited quantity of water has been used
- The magnitude of the setting expansion is approximately doubled for plaster.

Factors Controlling Setting Expansion

Antiexpansion Solutions

Combinations of accelerators and retarders, in solution, can control the setting expansion. These are known as **anti-expansion solutions**.

The altering of the powder-liquid system

Adding more water, the setting expansion is more.

Increasing the spatulation time

A longer spatulation time will increase the setting expansion.

The Setting Expansion may be Altered by

- Increased expansion — for example, calcium acetate can give over 1% linear setting expansion
- Decreased expansion — for example, potassium sulfate can reduce the linear setting expansion down to 0.05%.

11. Mention the composition and applications of any three types of gypsum. Describe their properties, ideal requirements and manipulation. Add a note on recent advances in gypsum.

COMPOSITION

Impression Plaster

Contains potassium sulfate, borax and coloring agents.

Cast and Die Materials

Are based on autoclaved calcium sulfate hemihydrate, plus additives to adjust the setting time and colored pigments.

Dental Casting Investment Materials

- Contain autoclaved calcium sulfate hemihydrate, to act as a binder
- Gypsum is calcium sulfate dihydrate, $CaSO_4$ $2H_2O$. When this substance is heated to a temperature to drive off some of the water, it is converted into calcium sulfate hemihydrate, $(CaSO_4)2\ H_2O$.

Plaster

- Calcium sulfate dihydrate is heated in an open vessel. Water is driven off and the dihydrate is converted into hemihydrate, known as calcined calcium sulfate or β-hemihydrate

- The resultant material consists of large irregular porous particles
- The usual water to powder ratio is 50 mL of water to 100 g of powder.

Dental Stone

- If the dihydrate is heated in an autoclave, the hemihydrate that is produced, consists of small, regular shaped particles which are relatively non-porous. This autoclaved calcium sulfate is known as α-hemihydrate
- Water-powder ratio is 20 mL water to 100 g of powder.

Investments

- Calcium sulfate hemihydrate forms dihydrate when it is boiled in the presence of calcium chloride and magnesium chloride. The hemihydrate particles that are produced are more compact and smoother than those of the dental stone
- Water-powder ratio is 100 gm of powder to 20 mL of water.

APPLICATIONS

- Impression plaster used for impression making in hyperplastic edentulous situations
- Dental stone used as models and dies
- Investment material used for making moulds and investing.

PROPERTIES

Strength

Factors that determine the strength of plaster and stone are as follows:

- Powder-water ratio
- Dryness of material
- Presence of pores within the set material.

Compressive Strength

- The compressive strength is altered by the powder-liquid ratio
- Less amount of water used for mixing gives a better compressive strength
- The use of an excessive amount of water decreases the compressive strength
- The dry strength is about twice the wet strength.

Tensile Strength

The wet tensile strength of plaster is very low (approximately 2MPa). This is due to the brittle nature of the material.

Hardness and Abrasion Resistance

The surface hardness of gypsum products is very low, so the material is highly susceptible to scratching and loss through abrasion.

IDEAL REQUIREMENTS FOR GYPSUM MATERIALS

- Ability to reproduce fine detail and sharp margins
- Dimensional accuracy and stability: should show little dimensional change on setting and should remain stable
- Compatibility with impression materials: there should be no interaction between surface of impression and cast or die
- Good color contrast with other materials
- Cheapness and ease of use.

MANIPULATION

- Correct water-powder ratio is advocated for proper mix
- During mixing, air incorporation should be avoided
- Mixing time of one minute is ideal
- Vibration is used to let the material flow well into the impression and it also helps to eliminate air bubbles
- A separating agent is applied to a stone die before preparation of a wax pattern on the die to facilitate removal of the pattern from the die.

RECENT DEVELOPMENTS

Impregnation of the gypsum by a polymer like polyester, polystyrene, acrylics and epoxy resin. Can be used as die materials because they possess good abrasion resistance and strength.

Incorporation of Wetting Agents

- Addition of wetting agents retard the setting time and increase the setting expansion
- 4% potassium sulfate, 0.4-1% borax and 0.04% alizarin red. This solution is called 'AE' or 'anti-expansion' solution.

Soluble Plasters

- Additives such as gum tragacanth, to improve the cohesive properties of the mixed plaster
- Starch, incorporated so that the set plaster will disintegrate due to the swelling of the starch.

Special Plasters

- *Alpha K*—a very hard type of plaster intended for high quality model and sculptural work.
- *Cerrostone plaster* is a fine particle medium strength plaster made in Germany formulated to be used as a strickling to produce a profile or pattern over the setting plaster.
- *Crystacal 'R' plaster* is a white alpha plaster with high strength and surface hardness. Used for study models in medical applications.
- *SP201 polymer for PMG* (polymer modified gypsum) used to produce composites and laminates. Other types as casting and flasking plasters are also available.

12. Enumerate the ideal properties of a denture base material. Describe the compression molding technique used in the processing of heat cure acrylic resin denture.

IDEAL PROPERTIES OF DENTURE BASE MATERIAL

(American Dental Association (ADA) Specification No. 12)

- It should be non-toxic and non-irritant
- It should be insoluble, non-absorbent and inert
- It should have adequate mechanical properties such as:
  - High modulus of elasticity, for greater rigidity, even in thin sections of material.
  - High proportional limit, so that the denture will not easily undergo permanent deformation when stressed.
  - Great strength
  - Sufficient resilience
  - High impact strength, to resist fracture if accidentally dropped
  - High fatigue strength
  - Good abrasion resistance, so that the material will not wear but retain a high polish
- The other physical properties required are:
  - The thermal expansion of the denture base should match to that of the tooth material
  - The thermal conductivity should be high
  - The density should be low, to assist in the retention of an upper denture
  - The softening temperature should be higher than the temperature of liquids and foods in the mouth
  - The material should be transparent or translucent and easily pigmented. The color should be permanent.
- Other considerations for denture base materials are:
  - Radio-opacity—easily located in X-ray if accidentally inhaled or ingested
  - A denture base material should be easy to process
  - It should be easy to repair
  - There should be no dimensional changes (expansion, contraction or warpage) either on processing the denture, or while it is in service
  - The material should be easy to clean.
- No known denture material adequately fulfils all these requirements.

COMPRESSION-MOLDING TECHNIQUE

- Flasking procedure

- Wax elimination
- Packing
- Deflasking procedure.

Flasking Procedure

- The cast with its trial denture is embedded in dental plaster on the lower portion of the flask
- When the dental plaster reaches its initial set, it is coated with an appropriate separator
- The upper portion of the selected denture flask is positioned atop the lower portion of the flask
- A surface tension-reducing agent is applied to the exposed wax surfaces and a second mix of dental stone is prepared. The dental stone is poured into the denture flask. Care is taken to ensure that the investing stone achieves intimate contact with all the external surfaces
- The investing stone is added until all surfaces of the tooth arrangement and denture base are completely covered. The stone is allowed to set and after which it is coated with separator
- An additional increment of dental plaster is mixed and the remainder of the flask is filled. The lid of the flask is gently tapped into place and the plaster is allowed to set.

Wax Elimination

- On completion of the setting process, the record base and wax is eliminated by immersing the denture flask in boiling water for 4 minutes
- The flask then is removed from the water and the appropriate segments are separated
- The prosthetic teeth remain firmly embedded in the investing stone of the remaining segment
- Any residual wax is removed from the mold cavity using wax solvent/hot water
- The mold cavity subsequently is cleaned with a mild detergent solution and rinsed with boiling water.

Packing

Selection and Application of a Separating Medium

Separating medium is applied onto the walls of the mold cavity, which prevents direct contact between the denture base resin and the mold surface of the dental stone.

Significance

- Water is prevented from passing from the mold surface into the denture base resin
- Water can affect the polymerization rate as well as the optical and physical properties of the processed resin
- If dissolved polymer or free monomer comes in contact with the mold surface, portions of the investing medium may become fused to the denture base.

Types of separating agent

- Thin sheets of tin foil
- Solutions containing alginate compounds
- Soaps and starches
- The most popular separating agents are water-soluble alginate solutions
- When applied, they evaporate leaving a thin, relatively insoluble calcium alginate films.

Rules for application

- A fine brush is used to spread the separating medium onto the exposed surfaces of a warm, clean stone mold
- The separating medium is carefully applied into the interdental regions
- Separator should not be permitted to contact exposed portions of acrylic resin teeth, as it can interfere with chemical bonding between acrylic resin teeth and denture base resins
- The separating medium is permitted to dry
- Three coats can be applied, each coat is applied after ensuring that the first coat is dry
- Pooling of a separating agent should be avoided.

Manipulation of Denture Base Resins

Polymer monomer ratio

- The powder consists of pre-polymerized polymethyl methacrylate beads, referred to as a polymer. The liquid contains unpolymerized methyl methacrylate and is termed as a 'monomer'
- The accepted polymer monomer ratio is 3:1 by volume
- Using a 3:1 ratio, the volumetric shrinkage may be limited to approximately 6% (0.5% linear shrinkage).

Polymer-monomer interaction

When monomer and polymer are mixed in the proper proportions, a workable mass is produced, which has five stages:

- Sandy
- Stringy
- Doughy
- Rubbery or elastic
- Stiff.

Sandy stage

Little or no interaction occurs on a molecular level. Polymer beads remain unaltered and hence described as 'coarse' or 'grainy'.

Stringy stage

- During this stage, the monomer attacks the surfaces of individual polymer beads
- Some polymer chains are dispersed in the liquid monomer
- These polymer chains uncoil, thereby increasing the viscosity of the mix
- This stage represents stringiness when the material is touched or drawn apart.

Dough-like stage

- On a molecular level, an increased number of polymer chains enter solution
- Hence, monomer and dissolved polymer are formed
- A large quantity of undissolved polymer also remains
- The pliable dough is not tacky and does not adhere to the surfaces of the mixing vessel or spatula

- The material should be packed into the mold cavity during the latter phases of the dough-like stage
- Resins reach a dough-like consistency in less than 10 minutes and remain moldable for at least 5 minutes
- Working time may be defined as the time for which a denture base material remains in the dough-like stage.

Rubbery or elastic stage

- Monomer is dissipated by evaporation and by further penetration into the remaining polymer beads
- Clinically, the mass rebounds when compressed or stretched.

Stiff

Monomer is evaporated and the mixture appears dry and is resistant to mechanical deformation.

Packing of Material into the Mold

- In trial closure, the pressure is applied until the major portions of the flask closely approximate one another
- The major flask portions are separated and the polyethylene packing sheet is removed from the surface of the resin with a rapid, continuous tug
- Excess resin is called flash. Using a rounded instrument, the flash or excess resin is gently removed
- A fresh polyethylene sheet is placed and trial closure is repeated until no flash is observed
- The mold sections are properly oriented and placed in the flask press
- The flask carrier maintains pressure on the flask assembly during denture base processing.

Deflasking

After the curing cycle, the flask is allowed to bench cool and then the denture is carefully removed without fracturing it.

13. Classify denture base materials. What are the stages in polymerization? Give the composition of heat cure acrylic resins and discuss the causes of porosity. Why is it objectionable? How would you avoid it in your denture prosthesis?

CLASSIFICATION

- Autopolymerizing resin
- Heat-activated resin
- Light-cured resin.

New Types of Denture Base Resins

- Reinforced resins
  - High impact resins
  - Fiber-reinforced
- Hypoallergenic resins
- Resins with modified chemical structure
  - Thermoplastic resins
  - Gum toning in denture bases.

STAGES IN POLYMERIZATION

- Induction
- Propagation
- Termination
- Chain transfer.

Induction/Activation and Initiation

- The polymerization of a vinyl compound requires the presence of free radicals
- Free radicals are formed when the decomposition of peroxide occurs
- A molecule of benzoyl peroxide yields two free radicals, which, in turn, decompose other peroxides to give other free radicals
- Before initiation, the initiator needs to be activated
- Activation can be achieved by decomposition of the peroxide by any one of the following:
  - Ultraviolet light, visible light or other electromagnetic radiation
  - Heat
  - Other chemicals, such as tertiary amines (e.g. N, N-dimethyl-p-toluidine).

Propagation

Free radicals react with monomer.

- This free radical, in turn, can react with another molecule of monomer
- Thus, the reaction proceeds, leading to the formation of a polymer chain.

Termination

This occurs when two free radicals react to form a stable molecule.

Steps in Termination

- Annihilation reaction
- Disproportionation reaction
- Transfer reaction.

Chain Transfer/Cross-linking

Many reactions can be used to prepare polymers with chemical bonds between different chains. These materials are said to be cross-linked.

Examples

- Dimethacrylate compounds can form methyl methacrylate by free-radical addition reactions
- These dimethacrylates may be:
  - Aliphatic, such as ethylene glycol dimethacrylate.
  - Aromatic, such as Bowen's resin.
  - Alicyclic.
  - Compounds with two epimine groups can be cross-linked by a benzene sulphonate ester.

COMPOSITION

Polymer (Powder)

- Polymethyl methacrylate, either beads produced by polymerizing methyl methacrylate in water, or irregular particles ground from a block of polymer
- Peroxide initiator—0.2–0.5% benzoyl peroxide
- Pigment, about 1%, ground into the polymer particles.

Liquid

- Monomer—methyl methacrylate
- A stabilizer (Inhibitor)—about 0.006% Hydroquinone to prevent polymerization on storage
- A cross-linking agent: ethylene glycol dimethacrylate
- Polymer-monomer ratio is usually 3-3.5/1 by volume, or 2.5/1 by weight.

POROSITIES AND CAUSES OF DISTORTION IN ACRYLIC

Monomer: Polymer Ratio

- If it is too high, all the polymers will not be wetted by monomer and the cured acrylic will be granular

- If too low, there is a shrinkage on polymerization of about 21% by volume for pure monomer
- In correctly proportioned acrylic dough, this is about 1%.

Manipulation Method

- The acrylic should be packed in dough stage and the correct proportions should be mixed
- The lower the molecular weight of the polymer, the faster is the dough formation
- Plasticizer, when present in some materials, reduces the dough time
- In refrigerated resins, dough formation is delayed
- The more the polymer-monomer ratio, the shorter is the dough time.

Incomplete Wax Elimination

Can cause lack of adherence between teeth and acrylic resin.

Separating Agent

- Used to prevent monomer penetrating into the mold material and polymerizing, which can produce a rough surface with adherent mold material
- To prevent water from the mold entering into the acrylic resin.

Packing

On polymerization, there is contraction which reduces the pressure in the mold. Underpacking can lead to shrinkage porosity.

Curing

- If the material is undercured, the denture may have a high residual monomer content leading to distortion
- The rate of temperature must not be above 100.3°C as the monomer boils at 100.3°C
- If the monomer vaporizes, it will lead to gaseous porosity
- Two alternative heating techniques are used:
  - Heat at 72°C for at least 16 hours or
  - Heat at 72°C for 2 hours and then the temperature is raised to 100°C and heating is continued for further 2 hours.

Cooling

- The flask should be cooled slowly on the bench, or in the oven or water bath
- Flask should not be cooled suddenly
- Slow cooling permits relief of these stresses by plastic deformation
- Materials cured at higher temperatures will have greater residual stresses and will be more likely to warp.

Deflasking

This has to be done with care to avoid flexing and breaking the denture.

Finishing and Polishing

Final polishing can be done by either wet polishing done with finely ground pumice in water used as a suspension on a wet soft mop. During dry polishing, if excess heat is used, it can distort the denture.

COMMONLY SEEN DEFECTS

- Polymerization shrinkage
- Porosity
- Water absorption
- Solubility
- Processing stresses
- Crazing.

Polymerization Shrinkage

Volumetric Shrinkage

- When methyl methacrylate monomer is polymerized to form polymethyl methacrylate, the density of the mass changes from 0.94 g/cm to 1.19 g/cm. This change in density results in a volumetric shrinkage of 21%
- A conventional heat-activated resin mixed at the correct powder-liquid ratio exhibits volumetric shrinkage of approximately 7%.

Linear Shrinkage

- Total dimensional changes occurring because of processing and service are in the range of 0.1 to 0.2 mm (as measured from second molar of right quadrant to second molar of left quadrant in upper denture.)
- Acrylic resin denture base exhibits a linear shrinkage of approximately 2%
- Thermal shrinkage of resin causes the linear shrinkage phenomenon in heat-activated systems
- Complete dentures constructed using chemically activated resins have less thermal shrinkage
- Processing shrinkage is measured as 0.26% for chemically activated resin, compared with 0.53% for heat-activated resin.

Porosity (Figs 3A to E)

Manipulation of Material

Porosity results from inadequate mixing of powder and liquid components. During polymerization, thick regions shrink more than adjacent regions and the localized shrinkage tends to produce voids.

Packing of Material

This type of porosity is caused by inadequate pressure or insufficient material in the mould during polymerization. Voids produced are irregular shapes. These voids may be so abundant that the resultant resin appears significantly lighter and more opaque than its intended color.

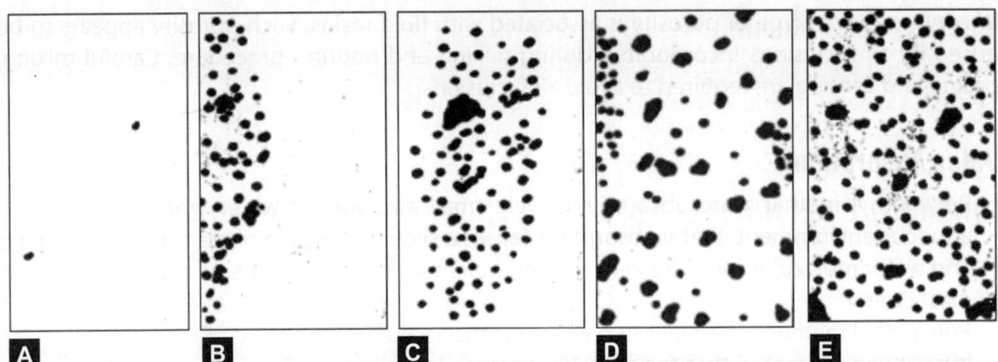

Figs 3A to E: Factors causing porosities in processed denture. (A) Properly polymerized—no porosity; (B and C) Rapid heating—relatively small subsurface voids; (D) Insufficient mixing of monomer and polymer, large voids resulting from localized polymerization shrinkage; (E) Insufficient pressure during polymerization—relatively large irregular voids

Temperature Rise

If the curing temperature increases or exceeds the boiling point of unreacted monomer (100.3°C), this increases the decomposition rate of benzoyl peroxide leading to internal porosity.

Excessive Thickness of Resin

Heat generated in a thick segment of resin cannot be dissipated due to its poor thermal conductivity. This results in a rise in the peak temperature of this resin above the boiling point of monomer leading to porosity within the processed denture base.

Polymerization Cycle

- Polymerization cycle should be controlled to avoid the effects of uncontrolled temperature rise, such as boiling of monomer and denture base porosity
- One technique involves processing the denture base resin in a constant-temperature water bath at 74°C (165°F) for 8 hours or longer, with no terminal boiling treatment
- A second technique involves processing the resin at 74°C for approximately 2 hours and then increasing the temperature of the water bath to 100°C and processing for 1 more hour.

Rapid Cooling

- The denture flask should be cooled slowly to the room temperature. If rapidly cooled, it can result in warpage of the denture base because of differences in thermal contraction of resin and investing stone
- The flask should be removed from the water bath and bench cooled for 30 minutes. Later it is immersed in cool tap water for 15 minutes.

Storage of Denture Before Delivery

To decrease the chances of dimensional changes, the denture should be stored in water until it is delivered to the patient.

Other types: A final type of porosity is associated with fluid resins. Such porosity appears to be caused by air inclusions incorporated during mixing and pouring procedure. Careful mixing, spruing and venting are required to avoid air inclusions.

Water Absorption

- Polymethyl methacrylate absorbs relatively small amounts of water when placed in an aqueous environment. Water absorption causes a slight expansion of the polymerized mass and water molecules interfere with the entanglement of polymer chains and thereby act as plasticizers
- Polymethyl methacrylate exhibits a water sorption value of 0.69 mg/cm^2
- It has been estimated that for each 1% increase in weight produced by water absorption, acrylic resin expands 0.23% linearly.

Solubility

Although denture base resins are soluble in a variety of solvents and a small amount of monomer may be leached, they are insoluble in oral cavity fluids. ADA Specification No. 12 states that the weight loss must not be more than 0.04 mg/cm^2 of specimen surface.

Crazing

- Stress relaxation may produce small surface flaws that adversely affect the aesthetic and physical properties of a denture. These microcracks are termed as 'crazing'
- Crazing is seen as small linear cracks that appear to originate at a denture's surface
- Crazing in a transparent resin imparts a 'hazy' or 'foggy' appearance. In a tinted resin, crazing imparts a whitish cast
- These surface cracks predispose a denture base to fracture
- Tensile stresses are often responsible for crazing in denture base
- Crazing also may be produced as a result of solvent action as with prolonged contact with ethyl alcohol
- Improved acrylic resin teeth and cross-linked denture base resins have decreased incidence of denture base crazing.

Porosities can be avoided by:
- Ensuring homogeneity of the resin mix
- The use of proper polymer monomer ratios and well-controlled mixing procedures
- Packing the material in dough stage.

14. Compare and contrast heat cure acrylic resin with self-cure acrylic resin with reference to:

a. Strength
b. Composition and chemical reaction
c. Color defects
d. Defects/porosities.

HEAT CURE ACRYLIC RESIN VS SELF-CURE ACRYLIC RESIN

SIMILARITIES

Strength

- Strength is decreased when the length of polymer chain is less
- Strength is decreased when the residual monomer content is more. (More in chemically activated resins)
- High levels of residual monomer present decreases, the strength and stiffness values.
- Creep phenomenon also decreases strength.

Creep: When a denture base resin is subjected to a sustained load, the material exhibits an initial deflection or deformation. If this load is not removed, additional deformation occurs over time. This additional deformation is termed creep.

Creep rate is increased by:

- Increases in temperature
- Applied load
- Residual monomer
- The presence of plasticizers
- The 'strength' of a denture depends on the design of the denture, stress concentration around a notch (e.g. the frenal notch) which can lead to midline fracture. Surface irregularities also lead to stress concentration.
- The strength of the acrylic depends on the molecular weight of the cured polymer, the residual monomer content, porosity and inclusions of foreign matter.

Composition and Chemical Reaction

- Free monomer released from the denture can irritate the oral tissues
- Residual monomer will act as a plasticizer and make the resin weaker and more flexible
- Processing at too low a temperature, or for too short a time, gives higher residual monomer values.

Color Defects

Control of Color

- The coloring pigment is usually incorporated in the polymer powder. If the coloring pigment is on the surface of the polymer beads, then it can get washed off by too rapid a contact of the monomer. In this case, the polymer should be added to the monomer slowly. Too little powder will produce lighter shade
- Amines with improved color stability, such as dihydroxy ethyl-p-toluidine DHEPT, may be substituted for DMPT.

Defects/Porosities

Porosity has undesirable effects on the strength and optical properties of the acrylic.

Factors Important for Accuracy

- The mold expansion on packing
- Thermal expansion of the acrylic dough
- Polymerization shrinkage — 7% by volume for the polymerization of the dough, or about 2% linear contraction
- Thermal shrinkage on cooling—the coefficient of thermal expansion of acrylic is 81 × 10~6/°C, there is 0.44% shrinkage on cooling from 75–20°C. This can cause palatal discrepancies in upper dentures
- Excess heat generated during polishing the denture can cause warpage due to release of stresses within the material.

DIFFERENCES

Strength

- The transverse strength of cold-cured PMMA is only 80% of the heat-cured material
- Creep rates for heat-activated and chemically activated resins are similar at low stresses (9.0 MPa), but creep rates for chemically activated resins increase as stresses are increased
- *The Charpy impact strength* for a heat-activated denture resin varies from 0.98 to 1.27 J and for a chemically activated resin, it is lower (0.78 J)
- *The Knoop hardness values* for heat-activated resins may be as high as 20, whereas chemically activated resin has values of 16 to 18.

Factors which Increase Strength of Heat Cure Denture Base Materials

- Materials based on rubber—PMMA copolymers
- Inclusion of carbon fibers
- Inclusion of polythene fibers or mats
- Wettable acrylics
- Radiopaque acrylics
- Polycarbonate denture bases.

Chemically activated resins shrink less than heat-activated resins because of a less complete polymerization. Hence, chemically activated resins have greater dimensional accuracy.

Rubber-modified resins

Beads of polymethyl methacrylate, to which are grafted a rubbery butadiene-silane layer, is coated with polymethyl methacrylate. These beads are then wet with monomer, which is composed of methyl methacrylate, a cross linking agent and an inhibitor. Rubber modified resins have better impact and fatigue properties.

Fiber-reinforced acrylic resins

To incorporate whiskers of alumina and carbon fibers to improve the strength properties.

Wettable acrylics

- A co-polymer of methyl methacrylate and hydroxyethyl methacrylate is easily wetted, so that enhanced denture retention is obtained
- But when the material is saturated with water, it has poorer mechanical properties than polymethyl methacrylate.

Radiopaque materials

Containing 8–10% barium sulfate in the powder. Greater quantity of the barium salt causes a deterioration of the mechanical properties of the material.

Polycarbonate denture bases

- Are linear polyesters of carbonic acid in which Aliphatic or Aromatic group is present
- These materials have good strength and dimensional stability as compared to resins
- Strength is further improved by adding 10 micron thick and 150 micron long glass fibers.

Modifications of Chemically Activated Denture Base Resins

Pour-and-cure resins

- These are cold cure resins that are so liquid when mixed that they can be poured into a mold made of a hydrocolloid
- They give excellent reproduction of surface detail but are inferior to both the heat- and cold-cured acrylics related to physical properties.

Visible light-cured resin

- It is composed of a matrix of urethane dimethacrylate that contains a small amount of colloidal silica to control the rheology. The filler consists of acrylic beads that become part of an interpenetrating polymer network structure when it is cured
- Available in light proof pouches as sheet or rope form
- Roll material is used as an index to place the arranged teeth after curing for 10 minutes
- The sheet material is used to make denture base.

Composition and Chemical Reaction

Composition

Heat-cured PMMA

Polymer

- Emulsion-polymerized beads of PMMA, of average molecular weight 10_5–10_6
- Plasticizer (dibutyl phthalate)

- Initiator benzoyl peroxide, 1%
- Pigments—Inorganic or organic, to color the denture base; may include HgS, CdS, Fe_2O_3.

Monomer-methylmethacrylate

- Cross-linking agent (e.g. glycol dimethacrylate, 1–2%)
- The cross-linking agent increases the surface hardness of the polymer and reduces the incidence of surface crazing
- Inhibitor (e.g. hydroquinone, 0.1%)
- Hydroquinone (is a colorless crystalline solid, soluble in MMA) can donate H atoms
- Readily to free-radical species (hydrogen abstraction)
- By heating to 70°C (heat-cured PMMA).

Molecular weight

Polymer powder is supplied up to 500,000 to 1,000,000.

- Of monomer, 100
- Of the cured polymer, up to 1,200,000.

Cold-curing PMMA

Polymer

- Emulsion-polymerized beads of PMMA, of average molecular weight 10_5–10_6
- *Plasticizer*: The polymer beads are more heavily plasticized than the heat-curing materials
- Initiator (dibenzoyl peroxide): 1%
- Pigments.

Monomer

- Methylmethacrylate
- Cross-linking agent (glycol-dimethacrylate) 0–10%
- Inhibitor (hydroquinone)
- Tertiary amine (DMPT)
- By chemical activation at room temperature (cold-curing).

Molecular weight

The size of the polymer beads is smaller than in the heat-cured resin. The average bead size of 150 μm has ease of dissolution in the monomer to produce a dough.

Chemical Reaction/Method of Activation

Heat-cured PMMA

- When heat activated monomer and polymer are mixed together, the polymerization of methylmethacrylate is activated by *dibenzoyl peroxide*, which decomposes to form phenyl free-radicals at a temperature of 70°C (through the use of dry heat, as in an oven, or *via* a heated water bath)
- The temperature should not rise above the boiling point of the monomer (100.3°C under 1 atm pressure).

Cold-curing or Auto-polymerizing Acrylic Resin

- Methylmethacrylate is polymerized through the chemical decomposition of dibenzoyl peroxide by a tertiary amine, as dimethyl-para-toluidine, (DMPT) at room temperature

- The peroxide is added to the polymer beads, as with the heat-processed material, while the amine is dissolved in the monomer
- Properties of the cold-curing materials are inferior to the heat-processed system
- Residual monomer for heat activated material, if properly cured, is 0.2 to 0.5%
- The residual monomer content of chemically cured is as high as 5% (wt).

Color Defects

- The color stability of chemically activated resins generally is inferior to the color stability of heat-activated resins
- The presence of tertiary amines within the chemically activated resins oxidizes and causes color changes that may affect the appearance of the resin
- Discoloration of these resins can be minimized by the addition of stabilizing agents that prevent oxidation.

Defects/Porosities

Heat Cure

Shrinkage porosity

Appears as irregular voids throughout and on the surface of the denture.

Gaseous porosity

Shows as fine uniform bubbles, particularly in thicker sections of the denture remote from the external heating source.

Dimensional stability is related to:

- Water absorption
- Relief of internal stresses
- Fracture if dropped on a hard surface, due to fatigue, from repeated bending of the denture in service.

Surface crazing

Cracks may appear on the surface of the resin due to tensile stresses causing separation of the polymer molecules.

Crazing results from:

- Mechanical stresses on repeated drying and wetting of the denture, causing alternate contraction and expansion. The use of tin-foil substitutes for mold lining permits the cured denture to contain water. Subsequent loss of this water leads to crazing
- Stresses due to differences in the coefficients of thermal expansion between porcelain teeth or clasps and the acrylic denture base; cracks may appear around the insert
- Solvent action—when a denture is being repaired, some monomer comes in contact with the resin and this can cause crazing
- Crazing has a weakening effect on a denture. Cross-linked resins are less prone to craze.

Water absorption

Water absorption can occur in a mold with tin-foil substitutes. Each 1% increase in weight of the resin due to water absorption causes a linear expansion of 0.23%. If the denture is not placed in water, drying out can cause shrinkage.

Cold Cure

- Is susceptible to distortion
- The lower molecular weight results in a lowering of the glass transition temperature (75–80°C), hence chances of warpage
- No external heat source is used to cure the resin and this produces lower build-up of internal strain
- The material is highly susceptible to creep, which can result in eventual distortion of the denture when in use.

RECENT ADVANCES IN DENTURE BASE RESINS

High Impact Resins

Rubber reinforced [butadiene-styrene polymethyl methacrylate (PMMA)] in which rubber particles are grafted to MMA for better bond with PMMA. They possess high impact strength and fatigue properties, e.g. Lucitone 199 and DPI Tuff. (Impact strength of DPI Tuff is more than Lucitone 199).

Fiber Reiforced Resins

Metal: Metal is prone to corrosion hence less used

Carbon/Graphite reinforced—65–70 mm length, 5% by weight treated with silane coupling agent are placed during packing.

Available as chopped, continuous, woven, braided and tubular but tubes of braided fibers provide a more even distribution of reinforcement.[1]

Disadvantage—Black in color

- *Aramid fiber reinforced*—Increases the strength but is unaesthetic and difficult to polish
- *Polyethylene fiber reinforced*—Polyethylene strands are cut to 65 mm length and surface treated with epoxy-resin to improve adhesion and are placed in resin during packing. Esthetic is good as they are invisible but difficult to polish
- *Highly drawn linear polyethylene fibers (HDLPF)*—Reinforcement done by a prepreg (layup) technique in which 2 layers of fiber are placed in lateral direction sandwiched between 2 layers at 45 degree from middle ones in maxilla and fibers are placed at right angle to ridge close to fitting surface in mandible.[2]
- *Glass fibers*: Are highly esthetic. Can be oriented within denture as continuous parallel fibers or randomly oriented fibers.
- *E-glass fibers*: Is computer impregnated with a porous PMMA and silane coupler that allows dissolution bonding to acrylic (e.g. Preat Perma Fiber). Available as mesh and fiber
- *Hypoallergenic resins*: Diurethane dimethacrylate, polyurethane, polyethylenterephthalate and polybutylenterephthalate. These materials have low monomer content.
- *Resins with modified chemical structure*: Hydroxyapatite or Al_2O_3 fillers are added to increase fracture toughness. The ratio of 2.2 :1 by weight of powder to liquid was found to be the best ratio.[3]
- *Thermoplastic resins*: A fully polymerized basic material is softened by heat (without chemical changes) and injected afterwards are used for making dentures. They are unbreakable, light weight and flexible.

- *Thermoplastic nylons*: Valplast and flexiplast are polyamides (nylon plastics). The Flexite Company also developed a tooth colored clasps known as Clasp-Eze, made of nylon material. Difficult to repair and polish.
- *Lucitone FRS Flexible Dental Resin*: Highly esthetic and is an injection molding system.
- *Thermoplastic polycarbonate/acrylics*: Flexite is a thermoplastic acrylic with high impact strength. Thermoplastic polycarbonates is a polymer chain of bisphenol—A carbonate. Used for provisional crown and bridges.[4]
- *Enigma Gum Toning*: Available in various colors such as ivory, light pink, natural pink, dark pink and light brown. By mixing these colors accurate gum tones can be obtained.

REFERENCES

1. Kostoulas IE, Kavoura VT, Frangou MJ, Polyzois GL. The effect of length parameter on the repair strength of acrylic resin using fibers or metal wires. Gen Dent. 2008;56(1):51-5.
2. Dixon L, Breeding Larry C. The transverse strength of three denture base resins reinforced with polyethylene fibers. J Prosthet Dent. 1992;67(3):417-19.
3. Ellakwa AE, et al. The effect of aluminium oxide on the flexural strength and thermal diffusivity of heat polymerized acrylic resin. J Prosthodont 2008;17(6):439-4.
4. Meda Negrutiu, Cosmin Sinescu, Mihai Romanu, Daniela Pop, Sorin Lakatos. Thermoplastic Resins for Flexible Framework Removable Partial Dentures. TMJ 2005;55(3):295-99.

15. Mention the various types of base metal alloys. Give the composition, advantages and uses of Cr-Co alloy along with its manipulation and recent advances. Give your reasons for alloying of metals for use in dental restoration work.

CLASSIFICATION OF BASE METAL ALLOYS

Base metal alloy	Uses
Gold alloys (high-content and medium-content)	Bridges; crowns; inlays; clasps; lingual bars; root canal posts; porcelain fused to metal
Cobalt-chromium	Framework of partial dentures
Nickel-chromium	Bridges; crowns; porcelain fused to metal
Silver-palladium	Bridges; crowns; porcelain fused to metal
High-content palladium	Porcelain fused to metal.

REVISED CLASSIFICATION SYSTEM FOR ALLOYS FOR FIXED PROSTHODONTICS (PUB 2003 IN ADA)

Classification Requirement

- High noble alloys noble metal content ≥ 60% (gold + platinum group) and gold ≥ 40%
- Titanium and titanium alloys titanium ≥ 85%
- Noble alloys noble metal content ≥ 25% (gold + platinum group)
- Predominantly base alloys noble metal content < 25% (gold + platinum group)

COBALT-CHROMIUM CASTING ALLOYS (STELLITE)

Co-Cr alloys were first introduced in 1930s and from then on have replaced Type IV gold alloys for the construction of partial denture frameworks.

Other Terms

Chrome-cobalt, chromium-cobalt or chrome alloys.

COMPOSITION

Cobalt	35–65%
Chromium	20–35%
Nickel	0–30%
Molybdenum	0–7%
Carbon	Up to 0.4%
Tungsten, manganese, silicon and iron	Traces

Functions of Constituents

- *Cobalt* is a hard, strong and rigid metal
- *Chromium* forms a solid solution with cobalt rendering the alloy corrosion resistant, due to a passivating effect
- *Nickel* can replace some of the cobalt
- *Molybdenum, tungsten, manganese and silicon* harden and strengthen the alloy *Molybdenum* reduces the grain size
- *Carbon* reacts with many of the other constituents to form carbides. In excess amount, they embrittle the alloy
- The carbon content of a cobalt-chromium casting depends on:
  - The quantity of carbon initially present before casting; and
  - Pick up of carbon from a heating flame.

ADVANTAGES

- Low cost
- High strength
- Rigid and corrosion resistant.

USES

Cast partial dentures:
- The modulus of elasticity of a Co-Cr alloy is typically 250 GPa. This high modulus of elasticity helps in forming thinner cross-sections with adequate rigidity
- Surgical implants.

MANIPULATION

The melting point of these alloys is in the range of 1250 to 1450°C. Hence, phosphate-bonded investments need to be used. These alloys are prone to oxidation on melting and the castings produced are hard and brittle. Shrinkage, on cooling, is (1.9% linear). Hence, dimensional accuracy is difficult to achieve.

Due to high melting range, either:
- *Oxyacetylene flame*: Too much acetylene will result in carbon pick-up by the alloy, which must be avoided.
- Induction heating is the ideal method to be used
- Polishing and finishing techniques:
  - Sand blasting is used to smoothen the surface of the casting and remove adherent investment materials
  - Electrolytic polishing is then applied.

RECENT DEVELOPMENTS

An alloy containing titanium has been introduced with 4 to 10% titanium, 5 to 15% chromium, 5 to 15% nickel, less than 3% molybdenum, with small quantities of silicon, manganese, iron and carbon and cobalt.

This alloy is more ductile than other cobalt-chromium alloys.

Special casting techniques are required.

REASONS FOR ALLOYING

Effect of Alloying Elements

Copper

- When copper is alloyed with gold, the melting point of the alloy is less than that of gold
- Solution hardening and order hardening occurs when alloys contain approximately 40 to 88% of gold, if the correct heat treatment is given
- Copper imparts a red color and also reduces the density of the alloy. (Its density is about half that of gold)
- Precipitation hardening occurs when copper is present in the alloy. Less amount of copper with at least 75% noble metals (gold, platinum and palladium) is required for complete corrosion resistance.

Silver

- Forms a solid solution with gold and there is partial solid solubility in the silver-copper system
- Silver increases the hardness and strength by solution hardening

- Molten silver can dissolve gases such as oxygen, leading to porosity in a casting
- It tends to whiten the alloy and overcome the reddening effect of copper.

Platinum

- Forms a solid solution with gold, but increases the tendency for coring to occur
- Precipitation hardening can occur by reaction with copper
- It increases the melting point of the alloy
- It helps the corrosion resistance of the alloy.

Palladium

- Is similar to platinum in its effects on dental gold alloys and is a less expensive metal.

Zinc

- Is a scavenger
- When the alloy is being melted prior to casting, oxidation of some of the constituents (e.g. copper) can occur. This copper oxide embrittles the alloy
- Zinc oxide can be removed as a slag from the molten alloy.

Nickel and Indium

- Indium helps to refine the grain structure of the alloy.

16. Classify noble metal alloy and their applications. What is casting shrinkage of gold alloys? Describe methods to compensate casting shrinkage.

CLASSIFICATION AND APPLICATIONS OF GOLD ALLOYS

Depending on the Use of Gold Alloy

Type I Alloys

- For inlays in low stress situations
- These alloys are relatively soft and easily deformed
- The low yield stress of these alloys allows the margins to be burnished easily as they are highly ductile
- Chances of fracture are less.

Type II Alloys

- For most inlays
- Those with thin sections should be avoided as deformation is still possible.

Type III Alloys

- Used for all inlays, onlays, full coverage crowns and short-span bridges, cast posts and cores because of their greater strength
- Difficult to burnish.

Type IV Alloys

Used for cast posts and cores, long-span bridges and in partial denture construction, particularly clasp arms.

Depending on the Content of Gold

- High gold alloys
- Medium gold alloys
- Low gold alloys.

High-gold Alloys

- Their high noble metal content must not be less than 75%
- They contain gold, silver, platinum and palladium.

Medium-gold Alloys

- In medium-gold alloys, the gold content varies from 40–60%
- Palladium and silver contents were increased to compensate for the reduced gold content
- Palladium is added to counteract the tendency of silver to tarnish
- Copper content is in the range of 10–15%
- The palladium, silver and copper form substitutional solid solutions, with gold producing a single phase structure.

Applications

- Long-span prostheses
- Implant-supported prostheses
- Posts and cores.

Low-gold Alloys

- Gold contents range from 15 to 20%
- Silver (40–60%) and palladium (up to 40%)
- Due to the reduced gold content, these alloys are white in appearance
- The matrix phase is essentially an Ag-Au solid solution with minor additions of palladium, indium and zinc.

Casting Shrinkage of Gold Alloys

- The gold alloys contract after casting

- Hence, to compensate for contraction of gold alloys, a mold that expands is used along with proper sprue design
- If this is not done, the final casting will be smaller in size.

COMPENSATION FOR SHRINKAGE

Setting Expansion of Gypsum

- Setting expansion occurs when a change from the hemihydrate to the dihydrate takes place
- Depending on the composition of the gypsum product, this linear expansion can be as low as 0.06% to as high as 0.5%
- Setting expansion occurs by the outgrowth of crystals from nuclei of crystallization that produces an expansion of the entire mass resulting in the production of micropores
- On drying, the excess water is lost and the void space is increased
- A setting expansion of approximately 0.12% can occur.

Control of Setting Expansion

Normal Setting Expansion

- The less the W: P ratio and the longer the mixing time, the greater is the setting expansion
- The setting expansion can be controlled by addition of chemicals.

Accelerators and Retarders

- The addition of an accelerator to dental plaster results in a fast set but reduces the working time
- To increase the working time, a retarder is also added
- Chemical accelerators and retarders regulate the setting time and reduce the setting expansion of the gypsum products.

Accelerators

- Sodium sulfate
- Potassium sulfate
- Sodium chloride
- Calcium sulfate dihydrate
- Accelerators increase the rate of solubility of hemihydrate, thus accelerating the reaction. Sodium sulfate has its maximum acceleration effect at approximately 3 to 4%. At greater concentrations, it becomes a retarder
- When hemihydrate reacts with accelerator potassium sulfate 2%, the reaction product is syngenite ($K_2Ca[SO_4]2\text{-}H_2O$), which crystallizes rapidly
- Decreasing the mixing time or adding more water slightly retards the mix.

Retarders

- Citrates
- Acetates
- Borates.
- Retarders form a coating on the hemihydrate particles and thus prevent the hemihydrate from going into the solution in the normal manner. This retards the reaction.

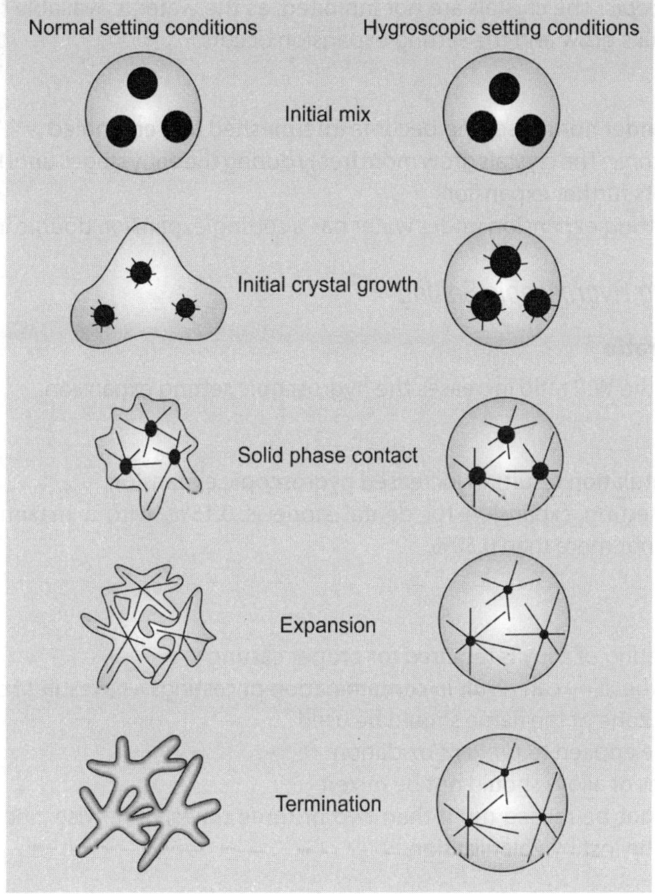

Fig. 4: Stages in hygroscopic expansion

Hygroscopic Setting Expansion

Theory of Hygroscopic Expansion (Fig. 4)

Stage I

Initial mix (showing three round particles of hemihydrate surrounded by water).

Stage II

- The reaction has started and the crystals of the dihydrate are forming and particles are drawn closer due to loss of water
- *Under hygroscopic:* The water of hydration is replaced and the distance between the particles remains the same. When the crystals of dihydrate grow, setting expansion begins.

Stage III

- Here the crystals grow and the contraction is opposed by the outward thrust of the growing crystals

- *Under hygroscopic:* The crystals are not inhibited, as the water is available from the outside. Here the crystals grow and the setting expansion occurs.

Stages IV and V

- The crystals under normal setting become intermeshed and entangled
- *Under hygroscopic:* The crystals grow more freely during the early stages until the intermeshing finally prevents further expansion
- Hence, the setting expansion under water has a setting expansion double in magnitude.

Factors Affecting Hygroscopic Setting

Water : Powder ratio

The reduction in the W:P ratio increases the hygroscopic setting expansion.

Spatulation

- Increased spatulation results in increased hygroscopic expansion
- The normal setting expansion for dental stone is 0.15%, with a maximum hygroscopic expansion of not more than 0.30%.

Precautions

- Complete heating of alloy is required for proper casting
- Overheating the alloy can result in contamination of castings as a result of oxidation
- The reducing zone of the flame should be used
- Flux should be applied to prevent oxidation
- Different types of alloys should not be mixed
- Alloy should not be reused more than two or three times, otherwise zinc (a scavenger for oxygen) may be lost by volatilization.

RECENT APPLICATIONS OF GOLD ALLOYS

- The process of electroforming for inlays was first introduced in 1961 and was reported in gold bulletin.[1]
- The electroforming baths contain a gold sulfite electrolyte.
- Electroformed pure gold has a hardness of 100 HV and fineness between 99.9 and 99.99% with crystal structure of a very fine grain size of less than 1 μm.
- In dentistry the process is used to form precise coping of pure gold, which does not change its dimensions during firing on porcelain, hence eliminating wax modeling.
- After firing on porcelain, recrystallization leads to a grain size of 50 μm.
- Also used in crown- and bridgework.
- Joining cast pontics with electroformed copings can be done by sintering, laser soldering and galvanizing techniques of which the sintering technique with electroformed bridgework is reported to be the most precise method.
- Presently researchers are focusing to develop electroformed gold with increased strength through dispersion strengthening by incorporating a suspension of ceramic particles.
- Deposition of multilayers by electrochemical structure modulation to increase strength is also reported.[2]

REFERENCES

1. 'Electroformed Gold Dental Crowns and Bridges' Matthijs MA. Vrijhoef, Adam J. Spanauf, Heinz H. Renggli, Gerard A. Somers and Horst L. Wismann, Gold Bulletin, 1984;17(1): 13-17.
2. Zielonka A, und Fauser H, 'Advanced Materials by Electrochemical Techniques', Z. Phys. Chemie 208(1999)195.

17. Classify dental waxes. Give the composition of dental casting wax and describe the properties of the same.

CLASSIFICATION OF DENTAL WAXES

According to their Use and Application

- Pattern wax
- Casting wax
- Base plate wax
- Boxing wax
- Utility wax
- Sticky wax
- Corrective impression wax
- Bite registration wax.

According to their Origin

Natural Waxes

- Mineral
- Plant
- Insect
- Animal.

Synthetic Waxes

- Gums
- Fats
- Fatty acids
- Oils
- Natural and synthetic resins.

The particular working characteristics of each of the dental waxes are achieved by the blending of appropriate natural and synthetic waxes and resins and other additives.

Natural Waxes

- Mineral
- Paraffin
- Microcrystalline
- Barnsdall
- Ozokerite
- Ceresin
- Montan.

Plant

- Carnauba
- Ouricury
- Candelilla
- Japan wax
- Cocoa-butter.

Insect

- Beeswax.

Animal

Animal waxes, such as spermaceti wax, obtained from the sperm whale, are mainly ester waxes. The spermaceti wax has been used as a coating in the manufacture of dental floss.

Synthetic Waxes

- Acrawax C
- Aerosol OT
- Castorwax
- Flexowax C
- Epolene N-10
- Albacer
- Aldo 33
- Durawax 1032.

Additives

- Stearic acid
- Glyceryl tin stearate.

Oils

- Turpentine.

Natural resins

- Rosin
- Copal Resin
- Gum Dammar
- Sandarac
- Mastic

- Shellac
- Kauri.

Synthetic resins
- Elvax
- Polyethylene
- Polystyrene.

CASTING WAX

Composition

- Little is known of the exact composition of these sheet and shape waxes
- The most common ingredients are paraffin, ceresin, beeswax, resins and other waxes being used. Hydrocarbon waxes, therefore, constitute the major portion of this formulation.

Shape and Gauge

- The pattern for the metallic framework of removable partial dentures and other similar structures is fabricated from the casting waxes
- These waxes are available in the form of sheets, usually of 28- and 30-gauge (0.40 and 0.32 mm) thickness, readymade shapes and in bulk
- The readymade shapes are supplied as round, half-round and half-pear-shaped rods and wires of various gages in approximately 10 cm lengths.

Uses

- The casting wax sheets are used to as wax patterns of major connector to produce the desired contour of the lingual bar
- The casting wax can also be used for postdamming of complete maxillary denture impressions, for checking high points of articulation, for producing wax bites of cusp tips and for the articulation of stone casts.

Properties of Casting Wax

Physical Characteristics (No ADA Specification, only Federal Specification)

- The casting sheets and prefabricated sheets possess tackiness, which helps to maintain their position on the cast and on each other during assembly of the pattern
- These patterns are sealed to the investment cast with a hot spatula
- Casting wax possesses high degree of toughness and strength, with a true gauge dimension and a minimum of dimensional change with change in temperature and the ability to be vaporized completely from the investment mold
- Casting wax need not exhibit low flow at body temperature
- The flow property of the casting wax shows a maximum of 10% flow at 35°C and a minimum of 60% flow at 38°C
- The requirement for ductility of the casting waxes is high. The federal specification requires that the casting wax be bent double upon itself without fracture at a temperature of 23°C and that the waxes be pliable and readily adaptable at 40° to 45°C

- Heating over a flame and the compression to adapt either the readymade shapes or the sheet casting wax can alter their thickness and contor because of their relatively high ductility and flow
- Casting wax must vaporize at about 500°C with no residue other than carbon. Pattern waxes are now replaced by preformed plastic patterns.

Properties of waxes

Important properties of waxes are melting range, thermal expansion, mechanical properties, flow, residual stress and ductility.

Melting range

- They contain several types of molecules, each having a range of molecular weights and, hence, possess melting ranges rather than melting points
- The melting range for paraffin wax is from 44° to 62°C and for carnauba wax, it is from 50°C to 90°C
- When a mixture of 75% paraffin and 25% carnauba wax was prepared, the melting range increased to 44°C, compared with 18°C for paraffin alone.

Thermal expansion

- Waxes expand when subjected to a rise in temperature and contract as the temperature decreases
- Dental waxes and their components have the largest coefficient of thermal expansion. The mineral waxes possess higher coefficients of linear thermal expansion than plant waxes
- The mineral waxes expand more because they have weak secondary valence forces
- Many waxes exhibit at least two rates of expansion between 72° and 52°C.

Mechanical Properties

Elastic modulus, proportional limit and compressive strength

- The elastic modulus, proportional limit and compressive strength of waxes are low compared with those of other materials
- Carnauba wax has the highest values and beeswax the lowest. The elastic modulus of carnauba wax decreased from 1790 to 759 MN/m^2 (260,000 to 110,000 lb/inch^2) from 23° to 37°C
- Paraffin wax showed a decrease in modulus from 310 to 276 MN/m^2 (45,000–4,000 lb/inch^2) between 23° and 30°C
- The proportional limit of carnauba wax decreased from 11.0 to 5.5 MN/m^2 (1,600–800 lb/inch^2) over the temperature range of 23° to 37°C.

Flow

- Flow is dependent on the temperature of the wax, the force bringing about the deformation and the time the force is applied
- The mineral waxes, paraffin, barnsdahl and ceresin, flow 50% approximately 20°C below their melting range
- Yellow beeswax, flows extensively at 24°C below its melting range (61°–63°C) with an 8°C temperature difference between 1% and 70% flow. Yellow beeswax flows 7% at 40°C.

Residual Stress

- When the wax is cooled, the atoms and molecules are forced closer together with restriction in molecules resulting in residual stress within the specimen
- When the same wax is heated, release of the residual stress is added to the normal thermal expansion and the total expansion is greater than normal, resulting in a dimensional change that is opposite to the thermal expansion.

Ductility

- The ductility increases as the temperature of wax increases. Waxes with lower melting temperatures have a greater ductility at any given temperature
- The ductility of a blended wax depends on the melting temperatures of the component waxes
- A blended wax with components having wide melting ranges has greater ductility than blended waxes having a narrow range
- Highly refined waxes are brittle. The lower melting point microcrystalline mineral type of waxes exhibit a high degree of ductility and high melting temperatures.

LATEST TYPES OF WAXES AND WAXING-UP TECHNIQUES IN DENTISTRY

- *Candulor Esthetic Color Wax-set*: For gingival wax set up available in three shades (53,55,57).
- Comes in a 3 well wax pot, and are able to be ready on demand for use at the desired temperature.
- Wax colors are also available to customize as to each patients gingival tone.
- *Wax less techniques*: 3 shape dental system from GEMCO (CAD CAM 2014): Are virtual computer aided wax up techniques.

18. Give the composition of phosphate-bonded dental investment and function of each component. Describe the chemical reaction and methods by which casting shrinkage is compensated. Add a note on the factors affecting working and setting time.

COMPOSITION

Refractory Fillers

- Silica, in the form of cristobalite, quartz, or a mixture of the two—approximately 80%
- Fillers provide high-temperature thermal shock resistance (refractoriness) and a high thermal expansion
- The particle size varies from a submicron level to that of fine sand.

Binder

- Initially phosphoric acid was used
- Later magnesium oxide (basic) and a phosphate, that is acidic in nature, was used
- Presently, mono-ammonium phosphate incorporated into the powdered investment is used.

Colloidal Silica

- 33% dilution of the colloidal silica is required
- Colloidal silica suspensions increase expansion of the investment more than water
- Colloidal silica liquid suspensions can freeze and become useless during winter but can regain use after they have been thawed out and shaken. Some suspensions are available as *freeze-stable* products
- Some phosphate investments are made to be used with water for the casting of many alloys.

Reducing Agents

Carbon

- It is added only when gold alloys are cast to produce clean castings and facilitate the *devastating* of the casting from the mold
- If carbon is used for base metal alloys, then they cause embrittlement.

Palladium

- Reacts with carbon at temperatures above 1504°C (2740°F)
- If alloy temperature exceeds this critical point, a phosphate investment without carbon should be used and a carbon crucible should not be used for melting the alloy.

Reaction of Phosphate-bonded Investment when Mixed with Colloidal Silica

- Magnesia and monoammonium phosphate, react to form magnesium ammonium phosphate. An excess of magnesia is present, which never fully reacts
- Hence, a predominantly colloidal multimolecular $(NH_4MgPO_4 \cdot 6H_2O)_n$ aggregate is formed around excess MgO and fillers.

On heating, the binder undergoes thermal reactions as:

$MgO + NH_4H_2PO_4 + H_2O$

↓ Room temperature

$(NH_4MgPO_4 \cdot 6H_2O)n$

MgO

$NH_4H_2PO_4$ > Colloidal-type particles

H_2O

↓ Prolonged setting at room temperature or dehydration at 50°C

$(NH_4MgPO_4 \cdot 6H_2O)n$

↓ Dehydrated at 160°C

$(NH_4MgPO_4 \cdot H_2O)n$

↓

Heated from 300-650°C

$(Mg_2P_2O_7)n$ → Non-crystalline polymeric phase

↓ Heated above 690°C

$Mg_2P_2O_7$

+MgO

↓ Heated above 1040°C

$Mg_3(PO_4)_2$

The final products are crystalline $Mg_2P_2O_7$ and MgO, along with unchanged quartz, cristobalite, or both. Some $Mg_3(PO_4)_2$ is formed if the investment is grossly overheated or when the molten metal contacts the mold cavity surfaces.

COMPENSATION FOR CASTING SHRINKAGE

Setting and Thermal Expansion

- Colloidal silica aids in expansion counterbalancing shrinkage
- When phosphate investments are mixed with water, they exhibit shrinkage at 200°C to 400°C [400°F to 750°F]. This contraction is eliminated when a colloidal silica solution is used
- Expansion can be decreased by increasing the liquid: powder ratio rather than by decreasing the concentration of the special liquid
- The early thermal shrinkage of phosphate investments causes a decomposition of the binder, magnesium ammonium phosphate, followed by evolution of ammonia

- For gypsum investments, the shrinkage is caused by the transformation of the calcium sulfate from the hexagonal to the rhombic configuration. This shrinkage is counterbalanced by the expansion of refractory filler, as cristobalite.

WORKING AND SETTING TIME

Factors Affecting Working and Setting Time

Temperature

The warmer the mix, the faster it sets. The setting reaction itself gives off heat accelerating the rate of setting.

Increased Mixing Time and Mixing Efficiency

- Determined by the type of mixing and speed of mixing, result in a faster set and a greater rise in temperature
- Mechanical mixing under vacuum is preferred.

Liquid: Powder Ratio

An increase in the liquid : powder ratio increases the working time.

Conclusion

- Increasing the special liquid: water ratio increases the smoothness but can lead to oversized extracoronal castings.
- Improvement in the techniques and the investment materials has led to fabrication of accurate castings.

19. Classify the investment materials. State the composition of gypsum-bonded investments. Mention the functions of each ingredient and add a note on the type of expansions occurring in investment materials.

CLASSIFICATION OF INVESTMENT MATERIALS

Type I (Gypsum Bonded)

Investments used for the casting of inlays or crowns when the alloy casting shrinkage compensation is accomplished by thermal expansion of the investment.

Type II (Phosphate Bonded)

Investments used for the casting of inlays or crowns, but casting shrinkage compensated by the hygroscopic expansion of the investment.

Type III (Ethyl Silicate Bonded)

Investments are used in the construction of partial dentures with gold alloys.

Classification Based on Silica Type

- Quartz investments
- Cristobalite investments.

Gypsum-bonded Investments

(ADA) Specification No. 2.

Composition

Alpha-hemihydrate of Gypsum

- Serves as a binder to hold the other ingredients together and to provide rigidity. The investment may contain 25 to 45% of the gypsum product
- All forms of silica shrink between 200°C and 400°C (392–750°F)
- A slight expansion then occurs between 400°C and approximately 700°C (1300°F), followed by contraction due to the decomposition and release of sulfur gases, such as sulfur dioxide
- This decomposition causes shrinkage and contaminates the castings with the sulphides of alloying elements, such as silver and copper
- Hence, gypsum-bonded investments should not be heated above 700°C (1300°F)
- For gypsum products containing carbon, the maximum temperature should be 650°C (1200°F).

Silica

- Silica (SiO_2) is added as a refractory during the heating of the investment and to regulate the thermal expansion
- During the heating, gypsum shrinks, addition of silica prevents contraction and aids in expansion.

Types of silica

- Quartz
- Tridymite
- Cristobalite
- Fused quartz.
- When quartz is heated, it inverts from a 'low' form, known as α-quartz, to a 'high' form, called β-quartz, at a temperature of 575°C (1067°F).
- Cristobalite and Tridymite undergo an analogous transition.

Modifiers

Boric acid and sodium chloride regulate the setting expansion and setting time. They also prevent shrinkage of gypsum when it is heated above 300°C (572°F).

Coloring Matter and Reducing Agents

Carbon and powdered copper are used. The reducing agents provide a nonoxidizing atmosphere in the mold when the gold alloy is cast.

TYPES OF SETTING EXPANSIONS

- Normal setting expansion
- Thermal expansion
- Hygroscopic setting expansion.

Normal Setting Expansion

- A mixture of silica and gypsum hemihydrate results in setting expansion greater than that of the gypsum product because the silica particles interfere with the intermeshing and interlocking of the crystals as they form. Thus, the thrust of the crystals is outward during growth and they increase expansion
- Type I investment permits a maximum setting expansion in air of only 0.6%
- The setting expansion of modern investments is approximately 0.4%
- Setting expansion can be regulated by retarders and accelerators.

Significance

- Normal setting expansion enlarges the mold to compensate for the casting shrinkage of the gold
- The normal setting expansion is measured as the linear dimensional change that occurs as the investment sets in a V-shaped trough
- The expansion can occur simultaneously along with thermal and hygroscopic setting expansions
- The setting expansion is effective only when exothermic heat is transmitted to the pattern
- The lower the water-powder ratio for the investment, the greater is the setting expansion
- As the investment sets, it eventually gains sufficient strength to produce a dimensional change in the wax pattern as setting expansion occurs
- If the pattern has a thin wall, then the effective setting expansion is greater than, that with thicker walls
- The softer the wax, the greater is the effective setting expansion.

Thermal Expansion

- The thermal expansion of a gypsum-bonded investment is directly related to the amount and type of silica present
- Approximately, 75% of quartz is required to counterbalance the contraction of the gypsum

during heating

- The thermal expansion depends on the particle size of the quartz, the type of gypsum binder and the resultant water-powder ratio
- Modern investments set initially in 9 to 18 minutes.

Cristobalite

Has more expansion than Quartz because of the inversion of the Cristobalite occurring at 200°C (392°F) and 270°C (518°F) from 'low', called α-cristobalite, to 'high', called β-cristobalite.

Tridymite

- Two inversions of tridymite occur at 117°C (243°F) and 163°C (325°F) respectively
- The allotropic forms are stable only above the transition temperature and an inversion occurs on cooling.

Fused Quartz

Is amorphous and glasslike in character and it exhibits no inversion at any temperature below its fusion point. Not used in dental investments.

- Quartz, cristobalite, or a combination of the two forms may be used in a dental investment.

Hygroscopic Setting Expansion

- Hygroscopic setting expansion is a physical phenomenon and is part of setting expansion
- This phenomenon occurs when the water within the crystal space is lost by hydration; and is replaced by immersion of the setting investment in water
- The immersion in water replaces the water of hydration and thus prevents the confinement of the growing crystals
- The quartz particles, present within the investment material increases the hygroscopic setting expansion
- The greater the amount of the silica or the inert filler, the more is the hygroscopic expansion.

Factors Controlling Hygroscopic Expansion

Effect of composition

- Depends upon the amount and type of silica content of the investment
- The finer the particle size of the silica, the greater is the hygroscopic expansion
- α-hemihydrate produces greater hygroscopic expansion in the presence of silica than the β-hemihydrate
- If adequate silica is not present, shrinkage occurs during drying of the set investment. At least 15% of binder is necessary to prevent drying shrinkage.

Effect of Water-powder Ratio

The higher the water: powder ratio, the lesser the hygroscopic setting expansion.

Effect of Spatulation

When the mixing time is reduced, the hygroscopic expansion is decreased.

Shelf life of the investment

The older the investment, the lower is its hygroscopic expansion.

Effect of time of immersion

The hygroscopic setting expansion is more when immersed before the initial set.

Effect of confinement

- The effect of hygroscopic setting expansion is less in proportion to the expected expansion than is the normal setting expansion.
- Immersion in room-temperature water reduces the effective expansion.

Effect of the amount of added water

The magnitude of the hygroscopic expansion is in direct proportion to the amount of water added during the setting period until a maximum expansion occurs.

RECENT ADVANCES IN INVESTMENT AND CASTING

Investment casting using ceramic shell: (Kalpakjian and Schmid 2008):
Ceramic shell is formed around the wax pattern by injection molding and later this waxed is burned out and the hollow shell is injected with molten metal.

Composition of ceramic shell slurry: Ceramic flour (refractory powder) Ceramic flour includes silica sand, aluminosilicates, alumina and zirconium silicate or zircon
Basic colloidal silica as a liquid binder.[1]

Modified composition: (Doles and Viers 2009)
In order to increase strength of ceramic shell the composition was modified as follows:
Major portion of the filler component comprised of finely divided silica, aluminum silicate, alumina or zircon.

Minor portion comprised of plate-like particles such as kaoline or needle-like particles like mullite, kyanite, halloysite and asbestos.

This modified investment casting slurry produced a shell of uniform thickness and fine casting compared with the fiber-containing slurry.

Disadvantage: Is expensive.[2]

Ceramic shell for super alloys: Super alloys as gamma titanium aluminides (-TiAl) can be casted using ceramic shell mold made of ZrO_2 and Al_2O_3, using a range of techniques.[3]

Ospennikova et al. (2010) prepared hydrolyzed ethyl silicate (ETS) as investing material to build perfect ceramic shells.[4]

Rapid Proto-typing in Casting

The process of employing rapid prototyping techniques to fabricate patterns for the investment casting process is known as rapid investment casting (RIC). The rapid prototyping processes convert a three-dimensional CAD model into a solid physical model .

Rapid Freeze Prototyping (RFP)

- Ice patterns are substituted for wax patterns.

- A new investment casting technology, called freeze cast process (FCP), utilizes the making of investment castings with ice patterns.
- A master model is obtained from silicone mold. Then the ice pattern is made by dropping water into the silicone mold and freezing it. This frozen ice pattern is then dipped into refrigerated ethyl silicate slurry and dried. This dipping and drying process is repeated until a ceramic shell is developed.[5]

REFERENCES

1. Kalpakjian S, Schmid S. Manufacturing Processes for Engineering Materials, 5th edn. Pearson Education Incorporation 2008.
2. Doles RS, Viers DS. Filler component for investment casting slurries. US Patent No. 7588633 B2 (September 15) 2009.
3. Jia Q, Cui YY, Yang R. A study of two refractories as mould materials for investment casting TiAl based alloys. Journal of Materials Science 2006;41:3045-49.
4. OspennikovaOG, Pikulina LV, Antipin LM. Application of a hydrolyzed ethyl silicate in investment casting. Neorganicheskie Materialy 2010;46(5):633-5.
5. Gannon P, Sofie S, Deibert M, Smith R, Gorokhovsky V. Thin film YSZ coatings on functionally graded freeze cast NiO/YSZ SOFC anode supports. Journal of Applied Electrochemistry. 2009;39(4):497-502.

20. Enumerate the die materials. What are the requirements of a die material? Write the advantages and disadvantages of each.

MATERIALS USED IN DIE PREPARATION

- Gypsum
- Epoxy resin
- Silicophosphate
- Amalgam
- Polymers
- Ceramic
- Electroplated dies.

REQUIREMENTS OF DIE MATERIALS

- It must reproduce all surfaces of the prepared teeth accurately without any bubbles or voids
- The remaining unprepared tooth structure 1 mm cervical to the finish line should be readily discernible on the die **(Fig. 5)**

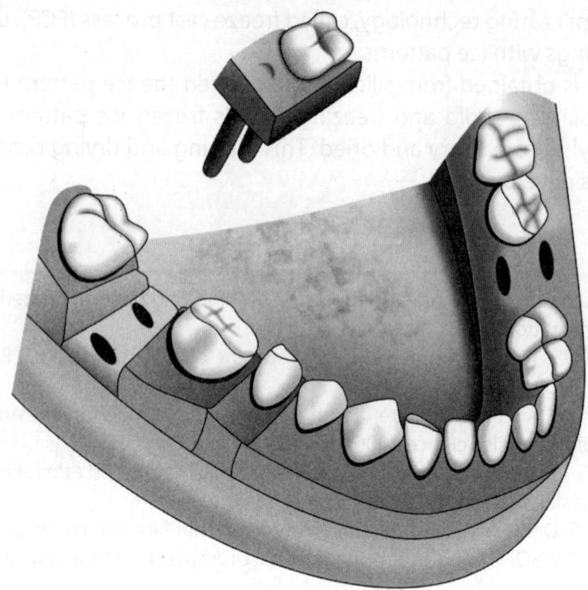

Fig. 5: Die and die pin

- Should be dimensionally stable
- Strong and resistant to abrasion
- Should be easily sectionable and easy to trim
- Should be compatible with the separating agent used
- Should color contrast with the wax used
- Should be easily wettable by the inlay wax
- Must be compatible with the impression material.

Gypsum

Advantages

- Inexpensive
- Easy to use
- Produces consistent results.

Disadvantages

- Decreased accuracy
- Decreased resistance to abrasion.

Variation of Technique

Impregnate the surface of the die with a low viscosity resin (cyanoacrylate) to improve abrasion resistance.

Epoxy Resin

Advantages

- Good strength
- Good abrasion resistance
- Can be cured at room temperature
- No complicated equipment required
- Dimensionally stable
- Retainers adapt better when made on epoxy dies
- Silicone and polyether are compatible with epoxy.

Disadvantages

- More expensive than gypsum
- Polymerization shrinkage
- Polysulfide and hydrocolloid are not compatible.

Variation

- Epoxy resin, which is heat-treated after setting, is also available.

Electroplated Die

Advantage

- Good abrasion resistance.

Disadvantages

- Silicone and polyether impressions are difficult to electroplate
- Polysulfide can be silver plated, but cannot be copper plated
- Silver plating uses cyanide solution, which is extremely toxic.

Technique

- Finely-powdered silver or graphite is brushed on to the impressions to make them conduct electricity
- The impression is then placed in the electroplating bath
- A layer of pure metal is deposited on the impression which is supported with type-IV stone or resin.

Silicophosphate Cement

This is similar to the filling and cementing material.

Advantage

- Harder than die stone.

Disadvantage

- Shrinkage on setting, loss of water on standing.

Amalgam

Advantages

- Produces a hard die
- Reproduces fine details and sharp margins.

Disadvantages

- Can only be packed into a rigid (for example, composition) impression
- Long time to reach maximum hardness
- High thermal conductivity, thus can cool a wax pattern rapidly, which may lead to distortion of the pattern—this can be overcome by warming the die
- A separating agent is needed as with stone dies.

Polymers and Filled Polymers

These are either self-curing acrylic materials, or polymeric materials (for example, epoxy resins, polyesters and epimines) with fillers (either metallic or ceramic fillers).

Advantages

- More abrasion resistant
- Not as brittle as die stones.

Disadvantage

- Shrinkage on polymerization may be a source of inaccuracy—fillers reduce this shrinkage.

Metal Sprayed Dies

A bismuth-tin alloy, which melts at 138°C, can be sprayed directly onto an impression to form a metal shell, which can then be filled with dental stone.

Advantage

- A metal-coated die can be obtained rapidly from elastomeric impression materials.

Disadvantage

- The alloy is rather soft; care is needed to prevent abrasion of the die.

Electroplated Dies

Some impression materials can be electroplated.

Copper Plating

- The surface of the impression is rendered conductive by coating it with fine particles of copper or graphite
- The coated impression is made the cathode (negative electrode) of a plating bath, with an anode (positive electrode) of copper
- The electrolyte is an acid solution of copper sulfate (about 250 g/L) along with organic constituents as alcohol or phenol which tend to increase the hardness of the deposited metal
- A current is passed, causing slow dissolution of the anode and movement of copper ions from anode to cathode, plating the impression. A current of 5 to 50 mamp/cm^2 of cathode surface is applied for approximately 10 hours
- Dental stone is then cast into the plated impression, when the stone has set, the metal covered die can be removed from the impression
- Not suitable for the elastomeric materials—it is not dimensionally stable in an acid solution.

Silver Plating

- Polysulfide and silicone impression materials can be silver plated by the same technique
- The impression is coated with silver or graphite powder
- The anode is silver
- The electrolyte is an alkaline solution of silver cyanide (with other constituents such as potassium cyanide and potassium carbonate)
- The current and time for plating is done according to the instructions supplied with the plating kit.

Precaution

Alkaline cyanide solution, releases HCN gas, which is a toxic; hence, silver plating is not often used.

Ceramic Die Materials

Two Ceramic Die Materials are Available

- A material for the production of dies on which porcelain restorations are to be fabricated, without the use of a platinum foil matrix. To form the dies heating to over 1000°C is necessary
- A ceramic material, supplied as a powder and liquid and mixed to a putty-like consistency. After 1 hour, the material is removed from the impression and fired at 600°C for 8 minutes to produce a hard strong die.

Other Die System

The Accutrac System

- Mainly used in the fabrication of laminate veneers.
- Involves the fabrication of two casts. Master cast is sectioned into dies and used to prepare the coping. After preparing the wax pattern, the sectioned dies are reassembled in the master cast.

- The first master cast is filled with wax to seal the crevices.
- The second cast refractory cast is duplicated from blocked out, die master cast using addition silicone. The second cast is poured using specially formulated stone, whose expansion compensates for the shrinkage porcelain when fired in the furnace.
- This is a working cast with removable die system.

Solid Die System: DVA Precision System

- This system needs no glueing of pins. Has a specially designed pin alignment and drilling machine, which determines dowel pin locations prior to the pouring of the model.
- Comes with premanufactured base plates; and specially designed dowel pins.

Zeiser System

From picodent is another single system with a premanufactured base.

21. Write briefly on casting failures and measures to avoid them.

GROUPED UNDER

- Distortion
- Surface roughness and irregularities
- Porosity
- Incomplete casting.

DISTORTION

Factors Causing Distortion

- Due to distortion of the wax pattern
- Uneven setting and hygroscopic expansions of the investment
- Configuration of the pattern, type of wax and thickness influence the amount of distortion caused by expansion of investment
- Distortion during the carving, pooling and removal of wax.

SURFACE ROUGHNESS AND IRREGULARITIES

- **Surface roughness** is defined as finely-spaced surface irregularities, whose height, width and direction establish predominant surface pattern
- **Surface irregularities** are isolated, generally caused by improper mixing technique.

Causes

Air Bubbles

- Air bubbles on margin of casting prevents proper seating
- This can be prevented by proper vacuum mixing, application of wetting agent and applying an initial layer of investment on pattern.

Water Films

- Appears as ridge or veins
- This occurs due to high water-powder ratio of investment material
- Application of wetting agent to wax pattern before investment can reduce water films.

Rapid Heating

- Seen as fins or spines
- When the invested material develops tensile stresses inside and compressive stresses outside, the investment cracks and forms fins.

Underheating

It is due to incomplete wax elimination.

Water-powder Ratio

Increased water-powder ratio causes rough casting and decreased ratio causes voids.

Prolonged Heating

This causes sulfur compounds that contaminate the surface of the casting.

High Temperature

Above 700°C causes breakdown of the investment and results in rough casting.

High Casting Pressure

Ideal casting pressure is 0.10 to 0.14 MPa (3-4 turns in the centrifugal casting machine).

Composition of Investment

If coarse silica is present, it can cause rough casting.

Foreign Bodies

Incorporated from rough crucible, sprue former, investment pieces, bits of carbon from flux.

Impact of Molten Alloy

Due to improper spruing.

Wrong Pattern Placement in the Casting Ring

Too many patterns placed together and patterns placed too close in the same ring should be avoided.

POROSITIES

Internal

- Solidification defects
- Microporosities
- Pin hole porosities
- Subsurface porosities
- Residual air in the mold.

External

- Surface roughnesses.

Solidification Defects

Solidification Shrinkage

Mainly occurs near sprue-cast junction.

Causes

- Incomplete feeding of molten metal
- Premature solidification of the sprue.

Suckback Porosities

- Near area of sprue
- This occurs when a hot metal, impinging from sprue channel on to a point on the mold wall, causes a hot spot. This hot spot causes local region to freeze last resulting in shrinkage of that area leading to a suckback porosity.

It can be prevented by:

- Flaring of the area of sprue attachment
- Lowering casting temperature by 30 degrees.

Microporosities (Fig. 6)

- Occurs when solidification occurs too rapidly before the microvoids can reorganize
- Prevented by lowering the mold temperature.

Pinhole Porosity (Fig. 6)

Spherical in shape whereas gas inclusion porosity is larger. During solidification absorbed gases are expelled leading to pinhole porosity.

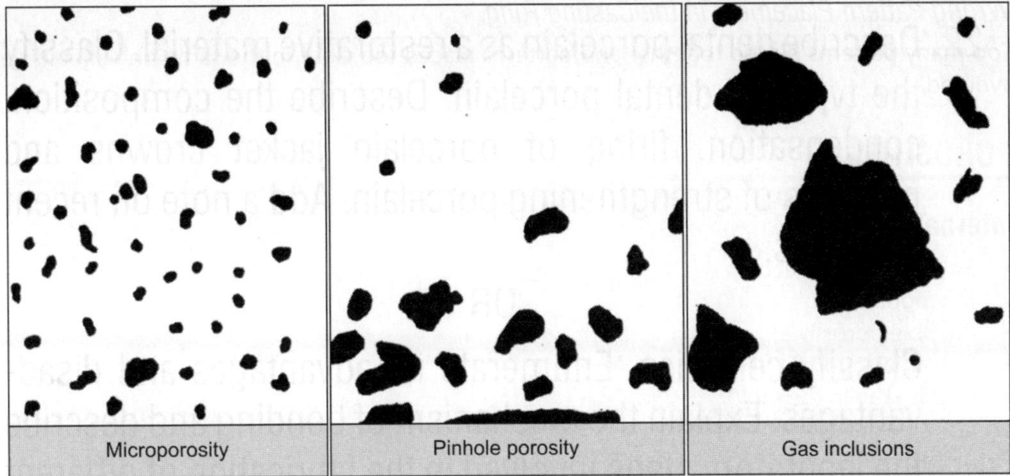

Fig. 6: Types of porosities

Subsurface Porosities

- Cause simultaneous nucleation of solid grains and gas bubbles as the metal freezes at the mold walls
- Can be decreased by controlling the rate of molten metal entry.

Residual Air in the Mold

- Causes back pressure porosity
- It occurs as a large concave depression due to the inability of air in the mold to escape.

Causes

- Dense investments
- Low mold temperature.

It can be prevented by:

- Proper burnout
- Adequate mold temperature
- Ideal casting pressure.

INCOMPLETE CASTING

Causes

- Insufficient venting
- Increased viscosity of fused metal
- Decreased casting pressure
- Incomplete wax elimination.

22. Describe dental porcelain as a restorative material. Classify the types of dental porcelain. Describe the composition, condensation, firing of porcelain jacket crowns and methods of strengthening porcelain. Add a note on recent advances.

OR

Classify ceramics. Enumerate its advantages and disadvantages. Explain the mechanism of bonding and describe the laboratory steps involved in the fabrication of different ceramics.

CLASSIFICATION

Depending on Use

Type 1

For denture teeth.
(Powders of feldspar, clay and quartz).

Type 2

For ceramometal applications.
(Potassium feldspar and glass).

Type 3

For all-porcelain restorations.
Porcelain jacket crowns, veneers and inlays.
(Feldspathic dental porcelain with increased amounts of aluminum oxide).

Depending on Fusion Temperature

- High fusing (1288–1371°C).
- Medium Fusing (1093–1260°C).
- Low Fusing (871–1066°C).
- Ultra Low Fusing (Below 850°C).

Based on Application

Core Porcelain

The core of porcelain jacket crown must have good mechanical properties.

Dentine or Body Porcelain

- More translucent than the above, this governs the shapes and color of the restoration
- Enamel porcelain forms the outer part of the crown and is translucent.

All Ceramic Restorations

Types

Conventional powder

Slurry ceramics
E.g.: Optec HSP, Duceram LFC.

Castable ceramics

E.g.: Picon, Dicor Plus.

Machinable ceramics

E.g.: Cerec vitablocs Mark I, Mark II, Dicor MGC, Celay.

Pressable ceramics

E.g.: IPS empress, OPTEC

Infiltrated ceramics

E.g.: INCERAM.

Advantages

- Highly Esthetic, can match the tooth color in translucency, color and intensity
- Special types of porcelain are available that can simulate all colors including gingival tones
- Life-like porcelain is achieved by glazing porcelain
- Glazed porcelain in contact with tissue surface is more biocompatible than metal
- All ceramic restoration has less failure rates
- Porcelain fused to metal prepared from foil copings uses thin metal copings (0.2–0.3 mm), which can increase bulk of porcelain.

DISADVANTAGES

- If there is difference in thermal matching between metal and porcelain, the porcelain fails at the margin
- More reduction of tooth structure to accommodate bulk of porcelain
- Brittle in nature and, if surface glaze is removed, cracks propagate leading to failure of porcelain
- Porcelain restorations do not give as close a marginal adaptation as metal marginal finish
- All-porcelain has lower tensile and shear strength, hence ideal to make a metal coping

- Porcelain shrinks during firing and if porosities are present the overall strength and translucency diminishes
- Ceramics and glasses have tensile strengths that are much lower than their compressive strengths
- Strength of ceramics reduces to 50% by sandblasting or by etching with hydrofluoric acid solution for 1 minute
- If tensile stresses or sub-microcracks are present on the surface, in presence of moisture may lead to stress corrosion
- Presence of a chemical environment decreases strength of porcelain.

FABRICATION OF METAL: CERAMIC RESTORATION

A. Condensation

Fine porcelain powder is mixed with water and condensed into the desired form.

Dense Condensation

1. Provides lower firing shrinkage.
2. Provides less porosity in the fired porcelain.

Methods of Condensation

1. Vibration

- Mild vibration to densely pack the wet powder upon the underlying framework
- The excess water is blotted with a clean tissue.

2. Spatulation

- A small spatula is used to apply and smoothen the wet porcelain.

3. Brush technique

- Dry porcelain powder is added to the surface with brush to absorb the water
- Porcelain must never be allowed to dry out until condensation is complete.

B. Firing

- The thermochemical reaction is complete during fritting.
- Firing is done to fuse the particles of powder together, a process called sintering.

Method

- The condensed porcelain mass is placed in a preheated furnace [approximately 650°C (1200°F)] for 5 minutes
- This removes the remaining water.

Stages in Firing

A low bisque (Low biscuit) firing

- In which the glass grains have softened and have started to flow.

A medium bisque (Medium biscuit) firing

- The glass grains have flowed to the extent that the powder particles exhibit complete cohesion.

In high bisque (High biscuit) firing

- The shrinkage is complete and the mass exhibits a smoother surface
- The lesser the firing cycles, the higher will be the strength and esthetics.

C. Glazing

Air-fired porcelain cannot be polished.

Application of overglaze/self-glaze

- Self-glazing, which was previously fired to a high bisque, is heated rapidly (10 to 15 minutes) to its fusion temperature
- It is maintained at that temperature for approximately 5 minutes before it is cooled
- Glass grains flow over the surface to form a vitreous layer
- Glazed porcelain is much stronger and reduces crack propagation than the unglazed variety.

D. Cooling

- Because of the low thermal conductivity of the porcelain, the differential between the thermal dimensional change of the outside and inside can introduce stresses, which embrittle the porcelain
- The ideal cooling method for a porcelain restoration from its firing temperature to room temperature is controversial.

OTHER TYPES OF PORCELAIN FABRICATIONS

A. Cast Coping

Requirements

- To be fusible to alloys, the porcelain has to be sufficiently low fusing
- It has to have a coefficient of thermal expansion that is considerably higher than ordinary porcelain
- The alloy should be sag resistant at the firing temperatures of porcelain
- It should be rigid to prevent fracture of porcelain
- There should be no pigmentation reaction produced between the porcelain and the alloy
- Further oxide formed should be soluble in porcelain and provide good wetting of the metal or metal oxide for attachment.

B. Bonded Platinum Foil Coping

- Makes use of tin oxide coatings on platinum foil
- The esthetics are improved with a thin platinum foil, which allows more room for porcelain
- The bonded foil reduces subsurface porosity and microcracks in the porcelain and increases the strength of the unit.

C. Swaged Gold Alloy Foil Coping

- Renaissance by the Williams Gold refining company is a laminated gold-alloy foil that is delivered to the use in a fluted shape
- This foil shape is swaged onto the die and flame sintered to form a coping
- An interfacial alloy powder is applied and fired and then coping is veneered with porcelain.

ALL CERAMIC MATERIALS

Conventional Powder-slurry Ceramics

Available as

- Powders to which water is added to produce a slurry
- Available in various shades and translucencies, with characterizing stains and glazes.

Manufacturing

- Leucite crystals are dispersed in a glassy matrix by controlling their nucleation and crystal growth
- The leucite and glassy matrix fuse together during the baking process
- The build-up and contouring of the crown can be done by using the powder-slurry technique on semipermeable die material.

Advantages

- Greater strength than conventional feldspathic porcelain due its leucite content
- Does not require a core as with aluminous porcelain jacket crowns
- The body and incisal porcelains can be pigmented to provide desired shade and translucency
- Does not require special processing equipment
- These restorations fit accurately.

Disadvantage

- Their high leucite content can cause increased wear to opposing teeth.

Other Types

Duceram LFC

- Hydrothermal low fusing ceramic
- Composed of an amorphous glass containing hydroxyl ions.

Advantages

- Greater density, higher flexural strength, greater fracture resistance and lower hardness than feldspathic porcelain
- No special laboratory techniques or equipment required.

Uses

- For fabrication of ceramic inlays, veneers and full-contour crowns.

Procedure

Base layer

Duceram Metal Ceramic (a leucite-containing porcelain) is placed on a refractory die using powder-slurry techniques and baked at 930°C.

Over base layer

Duceram LFC is applied using the powder-slurry technique and baked at a relatively low temperature (660°C).

Castable Ceramic Systems

Available as

- Solid ceramic ingots, which are cast using lost-wax and centrifugal casting technique
- Only one shade is available
- Staining is done to obtain proper shading of the final restoration.

Picon

- A polycrystalline glass-ceramic material, in which glass is heat-treated under controlled crystallization.

Procedure

- When solid ceramic ingots are cast at 1350°C, a transparent glass crown is obtained
- This crown is then heat-treated at 1075°C for 10 hours
- 'Ceramming' causes partial crystallization (55 percent) of tetra-silic-mica-like crystals.

Advantages

- Easier, as it is a lost wax technique
- The transparent crown after heat treatment at 1075°C for 10 hours forms an opaque crown, which increases fracture resistance and strength
- Less abrasive to opposing tooth structure
- For final restoration colorant stains are baked on the surface of the glass-ceramic material.

Dicor Plus

It is a shaded feldspathic porcelain veneer applied to the Dicor substrate **(Fig. 7)**.

Disadvantages

- Abrasive to opposing teeth
- Requires a special high-temperature, electric-heated casting unit
- Fracture of the restorations is common.

Machinable Ceramics

- Available as ceramic ingots in various shades
- Used in computer-aided design and computer-aided manufacturing (CAD-CAM) procedures
- The machined restorations are stained and glazed to the desired characterization.

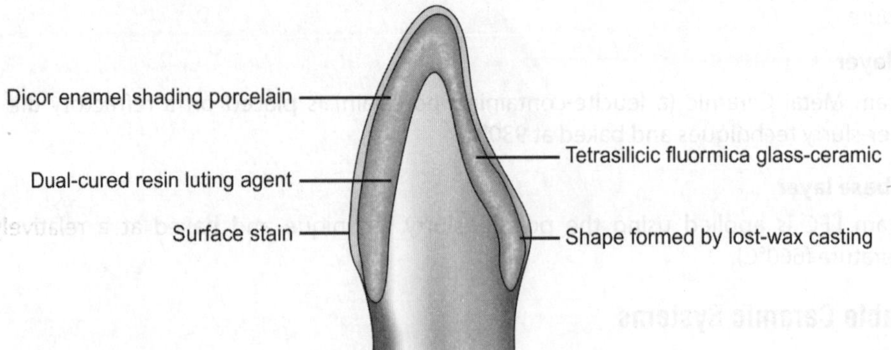

Fig. 7: Layers of Dicor glass ceramic crown

Cerec Vitablocs Mark I

- This is a feldspathic porcelain used with the Cerec system
- Composition and properties are the same as feldspathic porcelain used for porcelain-fused-to-metal restorations.

Cerec Vitablocs Mark II

This is a feldspathic porcelain of increased strength with less abrasive wear of the opposing tooth structure.

Dicor MGC

- Contains fluorosilicic mica crystals in a glass matrix
- It has greater flexural strength than the castable Dicor and Cerec
- Less abrasive wear of the opposing tooth structure than Cerec Mark I.

Celay

- Can be used for CAD-CAM-and copy-milling technique
- Identical in physical properties to Cerec Vitablocs Mark II.

Disadvantage

Marginal fit is not good.

Pressable Ceramics

- Available as ceramic ingots, which are melted at high temperatures and pressed into a mold created by lost-wax technique
- Can be made to full contour, or can be built up using feldspathic porcelain.

IPS Empress

- This is a feldspathic porcelain supplied in ingot form
- The ingots are heated and molded under pressure to produce the restorations.

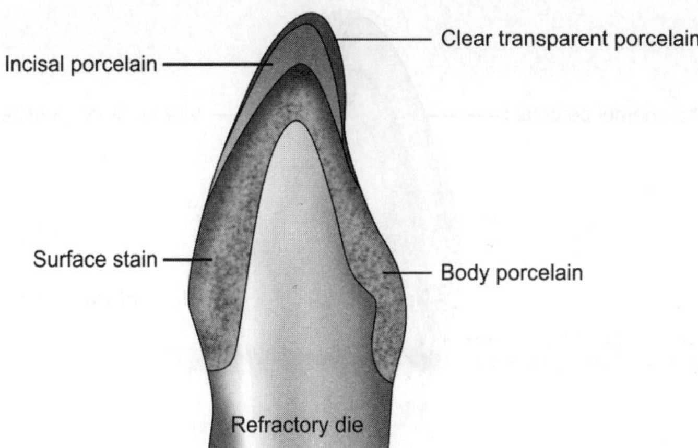

Fig. 8: Layers of an Optec HSP Crown

Procedure

- The ceramic ingot is placed under the plunger and heated to 1150°C
- The plunger presses the molten ceramic into the mold
- The final shade of the crown is done by staining or veneering (Cutback technique of wax pattern).

Optec Pressable Ceramic

This is a type of feldspathic porcelain with increased leucite content, processed by molding under pressure and heat **(Fig. 8)**.

Advantages of IPS and OPC

- Produce strong, translucent, dense and etchable ceramic restorations
- Useful in fabricating ceramic veneers.

Disadvantage

- Require special equipment to fabricate the restorations.

Infiltrated Ceramics

- Available as powder (aluminum oxide or spinel), which is fabricated into a porous substrate and a glass, which is infiltrated at high temperature into the porous substrate
- The infiltrated ceramic is then veneered using conventional feldspathic porcelain technique.

Inceram

- The spinel cores are more translucent than the aluminum oxide cores **(Fig. 9)**
- The core is made from fine-grained particles that are mixed with water to form a suspension referred to as a 'slip'.

Procedure

- The slip is placed on a gypsum die and baked at 1120°C for 10 hours to produce the opaque, porous core

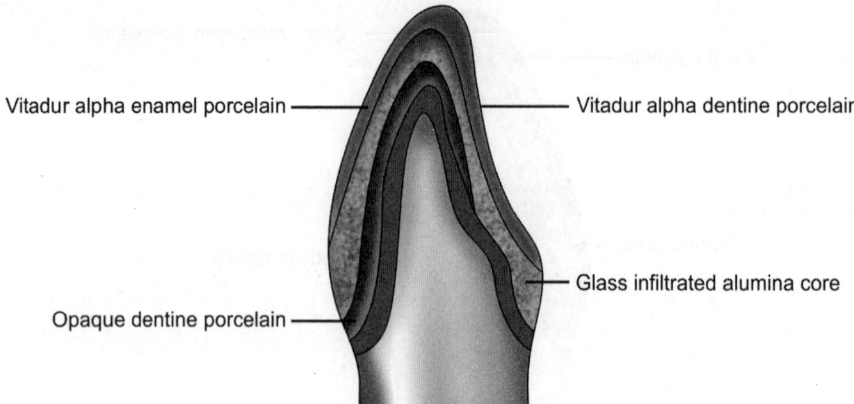

Fig. 9: Layers of an in-ceram crown

- An appropriate shade of glass powder is applied to the core, which is baked again at 1100°C for four hours
- During this process, the molten glass infiltrates the porous alumina core by capillary action.

Advantages

- Extremely high flexure strength
- The aluminum oxide or spinel crystals limit crack propagation and the glass infiltration reduces porosity
- Provide an accurate fit.

Disadvantages

- Cannot etch internal surface, hence, a resin cement such as Panavia 21TC is recommended
- Not as esthetic as other systems
- Requires specialized equipment to fabricate a restoration.

RECENT ADVANCES IN METAL-CERAMICS

- Pure titanium can be used as a coping and framework metal for metal ceramic restorations because of its excellent biocompatibility
- Copy milling is used to prepare duplicate dies of graphite and to machine the outer form of a titanium crown. The graphite die is then used as a positive electrode in a spark erosion system to serve as the pattern for removal of interior portion of the crown
- Other titanium-based products such as Tycast are melted in a specialized casting machine and cast using the conventional lost-wax technology. Ultra low fusing porcelain is used along with this.

METHOD OF STRENGTHENING PORCELAIN

Displacive Transformations

- Takes place where atoms become displaced, but no interatomic bonds are broken, when there is a temperature change

- These can occur for quartz, tridymite and cristobalite
- These strengthening mechanisms rely on the formation of a compressive surface layer.

Characteristics of Displacive Transformations

- They occur at specific temperatures
- The transformations are rapid
- The high-temperature form has a greater specific volume, thus the formation of the high-temperature material is accompanied.

Reconstructive Transformations

- Involve the breaking and remaking of Si-0 bonds. These processes need more energy.

Forms of Silica

- Quartz, with a hexagonal structure, is the instable form of silica
- When quartz is heated to 867°C, a reconstructive transformation to tridymite occurs
- At 1470°C, another reconstructive transformation takes place, to form cristobalite
- At over 1700°C, cristobalite melts and quartz, which is amorphous, is produced.

Ion Exchange

- It replaces smaller ions with larger ions via an ion-exchange mechanism. This process is carried out in a fused salt bath of the appropriate composition at a temperature of approximately 850°C
- An example of this is a glass ceramic placed in a solid solution of beta spodumene, where the exchange of lithium ions for the larger sodium ions leads to the formation of a surface compression layer during cooling, with a three-fold increase in the flexural strength.

23. Discuss the bonding of dental porcelain to casting alloys. Which types of alloys are suitable?

METAL-BONDED CERAMICS

Introduction

Elimination of microcracks forms stronger ceramics.

To Prevent Microcracks

- Glazing the internal fitting surface can eliminate microcracks
- Bonding the ceramic to a metal substrate can prevent microcracks

- Failure can occur at the junction of ceramic and metal due to a mismatch between the coefficients of expansion of the ceramic and the metal. If the mismatch is too great, then stresses will build up resulting in crazing or cracking of the ceramic.

BOND FORMATION

Mainly by Three Mechanisms

1. Mechanical retention
2. Compression
3. Chemical bonding.

Mechanical Bond

- Microscopic irregularities on metal surface are filled with porcelain; retention of the porcelain veneer by mechanical interlocking is achieved
- Mechanical retention occurs as the ceramic flows into the microscopic spaces in the surface of the metal.

Microscopic Spaces can be Created by

- Applying an alumina-air abrasive
- By grinding.

Increasing Mechanical Bond Strength

- Grinding or sand blasting
- Roughening by oxidation
- Electrochemical corrosion of the metal by molten glass
- Selective oxidation of grain boundaries
- Etching by acid in pre-treatment for fusing.

Compressive Stresses

- A very small degree of thermal mismatch between metal and porcelain leaves the porcelain in a state of compression
- This increases the bonding between metal and porcelain
- Before the ceramic is applied to the surface of the coping, the coping is subjected to a degassing cycle to burn off any remaining impurities
- On cooling, the metal will try to contract more than the ceramic due to its higher coefficient of expansion, which leaves the ceramic in a state of compression
- The mismatch in the coefficients of thermal expansion between ceramic and metal should be small; otherwise, the internal stresses created during cooling could cause the ceramic to fracture.

Chemical Bond

- True chemical bonding results from electron transfer between the oxygen of the glassy phase of porcelain and an oxidized metal surface

- During firing, the ceramic is heated above its glass transition temperature such that it can flow and fuse with the oxides on the metal surface by migration of the oxides into the ceramic
- In the case of gold alloy copings, small amounts of oxide forming elements are added to the alloy because gold does not form an oxide.

Increasing Chemical Bond

- By addition of tin, indium, iron to a noble metal casting alloy
- In nickel-chromium alloy, there is an indirect bond between glass and metal through an undissolved oxide formed on the metal surface
- Strong chemical bond is created between the ceramic and the oxide coating on the metal.

PROCEDURE FOR METAL CERAMIC BONDING

Preparation of the Metal Surface for Mechanical Bonding

Surface preparation is done in a metal to remove any contaminants and to produce a surface oxide layer of the correct composition for the ceramic to fuse to **(Fig. 10)**.

The various stages can be identified as:

- Surface grinding
- Heating under partial vacuum
- Acid pickling
- Heating in air.

Surface Grinding

The grinding process is done to remove all of imperfections, unwanted oxides, small porosities and fine projections, the surface roughness caused by grinding aid in the retention of the ceramic by micromechanical interlocking.

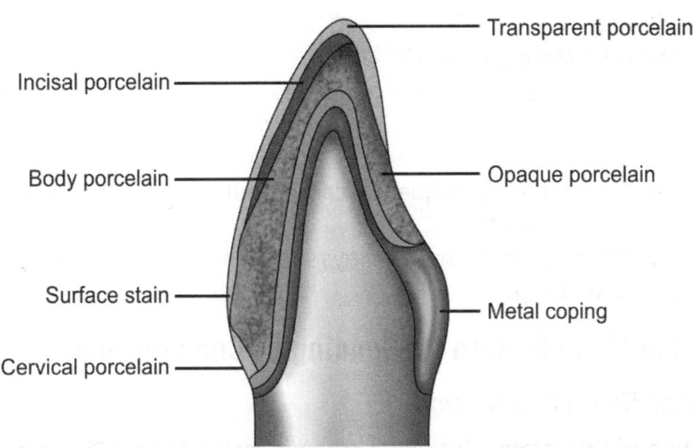

Fig. 10: Layers of a metal ceramic crown

Points to note

- If proper abrasives are not used, deep fissures can result which prevents proper wetting of ceramic
- The presence of trapped air and contaminants results in the presence of gas bubbles at the interface between the metal and the ceramic, decreasing the bond strength
- Surface contamination in the casting can be cleaned in an organic solvent (e.g. carbon tetrachloride) in a sealed ultrasonic bath.

Abrasives used

Fissure burs or carbide burs.

Heating Under Partial Vacuum

An oxide film can be formed by heating the casting at a temperature near to the firing temperature of the ceramic. This has the effect of allowing the metallic elements that are incorporated in the alloy to migrate to the surface and form an oxide surface layer.

Incorrect heating cycle

- Short heat treatment results in the formation of a thin or partial oxide coating—bonding of ceramic to metal is poor
- Long heating cycle results in the depletion of the oxidizing elements from the surface layer of the gold alloy
- Heat treatment under reduced pressure removes gases absorbed by the metal during the casting process.

Acid Pickling

- The heat treatment of gold alloys will produce tin oxide and other unwanted oxides on the surface which are removed by acid pickling procedure
- Acid pickling lightens the dark surface of the alloy from gray to white due to increased concentration of tin oxide on the alloy surface.

Acids used

- 50% hydrofluoric acid
- 30% hydrochloric acid (More preferred)
- Base metal alloys do not require these procedures.

Heating in Air

- A further heat treatment in air is frequently carried out in order to form an oxide coating of the correct thickness and quality
- The optimal oxide film on precious metal alloys should have a mat, greyish white appearance, composed mainly of tin oxide.

Preparation of the Metal Surface for Bonding by Compression

The Importance of Thermal Expansion

- The composition of the ceramic for metal-ceramic restorations is different from that of the ceramic used in porcelain jacket crowns. Thermal expansion of porcelain jacket crown is 8 ppm/°C

- Coefficient of thermal expansion of alloys is in the region of 12 ppm/°C. The thermal mismatch between the metal and ceramic used in metal ceramic should be minimal
- The ceramic loses its thermoplastic fluidity once it is cooled below its glass transition temperature (i.e. 600–700°C)
- The metal will attempt to shrink more than the ceramic and this places the ceramic in a state of compression. Since the tensile strength of the alloys used is quite high (500–1000 MPa), the interface bond strengths do not fail
- The coefficient of expansion of the ceramic is only slightly lower than that of the metal
- Multiple firings will increase the coefficient of thermal expansion, which can result in failure of the bond between metal and ceramic.

CHOICE OF METAL-CERAMIC ALLOYS

High-Gold Alloys

- For the high-gold alloys, the melting temperature is raised by the addition of platinum and palladium
- The high-gold alloys have good bond between the ceramic and the metal and is highly reliable
- Disadvantages of high-gold alloys are their low melting temperatures, susceptibility to creep at high temperatures and their low elastic moduli. A minimum coping thickness of 0.5 mm is required with their use
- In some areas, it can result in overcontouring to mask the metal color.

Gold-Palladium Alloys

- Introduced in 1970s due to rising cost of gold
- Their performance is comparable to that of the high gold alloys in terms of castability, accuracy of fit and corrosion resistance
- Some of them have mismatch in thermal expansion characteristics.

High-Palladium Alloys

- These alloys are palladium, with small additions of other elements, such as copper, gallium and tin
- The copper in palladium alloys do not cause discoloration. Copper can be present in amounts up to 15%
- As their sag resistance is poor, they are contraindicated for long-span bridges.

Palladium-Silver Alloys

- The Pd-Ag alloys have the most favorable elastic modulus of all of the precious metal alloys
- They produce castings with low flexibility and a reduced tendency to sag on porcelain firing
- Due to the presence of high amounts of silver, porcelain discoloration may occur
- Multiple firings should be kept to a minimum and overheating of the alloy should be avoided.

Nickel-Chromium Alloys

- The Ni-Cr alloys are very stiff and their elastic modulus can be 2–5 times higher than that of the high-gold alloys
- Hence, coping thickness can be reduced from 0.5 mm to 0.3 mm, which lessens the problem of overcontouring
- They are good for the construction of long-span bridges, as they provide greater rigidity and, because of the high melting temperature, there is less potential for sag during firing.
- The disadvantage with these alloys is that casting is difficult and the higher casting shrinkage can cause poor fit
- Bonding between ceramic to metal is not as reliable as for the other alloys
- The low cost of the alloy is an advantage.

Latest in Bonding

- Various surface treatments for ceramics have proved to increase the bond strength.
- Surface treatments include abrasion/sand blasting, sand paper disks, lasers, etching, atmospheric plasma, UV and treatment with ceramic primer.[1,2]

REFERENCES

1. Noro A, Kameyama A, Haruyama A, Takahashi T. Influence of hydrophilic pre-treatment on resin bonding to zirconia ceramics. Bull Tokyo Dent Coll. 2015;56(1):33-9.
2. Paul P, Reddy SND, RK Alla, Rajasigamani K, Chidambaram. Evaluation of shear bond strength of stainless steel brackets bonded to ceramic crowns etched with Er; Cr: YSGG Laser and Hydrofluoric acid: An in vitro study. Brit J Medical Med Res. 2015;7(7):550-60.

24. What are the ideal properties of the casting alloys? Discuss the various types of casting alloys, their properties and uses.

INTRODUCTION

The lost wax technique was introduced by Taggart in 1907 for casting inlay restorations.

IDEAL PROPERTIES OF CASTING ALLOYS

Cost

Cast gold alloys are expensive than base-metal alloys.

Biocompatibility

Gold alloys have good resistance to corrosion and tarnish than base-metal alloys.

Stiffness

Gold alloys have low modulus of elasticity compared to base-metal alloys and cannot be used for long span bridges, cast posts and long span partial dentures.

Resilience

For metal ceramic alloys, deflection under stress should be negligible to support the brittle porcelain.

Compatibility

Compatibility to porcelain: Elastic modulus, thermal expansion coefficient and heat conductivity are important for porcelain metal compatibility.

Tarnish Resistance

Good for gold alloy compared to base metal alloys.

Fatigue Resistance

Ability to withstand repeated deformation in the elastic region.

Sag Resistance

Ability of dental alloy to resist plastic and creep flow under its own weight during porcelain firing and soldering.

Fit

Is the ability of a casting to reproduce the pattern precisely.

Ease of Casting

The melting range and casting temperature of alloys are important for ease of casting.

Ease of soldering

Ease of burnishability

The Density of the Alloy

The higher the density of the alloy, the easier it is to force the air out of the mold space and to fill the space completely with alloy.

Casting Shrinkage and Cooling Contraction

Accounts for the size of casting

Types of Alloys Used for Casting

- Cast gold alloys
- Cast base metal alloys.

CAST GOLD ALLOYS

(Classified by Bureau of Standards)

Type I: Soft
83% of noble metals.
Type II: Medium
78% of noble metals.

Type III: Hard
78% of noble metals.

Type IV: Extra hard
75% of noble metals.

Composition of Cast Gold Alloys

Type	Gold %	Silver %	Copper %	Palladium %	Platinum %	Zinc %
I	79–92.5	3–12	2–4.5	0–0.5	0–0.5	0–0.5
II	75–78	12–14.5	7–10	1–4	0–1	0.5
III	62–78	8–26	8–11	2–4	0–3	1
IV	60–71.5	4.5–20	11–16	0–5	0–3.5	1–2

Composition of Modern Noble Metal Alloys

Types	Content	Gold %	Copper %	Silver %	Palladium %	In, Sn, Fe, Zn, Ga %
I	Yellow gold	83	6	10	0.5	Balance
II	Yellow gold	77	7	14	1	"
III	Yellow gold	75	9	11	3.5	"
III	Low gold	46	8	39	6	"
III	Silver-Palladium			70	25	"
IV	Yellow gold	69	10	12.5	3.5+3.0Pt	"
IV	Low gold	56	14	25	4	"
IV	Silver-Palladium	15	14	45	25	"
Metal ceramic	White gold	52			38	"
Metal ceramic	Palladium-Silver			30	60	"
Metal ceramic	Yellow gold	88		1	6.5+4.0%	"

ALLOYING ELEMENTS IN DENTAL GOLD ALLOYS

Major composition of gold alloys is gold, with lower amounts of silver and copper. Some contain very small amounts of platinum, palladium and zinc.

Silver

Strengthens the alloy and counteracts the reddish tint of the copper.

Copper

- Increases the strength, particularly of the Type III and IV gold alloys and reduces the melting temperature (16%)
- Addition of copper produces order-hardening.

Procedure

- The alloy is homogenized at approximately 700°C to ensure a uniform composition throughout the casting
- Then the alloy is reheated to 400°C and held at that temperature for approximately 30 minutes. At this temperature, the copper atoms arrange themselves in little ordered clusters
- This ordered structure prevents slippage of the atomic layers, raising the yield stress and the hardness of the alloy
- There must be at least 11% copper in the gold alloy for order hardening to occur, so it cannot occur in Type I and Type II gold alloys.

Platinum

Increases both the strength and the melting temperature.

Palladium

Has the same effect as platinum, but is cheaper.

Zinc

Acts as a scavenger during casting, preventing oxidation and improves the castability.

Other Elements, such as Indium and Ruthenium (<0.5%)

Have very high melting temperature and act as nucleating sites during solidification, thus helping to produce a fine grain size.

GOLD ALLOYS

Depending on function, these are classified as follows:

Type I Alloys

For inlays in low stress situations as these alloys are relatively soft and easily deformed. These alloys are highly ductile and can be burnished easily. They are less fracture prone.

Type II Alloys

For most inlays. However, those with thin sections should be avoided as deformation can occur.

Type III Alloys

Used for all inlays, onlays, full coverage crowns and short-span bridges, cast posts and cores because of their greater strength. They are difficult to burnish and have a higher potential for fracture compared to type I and type II.

Type IV Alloys

Used for cast posts, cores, long span bridges, in partial denture construction and clasp arms. The low elastic modulus and high yield strength of the gold alloy provide a high degree of flexibility to clasp arms.

Properties and Applications

- The medium-gold alloys can be used for long-span prostheses, implant-supported prostheses and posts and cores
- The low-gold content alloys are used for posts and cores, where the white color does not present a problem as the casting will be covered with another material
- The removal of copper and the addition of indium produces alloys with properties similar to those of the type III gold alloys, but with a yellow color. These alloys are difficult to cast
- The biocompatibility of these alloys is good.

MODERN NOBLE METAL ALLOYS

Silver-Palladium Alloys ('White Gold')

Composition

- 45% silver
- 24% palladium
- 15% gold
- 15% copper
- 1% zinc.

Palladium

- Improves the resistance to corrosion and helps to prevent tarnish. These alloys were introduced in the 1960s as an alternative to the high-gold alloys and are commonly called 'white golds'
- High casting temperatures require use of phosphate-bonded investments
- They are highly biocompatible, but tarnishing can occur with these alloys.

Properties

- Less expensive, hence can substitute gold alloys
- Their proportional limit and ultimate tensile strength are inferior to type IV gold alloys

- Silver-palladium alloys work-harden rapidly, so that if a clasp has to be adjusted, fracture is liable to occur
- Both silver and palladium dissolve oxygen when molten, leading to porosity of the casting
- Heat treatment can be carried out, but this reduces the percentage elongation and makes the alloy brittle.

BASE METAL CASTING ALLOYS

Cobalt-Chromium Alloys

Co-Cr alloys were first introduced to the dentistry in the 1930s.

Applications

- For the construction of partial denture frameworks
- As metal ceramic alloys.

Composition

- *Cobalt*: 35–65%
- *Chromium*: 20–35%
- *Nickel*: 0–30%
- *Molybdenum*: 0–7%
- *Carbon*: up to 0.4%

Tungsten, manganese, silicon and iron may also be present in small quantities.

Functions of Components

Chromium

The more the chromium content, the better is the corrosion resistance of the alloy. Chromium is added without introducing the brittle second phase.

Molybdenum

Is present in order to refine the grain size by providing more sites for crystal nucleation during the solid solidification process.

Iron

Increases strength.

Carbon

- Content can significantly alter the strength, hardness and ductility of the alloy
- If the patient is allergic to **nickel**, a nickel-free Co-Cr alloy is used
- The mechanical grinding and polishing process causes the release of beryllium, which is a known carcinogen.

Properties

- They must be heated to high temperatures before they can be cast
- Accuracy is compromised at high temperatures, hence limits the use of these alloys to partial dentures

- The high hardness of these alloys makes them difficult to polish mechanically
- Electrolytic polishing is used for the fitting surfaces, so as not to compromise the quality of fit, but nonfitting surfaces are still mechanically polished
- These alloys are also prone to casting porosity
- The modulus of elasticity of a Co-Cr alloy is typically 250 GPa, whereas for other alloys, the modulus is in the range of 70–100 GPa
- This high modulus of elasticity is of use to make thinner sections of the material whilst maintaining adequate rigidity
- The addition of chromium makes this a highly corrosion-resistant and biocompatible alloy.

Nickel-Chromium Alloys

Composition

- 75% nickel and 20% chromium.

Applications

- Resin-bonded techniques
- Porcelain bonding.

Manipulation

The casting technique for base metal alloys is similar to that of gold alloys, except that:

- The melting point of these alloys is in the range 1250–1450°, hence silica-bonded or phosphate-bonded material should be chosen. For gold alloys, gypsum-bonded investment is used
- Because of the high melting range, oxyacetylene flame/induction heating is used to melt alloy. Gold alloys can be melted using blowtorches.

BASE METAL VS GOLD ALLOYS

- The proportional limit and ultimate tensile strength of cobalt-chromium alloys is less than that of the hardened gold alloys
- The cobalt-chromium alloys have a modulus of elasticity about twice that of gold alloys. Hence, sections of cobalt-chromium alloys of about half the thickness of gold alloys can be used to achieve the same degree of rigidity
- The cobalt-chromium alloys are more brittle (lower percentage elongation)
- The cobalt-chromium alloys have high melting range and greater hardness
- The casting shrinkage of cobalt-chromium alloys is greater than that of the gold-containing materials
- The density of cobalt-chromium is about half that of gold.

25. What are abrasive and polishing agents? Give their desirable characteristics with examples.

ABRASION

The process in which hard sharp particles of an abrasive are moved over the surface by which the rough surface is made smooth.

Process of Abrasion

- The abrasive used produces a cutting groove in the surface of the article under treatment
- The surface leaves scratches depending on the particle size of the abrasive
- These scratches are smoothed by finer abrasives. Before changing to a new abrasive, the article should be washed well
- The abrasive particles must be harder than the surface being abraded
- The abrasive particles may be bonded together, as in a grinding wheel, disc or strip, or they may be carried across the surface by a brush or buff
- Heat is generated which can be reduced by water-spray as in tooth preparation
- Excessive heat should be avoided in abrading polymeric materials, as it can cause stress relief and warpage.

Factors Influencing the Efficiency of Abrasives

- Hardness of the abrasive particles. Diamond is the hardest material, whereas pumice, garnet, etc. are mild abrasives
- Abrasive particles with sharp edges will be more efficient than those with obtuse angles
- Abrasives with larger particles will cut deeper grooves
- If the abrasive material breaks, it should form a new cutting edge
- Slower abrasion produces deeper scratches
- If a large pressure is applied, the abrasive may fracture and increase the heat of friction evolved
- A brittle material can be abraded rapidly, whereas a malleable and ductile material will flow instead of being removed.

Materials Used for Abrasion

- **Diamond** is the hardest known abrasive and can be embedded in a ceramic or metallic holder as in dental burs
- **Tungsten carbide** is used mainly in the form of burs and abrasive wheels
- **Silicon carbide** may be supplied as a powder and bonded with rubber to form the stones and wheels used in the dental laboratory
- **Alumina** is used similarly to silicon carbide
- **Emery** is a mixture of alumina and iron, which is supplied as an abrasive coating on cloth or paper

- **Sand (silica)**—sandpaper, as abrasive paper discs
- **Garnet** is a milder abrasive, containing magnesium aluminum silicate and used as a coating paper disc
- **Cuttlefish** bone has similar uses to garnet
- **Pumice** is prepared by crushing pumice stone or porous volcanic rock and is used as a suspension in finishing of acrylic resins
- **Tripoli** is a ground porous rock, which is used with a wax to form a 'brick' of material.

POLISHING

Polishing does not cut grooves in a material, but rather reduces irregularities. For materials like thermoplastic polymers, the surface flows to fill in any scratches as the surface becomes heated.

Significance of Polishing

- If dental restorations and appliances do not have a smooth surface, food debris will be deposited on rough surfaces, which can cause corrosion of metallic materials
- Rough surfaces are not comfortable for the patient.

Polishing Materials

- Whiting (or precipitated chalk) is used as a suspension in water for polishing plastics, such as acrylic
- Zinc oxide in alcohol can be used for polishing amalgam restorations
- Iron oxide (rouge) is supplied in a soap base for polishing gold alloys. Cannot polish chromium-containing alloys
- Chromium oxide is also used in a soap base and is supplied for polishing stainless steel and cobalt-chromium alloys.

Electrolytic Polishing

- This is the reverse procedure to electroplating
- The alloy to be polished is made the anode of an electrolytic cell
- As the current is passed, some of the anode is dissolved leaving a bright surface
- This is an excellent method for polishing the fitting surface of a cobalt-chromium alloy denture, so little material is removed that the fit of the denture is unaltered.

Polishing Techniques for Titanium Alloys in Dentistry

- Sandblasting with 110 μ aluminium oxide for 30–60 sec at 4.5 Mpa pressure with a nozzle distance of 10–20 mm.
- Chemical dipping in 3–5% hydrofluoric acid and 30% nitric acid for 60–90 sec at 50–60°.
- Mechanical polishing with carborundum, diamond or carbon boron grinding materials
- Barrel polishing in which alumina is shaped as Trigon and polishing done at 450–650 rpm.
- Electrochemical
- Anodization techniques.

26. What are tarnish and corrosion? Describe the types of corrosion. What precautions would you take while making silver amalgam restoration in order to reduce tarnish and corrosion?

DEFINITION

Tarnish

- Tarnish is a process by which a surface loses its luster or becomes discolored due to a chemical film (sulfide, oxide or chloride film)
- Tarnish is often an indication of corrosion because of a film that is deposited which gradually accumulates elements that chemically attack metallic surface.

Corrosion

Corrosion is an electrochemical process through which a metal is attacked by natural agents like water or air resulting in complete or partial dissolution or weakening of the metal.

FACTORS CAUSING CORROSION

- Disintegration of metal occurs due to air, moisture, acids, alkaline solutions or certain chemicals
- Surfaces under stress or with intergranular impurities are more prone to corrosion
- Sulfides like H_2S or $(NH_4)_2S$ and H_2O, O_2, Cl ions present in saliva corrode silver and mercury present in alloys and amalgam
- H_3PO_4, lactic acid, acetic acid at proper concentration and PH also lead to corrosion.

TYPES OF CORROSION

Dry Corrosion/Chemical Corrosion

- Chemical corrosion is due to direct combination of metallic and nonmetallic elements. It is also referred to as dry corrosion, because it occurs in the absence of water or other fluid electrolytes
- For example, oxidation of alloy particles in dental amalgam.

Wet Corrosion/Electrochemical Corrosion

- It is known as wet corrosion as it requires the presence of water or other fluid electrolytes. It also requires a pathway for the transport of electrons, an electric current, for the process to continue
- Anode is a surface where positive ions are formed. This metal surface corrodes due to loss of electrons or oxidation reaction

- At the cathode, reduction reaction takes place to consume free electrons produced at the anode
- The metal with lowest electrode potential corrodes. The more active metal acts as the anode and corrodes and the more noble metal becomes the cathode.

Types of Electrolytic Corrosion

Galvanic corrosion

- Galvanic corrosion occurs when dissimilar metals lie in direct physical contact with each other. Saliva with its salts provides a weak electrolyte
- If gold restoration comes in contact with an amalgam restoration, amalgam forms anode and starts corroding
- Because both the restorations are wet with saliva, an electrical couple exists with a difference in potential between dissimilar restorations
- When the two fillings are brought into contact, the potential is suddenly short-circuited through the two alloys. The result is a sharp pain. This is called galvanic shock **(Fig. 11)**
- The electric currents between a gold crown and an amalgam restoration in the same mouth, but not in contact, is approximately 0.5 to 1μA with corresponding EMF of approximately 500 mV
- It usually occurs immediately after insertion and can be minimized by painting a varnish on the surface of the amalgam restoration
  Hence, it is better to avoid dissimilar metals in contact.

Heterogeneous compositions

- Heterogeneous compositions can cause galvanic corrosion

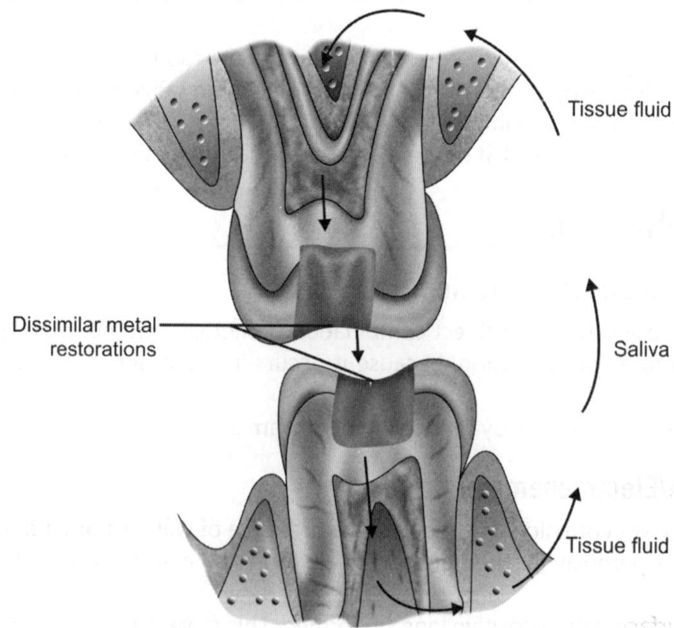

Fig. 11: Path of galvanic current in the mouth

- When an alloy containing eutectic is immersed in an electrolyte, the metallic grains with the lower electrode potential are attacked and corrosion results
- In a cored structure, differences in the composition within the alloy grains are found
- Thus, part of a grain can be anode and part cathode. Homogenization improves the corrosion resistance of the alloy
- In metals or alloys, the grain boundaries may act as anodes and the interior of the grain as the cathode
- Solder joints may also corrode due to the inhomogeneous composition
- Impurities in any alloy enhance corrosion.

Stress corrosion

- Any cold working of an alloy by bending, burnishing or malleting localizes stress in some parts of the structure
- Combined with an oral condition that promotes corrosion, the stressed appliance develops stress corrosion
- Slight surface irregularities at that point, such as notch or pit, can accelerate the process. When a couple composed of stressed metal is formed, the stressed area is readily dissolved by the electrolyte resulting in corrosion.

Concentration cell corrosion or crevice corrosion

Electrolyte concentration cell: In a metallic restoration which is partly covered by food debris, the composition of the electrolyte under the debris will differ from that of salvia and this can contribute to the corrosion of the restoration.

Oxygen concentration cell: Difference in oxygen tension in between parts of the same restoration causes corrosion of the restoration. Greater corrosion occurs in the part of restoration having lower concentration of oxygen.

PROTECTION AGAINST CORROSION

Passivation

- Certain metals like Cr, Ti and Al form strong adherent oxide film on their surface. Since, this film formed is passive to oxidative chemical attack, its formation is called passivation
- If more than 12% Cr is added to iron or cobalt, stainless steel or Co-Cr alloys are formed, which are highly corrosion resistant.

Increasing Noble Metal Content

- Alloy with noble metal content below 65% may tarnish. At least 50% of atoms in a dental alloy should be gold, platinum or palladium to ensure against corrosion
- Noble metals resist corrosion because their EMF is positive with regard to any of the common reduction reactions found in the oral environment.

Polishing

Polishing metallic restoration like amalgam and cast metal to a high lustre minimizes corrosion. The patient should also maintain good oral hygiene.

Precautions in Silver Amalgam

- Dissimilar metal restoration should be avoided
- Avoid using a high mercury containing amalgam, as it is more susceptible to corrosion
- Mercury tarnishes gold and care must be taken during manipulation of amalgam.

Methods to Prevent Tarnish and Corrosion

In Amalgam Restoration

- Finish restoration to high mirror like polish without any scratch or defects on surface.
- To prevent galvanic corrosion apply varnish to dentinal walls before amalgam placement.

For Other Metals/Alloys

- A coat of noble metal can be applied over base metal
- Paint or coat inorganic non-conductive coating
- Passivation procedure as in chromium based alloys

Electroplating with nickel followed by chromium in stainless steel.

27. Classify dental amalgam. Write in detail about the composition, advantage and disadvantage of each ingredient and the uses of dental amalgam.

An amalgam is an alloy of two or more metals, one of which is mercury. Dental amalgam is an alloy made by mixing mercury with silver, tin, copper and, sometimes, zinc.

CLASSIFICATION

Based on the SHAPE of the Alloy Particle

- Lathe cut (irregular)
- Spherical
- Spheroidal.

Based on the SIZE of the Alloy Particle

- Regular cut
- Fine cut
- Micro fine cut.

Based on ZINC Content

- Zinc containing (contains more than 0.01% Zn).
- Non-zinc containing.

Based on the NUMBER of Alloyed Metals

- Binary alloys, e.g. silver – tin
- Ternary alloys, e.g. silver – tin – copper
- Quaternary alloys, e.g. silver – tin – copper – zinc.

Based on the CHRONOLOGY

- I generation
- II generation
- III generation
- IV generation
- V generation
- VI generation.

Based on COPPER Content

- Low copper alloy (Less than 6% copper)
- High copper alloy (More than 6% copper).

High Copper Alloy

Unicompositional

- 13–30% copper
- Spherical particles of the same composition.

Admixed

- 6–20% copper
- Mixture of irregular (Lathe cut) and spherical particles of different composition.

Pre-amalgamated Alloys

- Manufacturer treats the alloy powder with 3% $HgCl_2$
- This reduces the final mercury content and improves the amalgamated reaction.

COMPOSITION OF VARIOUS SILVER ALLOYS

Particle shape	Low copper	High copper		Unicompositional
		Admixed		
	Lathe cut or spherical	Lathe cut 2/3	Spherical 1/3	
Silver	63–70%	40–70%	40–65%	40–60%
Tin	23–26%	26–30%	0–30%	22–30%
Copper	2–6%	2–30%	20–40%	13–30%
Zinc	0–2%	0–2%	0	0

Advantages and Disadvantages (Roles) of each Ingredient

Silver

Produces the characteristic silver color of the alloy.

Increases

- Strength
- Hardness
- Corrosion resistance
- Setting expansion.

Decreases

- Setting time

Tin

Decreases

- Strength
- Hardness
- Corrosion resistance
- Setting expansion.

Copper

Helps to cut alloy into fine particles during manufacturing.

Increases

- Strength
- Hardness
- Setting expansion
- Corrosion resistance.

Zinc

- Zn in liquid condition can dissolve O_2 and combine with it to form ZnO_2
- Since the affinity of Zn to O_2 is more than that of other metals, Zn gets oxidized preferentially and then prevents oxidation of other metals
- ZnO floats on the surface and can be easily removed
- Hence called as a deoxidizer or scavenger
- May cause delayed expansion if contaminated by moisture during amalgam manipulation.

Palladium

Whitens the alloy and improves mechanical properties.

Platinum

Hardens the alloy and improves resistance to corrosion.

Indium

Lowers creep, improves strength, and reduces mercury content.

Mercury

- Forms the matrix phase to hold the alloy particles together
- Concern for health hazard.

USES

Non-Zn-containing alloys can be used in conditions where moisture control is difficult.

- Pediatric restoration
- Retrograde filling.

28. What are low copper and higher copper amalgam alloys? Write in brief about the types of low copper alloys and add a note on high copper alloys.

Low Copper Alloys

- Lathe cut
- Spherical.

High Copper Alloys

- Admixed/blended
- Unicompositional.

Copper enriched alloys have become available since the 1970s.

Basic ingredients are same as the conventional silver amalgam, although they contain much more copper, (10–30%) compared to less than 6% in the conventional alloys.

LOW COPPER ALLOYS

Lathe Cut vs Atomized Spherical Powder

- Spherical alloys require less mercury than typical lathe-cut alloy because spherical alloy powder particles have a smaller surface area per volume than do the lathe-cut alloy particles
- Amalgams with low mercury content generally have better properties. The tensile strength of low copper is 48–70 MPa.

Spherical Alloys

- Atomized powder is made by melting together the desired elements
- The liquid metal is atomized into fine spherical droplets of metal
- If the droplets solidify before hitting a surface, the spherical shape is preserved
- These atomized powders are called spherical alloy powders.

Composition

- Ag: 63–70%
- Sn: 26–28%
- Cu: 2.5%
- Zn: 0.2%

Properties

Compressive strength

- The early compressive strength after 1 hour for the low copper spherical alloy is 141 Mn/m^{2}.
- For lathe-cut amalgam, compressive strength is 318 Mn/m^{2}.

Particle size

- The average particle size of modern powders ranges between 15 μm and 35 μm
- Parameter of the atomizing process is controlled to produce the desired particle sizes of spherical alloys
- The present trend in amalgam technique favors the use of a small average particle size, which tends to produce rapid hardening of the amalgam with greater early strength.

HIGH COPPER ALLOYS

Admixed

- Spherical Ag-Cu eutectic alloy particles are added to lathe-cut low Cu amalgam alloy particles
- Admixed alloy contains 30–55% spherical high-copper powder in which copper content ranges from 9% to 20%.
- The spherical silver-copper alloy consists of a silver-rich phase and a copper-rich phase with the crystal structure of pure silver and pure copper
- In the admixed type, the γ_2 forms around the Ag-Sn (lathe-cut) particles and is eliminated around the Ag-Cu (spherical) particles.

Dispersion Alloys

- A strengthening that is observed in metals when a large volume of ultra fine particles less than 1 mm is dispersed throughout the metal
- The spherical silver-copper particles are intended to dispersion harden and are made from the admixed powder, and are often called dispersion or dispersant amalgam alloys.

Advantages of dispersion amalgams

- The silver copper particles in admixed amalgams are small and closely spaced to produce dispersion hardening

- The hardening of admixed amalgams is due to the strength of the silver-copper particles
- Here the Ag-Cu particles act as strong fillers, strengthening the amalgam matrix
- Dispersion amalgams proved to be superior to low copper amalgam restoration for resistance to marginal breakdown.

Unicompositional

- The particles at the start of the reaction function like Ag-Sn particles of the admixed types
- Later the same particles function like the silver-copper particles of the admixed type, eliminating γ_2 phase.

29. What is high copper amalgam? Enumerate its advantages over conventional silver amalgam. What is the percentage of copper present in high copper amalgam? Add a note on the steps in the manipulation of amalgam.

HIGH COPPER ALLOYS

- Admixed/blended
- Unicompositional

Copper-enriched alloys have become available since the 1970s.

Basic ingredients are the same as the conventional silver amalgam, although they contain much more copper (10–30%) compared to less than 6% in the conventional alloys.

ADMIXED

- In the 1960s, attempts were made to increase the strength of dental amalgam by increasing the copper content of the alloy (6–12%)
- A spherical alloy (silver and copper) with a high copper content was added to the conventional lathe-cut alloy
- The increase in copper content of the alloy resulted in a modification of the setting reaction, which was beneficial (dispersion-strengthening agent).

Sequence of Reactions

- The function reaction is the same as that for the traditional alloys:

$$\underset{(\gamma)}{Ag_3Sn} + \text{(Ag-Cu) eutectic} + Hg \longrightarrow \underset{(\gamma_1)}{Ag_2Hg_3} + \underset{(\gamma_2)}{Sn_{78}Hg} + \text{Ag-Cu (unreacted particles)}$$

- This is followed by a second reaction:
  $$\underset{(\gamma_2)\ \text{eutectic}}{Sn_{78}Hg} + Ag\text{-}Cu \longrightarrow \underset{(\eta')}{Cu_6Sn_5} + \underset{(\gamma_1)}{Ag_2Hg_3}$$
- Thus, the final amalgam contains little or no γ_2.

The advantages over conventional amalgam are:

- Higher compressive strength
- A more rapid set to full strength
- A more reduction in creep
- A reduced susceptibility to corrosion.

UNICOMPOSITIONAL

- This is a single-composition high copper amalgam
- This single composition can either be all spherical or all lathe-cut
- Copper content ranges between 13% and 30%
- Its setting reaction produces no γ_2 phase. Hence, it is also called as non-γ_2 amalgam.

Setting Reaction

$$\underset{(\gamma)}{Ag_3\text{-}SnCu} + \underset{(\varepsilon)}{Cu_3Sn} + Hg \longrightarrow \underset{(\gamma_1)}{Ag_2Hg_3} + \underset{(\eta')}{Cu_6Sn_5} + \gamma_1$$

Advantages and Disadvantages

Admixed high copper	Spherical high copper
Longer working time	Less working time
Adapts better to cavity walls and adjacent teeth	Less adaptable
Slower set	Faster set
More mercury mix	Less mercury mix
Less early strength	Higher early strength
Higher creep during condense	Lower creep
Difficult to finish	Low condensation pressure

STEPS IN THE MANIPULATION OF AMALGAM

- Selection of alloy
- Proportion of Hg and alloy
- Trituration
- Condensation
- Carving, polishing and finishing.

Selection of Alloy

Particle size

- Smaller particles are used because they give better condensation, greater strength, easy carving, smooth finish, less marginal failures, faster setting time, easy to adapt and condense
- Large particles from porosity lead to decreased strength.

Shape of alloy

- Spherical alloys are preferred because they give better finish, good marginal adaptation, better condensation, high strength, easier carving, less Hg needed.

Composition

- High Cu amalgams are preferred since they produce less γ_2, phase in the setting reaction.

Proportioning of Alloy and Mercury

- The proportioning of alloy and mercury aids in forming a suitable mass of amalgam for placement into the prepared cavity
- Alloy/Mercury ratios vary between 5:8 and 10:8
- Those mixes containing greater quantities of mercury are 'wetter' and are generally used with hand mixing
- Those mixes containing smaller quantities of mercury are 'drier' and are used in mechanical mixing
- For optimum properties, the final set amalgam should contain less than 50% mercury
- Mercury consumption is also dependent on the size and shape of the alloy particle

  Lathe cut – 50%
  Spheroid – 43%
- Any excess mercury in the mix following trituration may be squeezed out using a squeeze cloth (Squeeze Cloth Technique).

Incremental dryness technique/increasing dryness technique

- Final mercury content is condensed in increments
- Condensation of each increment brings the excess mercury to the surface layer, which may be scraped out
- Thus, each increment is dried of excess mercury and only then subsequent increment is condensed
- Disadvantage is the chance of lack of bonding between two increments if too much of mercury is removed. This is known as Lamination.

Eames' technique

- Mercury content in the final set amalgam is minimized by reducing the initial mercury content
- Mixing alloy powder and mercury in the ratio of 1:1 parts by weight is known as Eames' technique
- This is also known as 'no squeeze cloth technique'.

Trituration Methods

- Volumetric dispensers
- Preweighed pellets or tablets
- Pre-proportioned capsules
- The most accurate method is to weigh the Hg and alloy components using a balance. But, this is rarely done and both are commonly proportioned using volume dispensers.

Volumetric dispensers

- Dispensing by volume is unreliable because it is affected by particle size
- Since medicines or coarse-grained alloys tend to produce erratic mixes, the choice of alloy is limited to fine-grained type

- The dispenser should be held vertically to ensure consistent spills of mercury
- Tilting the bottle to a 45° angle results in unreliable mercury-to-alloy ratio
- The dispenser should be at least half full, if not, then the weight of mercury dispensed may be erratic
- Entrapment of contaminants (air/voids) in the dispensers may result in incurred delivery of mercury.

Preweighed pellets/tablets

Manufacturer compresses alloy powder into tablets of uniform weight, which is used with the measured amount of mercury.

Pre-proportioned Capsules

- They contain alloy either in pellet form or in preweighed powder form, with the correct amount of mercury in compartment separated by a membrane
- Just before mixing, the membrane is broken by compression of the capsule or is automatically activated when placed in an amalgamator.
- The capsules may be:

  A i. Reusable
  ii. Disposable
  B i. Containing pestle
  ii. Not containing pestle

The final rule by FDA after mercury controversy

- Dental amalgam reclassified from Class1 to Class II
- This includes the fact that various additional tests are required for approval
- Additional tests required are particle size distribution assays, biocompatibility testing and corrosion testing.

  Extralabeling guidance as the composition, performance data, and contraindications.

These added guidelines is supposed to give patient a clear picture of the material and to restrict usage to an extended limit.

BIBLIOGRAPHY

1. FDA's "Class II Special Controls Guidance Document: Dental Amalgam, Mercury, and Amalgam Alloy." See § 872.1(e) for the availability of this guidance document.

30. What is a creep? How do you measure an amalgam creep? What is the significance of creep with respect to amalgam performance? Write in detail about the dimensional changes that occur in the use of amalgam and its control.

DEFINITION

- Creep is the time-dependent strain or deformation that is produced by a stress. The creep process can cause an amalgam restoration to extend out of the cavity preparation, thereby increasing its susceptibility to marginal breakdown
- The viscoelastic properties of amalgam are also reflected by the creep or permanent deformation under static loads, even after complete setting.

TYPES

- Static creep
- Dynamic creep.

Static Creep

Is a time dependent deformation produced in a completely set solid subjected to a constant stress.

Dynamic Creep

Produced when the applied stress is fluctuating, such as in fatigue-type test.

IMPORTANCE

Dental amalgam has components with melting points that are slightly above room temperature and the creep produced can be very destructive to the restoration.

MEASURING CREEP

The set dental amalgam is subjected to a continued application of force in compression.
This viscoelastic property is measured under static loads over a period of time.

CREEP VALUE

- Creep value for low copper cut alloy is 6.3%, which is the highest value, and the creep values are determined by an instrument
- Low creep values of high-copper amalgam increase the brittleness of the amalgam and decrease the relief of stresses at contact areas under load

- A high-modulus base under a high copper-amalgam is essential to minimize the development of tensile stresses at the amalgam cement base interface.
- According to ADA Specification No. 1, creep should be below 3%
- *Low copper*: 0.8–8.0%
- *High copper*: <0.1%

FACTORS AFFECTING CREEP

Influence of Microstructure on Creep

- The γ_1 phase (Ag_2Hg_3) has influence on low-copper amalgam creep rates. Creep rates increase with higher γ_1 volume fractions and decrease with larger grain sizes
- The presence of γ_2 phase is associated with higher creep rates
- Single composition high copper amalgams have very low creep rates, due to absence of γ_2 phase and due to the presence of $\eta'(Cu_6Sn_5)$ rods, which acts as barrier to deformation of the γ_1 phase.

Effects of Manipulative Variables on Creep

- Low creep and high compressive strength are closely related
- Mercury/Alloy ratio should be minimum
- Condensation pressure should be maximum for lathe cut or admixed alloys
- Overtrituration of alloys increases creep of dental amalgam and undertrituration lowers it.

DIMENSIONAL CHANGES

- Following, trituration, there is an initial contraction after first twenty minutes associated with solution of mercury in alloy particles
- After this period, expansion occurs due to the reaction of mercury with silver and tin and the formation of inter-metallic compounds
- This expansion continues as long as the crystals are forming until it reaches grain boundaries
- Maximum dimensional change permitted is ± 20 µm/cm
- The dimension becomes constant after 6–8 hours.

Factors Affecting Dimensional Change

Dimensional Change in Manipulation Factors

Manipulation factors that result in excess mercury leading to a net final expansion	Factors that cause net shrinkage
High mercury : alloy ratio	Low mercury : alloy ratio
Improper trituration	Trituration with sufficient force
Not squeezing out excess Hg	Squeezing out excess Hg
Not applying sufficient pressure during condensation	Applying sufficient condensation pressure

The newer high copper unicompositional amalgams show a net contraction due to a low mercury : alloy ratio.

Expansion Resulting from Moisture Contamination in Zn Containing Alloys

- Moisture contamination during trituration or condensation of Zn containing amalgam leads to the production of ZnO and H_2 gas
- This H_2 gas does not react with any other ingredients in the restoration nor is it able to escape from the restoration
- Thus, it applies force on the restoration, which results in expansion after 48–72 hours. This is known as delayed expansion
- $H_2O + Zn \rightarrow ZnO + H_2$
- This can be prevented by proper isolation technique during manipulation technique.

Expansion Resulting from Corrosion Products in Low Copper Amalgam

Over a period, the tin-mercury phase γ_2 in low copper amalgam reacts with atmospheric O_2 to form tin oxide and tin oxychloride releasing mercury.

This free mercury reacts with the unreacted alloy particles γ phase to form Silver-Mercury (γ_1) and Tin-Mercury (γ_2) phase again, which results in expansion.

$$\underset{(\gamma)}{Ag_3Sn} + Hg \rightarrow \underset{(\gamma_1)}{Ag_2Hg_3} + \underset{(\gamma_2)}{Sn_{78}Hg} + \underset{(\gamma)}{Ag_3Sn}.$$

$$Sn \text{---} Hg + O_2 + Cl \rightarrow SnO + SnOCl + Hg.$$

$$Hg + AgSn \rightarrow AgHg + SnHg + Ag_3Sn.$$

This expansion is called as mercuroscopic expansion.

Jorgensen Expansion

High copper amalgams also undergo corrosion, but the phase undergoing corrosion is the copper-tin phase. This corrosion does not result in release of free mercury, as the products formed are CuO and $CuCl_2$.

Dimensional Change Due to Creep

- The viscoelastic properties of amalgam are also reflected by the creep or permanent deformation under static loads
- Under a continued application of force in compression, an amalgam shows a continued deformation, even after the mass has completely set
- Maximum creep is seen with low copper amalgam (proportional to the amount of γ_2 phase)
- High copper amalgam shows minimum creep.

Factors affecting creep

1. More mercury—more creep
2. More γ_2—More creep.

Measures to Minimize Dimensional Change

- Choose spherical, high copper alloy powder (minimal Hg)
- Use the optimum mercury : alloy ratio
- Sufficient trituration pressure

- Squeezing out excess mercury
- Adequate condensation pressure
- Avoid moisture contamination during manipulation to prevent delayed expansion
- Use high copper amalgam to minimize corrosion and creep.

Creep of Acrylic Denture Base Resins

- Denture resins are viscoelastic, when subjected to a constant load so that strain can be observed as a function of time
- Acrylic resins show primary and secondary creep following the initial instantaneous elastic strain
- The secondary creep rate increases with increase in temperature, stress, residual monomer, plasticizers and cross-linking agents
- The creep rate for self-curing resins increases with stress more rapidly than for heat-cured resins.

Creep of Noble Metal Alloys for Metal Ceramics

- Some flow or creep of gold alloy occurs when it approaches 980°C (1800°F)
- When heated to 980°C, a second phase is precipitated which can produce hardening or strengthening of the alloy
- Such creep can be decreased in some commercial alloys but cannot be totally eliminated.

31. What is direct filling gold? Enumerate various forms of direct filling gold and its fabrication. Classify direct filling gold. Describe its physical properties, manipulation, advantages and disadvantages.

INTRODUCTION

- Gold can be used as a restorative material
- It is a noble metal with good resistance to tarnish and corrosion in the oral cavity
- Gold can be welded at room temperature if its surface is free from absorbed gases or other impurities, hence useful as a direct filling material in prepared cavities.

MAIN APPLICATIONS

- Pit and small class I restorations
- For repair of casting margins
- For class II and class V restorations.

CLASSIFICATION

Foil

- Sheet
  - Cohesive
  - Non-cohesive
- Ropes
- Cylinder
- Laminated foil
- Platinized foil.

Electrolytic Precipitate

- Mat gold
- Mat foil
- Gold-calcium alloy.

POWDERED GOLD

Physical Properties

Strength

Bending strength is taken because it reflects three types of stress:

1. Compressive strength.
2. Tensile strength.
3. Shear strength.
   - Any failure can propagate from area of weakness
   - Usually tensile stress causes failure
   - This is because of incomplete cohesion
   - Hence, binding strength of direct filling gold (DFG) represents cohesive strength
   - They cannot withstand masticatory stress.

Hardness

- Hardness indicates the overall quality of compacted gold
- Low hardness represents the presence of porosity
- The use of mechanical condenser improves hardness when mat gold and powder gold are used.

Density

- Exact density cannot be measured because of the presence of voids
- Density is greater in gold foil
- This implies better compaction of foil.

Tarnish and Corrosion Resistance

- They are more resistant to tarnishing in the oral cavity
- They have very little marginal leakage between the filling and cavity walls, if compaction is good.

FOIL GOLD

Manipulation of direct filling gold includes two steps:
1. Desorbing (Degassing)
2. Compaction.

Desorbing

- Gas can adsorb on the surface of gold during storage and packaging
- This adsorbed gas on the surface of gold prevents it from cohesing
- Hence, the foils or pellets are heated immediately before they are carried into the prepared cavity
- This process of removal of gas on the surface of gold to make it a clean surface is termed as desorption
- It is essential to the achievement of cohesive mass and maximal physical properties in restoration
- Desorption is done by heating the gold foils/pellets for long time at a temperature that removes gases.

Procedure

- Desorption is accomplished by heating the gold on a mica tray over a flame on an electric annealer
- Each piece of gold may be heated over a pure ethanol.

Precautions when using an electric annealer

- When heating in bulk on a tray, excessive amounts should be avoided
- Care should be taken to handle pieces with stainless steel wire points, or similar instrument will not contaminate gold
- Electric annealer is maintained at a temperature between 340°C and 370°C
- Time requires varies from 5 minutes to 20 minutes
- Temperature below 315°C is not adequate to attain optimum hardness.

Disadvantages of electric annealing

- Adhesion of pellets together
- Air currents may affect uniformity of heating over sintering
- Greater exposure to contamination
- Size selection among desorbed gold is limited.

Flame Desorption

- This consists of picking up each piece individually, heating directly in the open flame and placing it in the prepared cavity

- The fuel for the flame may be alcohol or gas
- Mostly alcohol is preferred (pure methanol or ethanol without colorants or other additives).

Advantages of flame desorption

- Selecting a piece of appropriate size is allowed
- Desorption of only those pieces used
- Less exposure to contamination.

Effects of Underheating and Overheating

Underheating

- Does not remove impurities properly
- Incomplete cohesion.

Overheating

- Excessive sintering occurs
- Incomplete cohesion, poor compaction
- Material becomes stiffer, less ductile and more difficult to condense.

Compaction

All direct filling gold must be compacted during insertion into cavity preparation.

Two fundamental principles involved in compaction:

1. Welding
2. Wedging.

Welding

Refers to the process of forming atomic bonds between pellets, segments or layers as a result of condensation.

Wedging

Refers to pressurized adaptation of the gold form within the space between tooth structure walls or corners that have slightly deformed elastically.

Instruments used for Compaction

- Hand mallet
- Pneumatic vibratory condensers
- Electrically driven condensers.

Condensers

- Condensers are used to deliver forces of compaction
- Original foil condensers had a single pyramid-shaped face
- But now they have a series of small pyramids or serrations on the face
- These act as swaging tools that exert lateral force on their inclines.

Size of condenser tip

- Size of condenser tip is an important factor in determining the effectiveness of compaction

- Small condenser tips give good compaction without using much force that might damage oral structures
- The diameters of circular tip should be 0.5–1 mm.

Pressure application

- Condensation pressure can also be applied by hand using a mallet.

Compaction Technique

- A piece of gold is placed in cavity preparation
- The gold is first pressed to place by hand
- A condenser is used to begin malleting in the center of the mass
- Each increment of gold must be carefully stepped by placing the condenser point in successive adjacent position as compacting force is applied
- This permits each piece to be compacted over its entire surface so that voids are not bridged
- The most efficient compaction occurs directly under nib face.

Result of Compaction

- To remove void space from within each increment of gold
- To compact the gold into cavity line angle and point angles and against walls
- To attach it to previously placed gold via cohesion.

Advantages

- They are more resistant to tarnish and corrosion
- Biocompatible
- Produces only a minimal pulp response
- Provides a reasonably long clinical service.

Disadvantages

- Very expensive
- Not esthetic, hence, cannot be used in anteriors
- Needs technical skill for manipulation.

ELECTROLYTIC PRECIPITATED GOLD

It is a crystalline gold powder formed by electrolytic precipitation.

Manufacturing

- The powder is formed into shapes by sintering at elevated temperature well below the melting point of gold
- This sintering causes self-diffusion between particles where they are in contact
- This self-diffusion causes particles to grow together.

Types

- Mat gold
- Mat foil
- Alloyed electrolytic precipitate.

Mat Gold

- It is a crystalline, electrolytically precipitated gold form that is formed into strips
- These strips can be cut into desired size.

Advantages

- It is easy to use in building up internal bulk of the restoration
- It can be easily compacted
- It can be easily adapted to retentive portions of prepared cavity.

Disadvantage

It is loosely packed; hence, it contains numerous void spaces between the particles.

Uses

They are used along with foil for the external surface of restoration.

Two-material technique

- Here the mat gold is covered with veneer of foil
- This is done because mat gold contains numerous voids that may be seen as pits form if it is used on the surface of restoration
- Hence, gold foil is used on external surface.

Mat Foil

- It is a sandwich of electrolytic precipitated gold powder between sheets of No. 3 gold foil
- The sandwich is sintered and cut into strips of differing widths
- It can be cut to desired lengths
- The purpose of sandwiching mat gold between foil sheets was to try to eliminate the need to veneer the restoration.

Alloyed Electrolyzing Precipitate (Electralloy)

- The newest form of electrolyte gold is an alloy of gold and calcium
- Here calcium 1–0.5 % wt is wrapped in a No. 4 foil
- This product is called electralloy
- The purpose of calcium is to give the product increased hardness strength
- Calcium produces stronger restoration by dispersion strengthening which locks in cold work strengthening
- It is available in strips and cut to desired length before insertion in a cavity preparation.

Powdered Gold

- It is a form of direct-filling gold
- It is a chemically precipitated gold powder, which has been available in agglomerated form
- The agglomerates were provided with a liquid such as alcohol or dilute carbolic acid, which held the agglomerate together until it was compacted
- The agglomerates disintegrated when compaction was attempted
- Hence, the gold powder was enclosed in a No. 3 gold foil.

Manufacturing

- Fine powder is formed by chemical precipitation or by atomizing the metal
- This powder is a mixture of powders of varying particle sizes
- The particle size is 15 μm
- The pellets are mixed with soft wax and then wrapped with gold foil (No. 3) rather than sintering the mass, like for mat gold
- The foil acts as an effective container for the powdered metal and acts as a matrix throughout the mass, while it is condensed
- The powdered gold pellets have a cylindrical or irregular shape and diameter of 1–2 mm
- The ratio of gold foil to powder varies from 1 to 3 for the smallest pellets to approximately 1–9 for the target
- Pellets of powdered gold increase cohesion during compaction and reduce the time required for placing the restoration.

32. Classify gold foils. Give the rationale and technique of fabrication of gold foil. Add a note on their properties.

GOLD FOIL

- It is the oldest of all products
- Gold is malleable and, hence, can be reduced to a thickness almost to transparency.
- This property enables gold to be used as **gold foil** in dentistry.

CLASSIFICATION

Gold Foil is of Five Types

1. Sheet
   - Cohesive
   - Non-cohesive
2. Ropes
3. Cylinder
4. Laminated foil
5. Platinized foil.

AVAILABILITY

- Gold foil is supplied as sheets of varying thickness
- For example, No. 4 thickness → wt. 4 grains → supplied as (0.259 grams) 4 × 4-inch sheet

- The numbering refers to the weight of a standard sheet and the thickness
- No. 3 gold foil is used in manufacturing of electrolytic and powder products
- Each sheet is cut into portion varying size for different applications—1/8, 1/16, 1/32, 1/64 and 1/128 of a sheet
- Each piece is formed into a pellet of gold, ready for clinical use.

GOLD FOIL SHEET

- Gold foil is manufactured by rolling and beating the material to form the required thickness of foil
- This work hardens the metal
- Gold foil sheet is annealed, recrystallized, to increase its ductility and malleability
- Of all the gold foils, only the sheet form is supplied in both cohesive and noncohesive forms.

Cohesive Gold Foil

- Gold should have a clean surface free from impurities
- Gold attracts gases, such as oxygen, to its surface and any adsorbed gas film prevents the cohesion of individual increments of gold during their compaction
- Gold free of surface contaminant, which is cohesive, is called cohesive gold foil.

Non-cohesive Gold Foil

- These foils are subjected to a volatile agent such as ammonia, which is adsorbed on the surface of the gold. This volatile substance acts as a protective film to prevent the absorption of non-volatile materials and premature cohesion of pellets in their container
- The ammonia treated foil is called non-cohesive foil
- The volatile film is readily removed by heating thereby restoring the cohesive character of the foil.

GOLD FOIL CYLINDERS

They are formed by rolling cut segments of No. 4 foils into desired width using a modified No. 22 tapestry needle.

PREFORMED GOLD FOIL

- They are made from No. 4 foil that has been carbonized or corrugated
- The ropes and cylinders are rolled in various diameters and then cut to various lengths to provide many sizes of increments for filling the preparation
- The laminates are not available as preforms but they can be made in dental office by placing a number of sheets on top of each other and then cutting the laminate into pieces of a desired size.

PLATINIZED GOLD FOIL

- Platinum foil is sandwiched between two sheets of pure gold foil

- Layers of platinum and gold are bonded together by a cladding process during the rolling operation
- Thus, the sandwich is already welded together before beating begins
- The need for adding platinum foil to gold foil is to increase the hardness of the restoration.

Uses

Class III and Class V cavities and not in situations subjected to direct masticatory stresses.

MANIPULATION

Degassing

- Before insertion of gold foil into a cavity, it is heated to remove absorbed gases as oxygen, from the metal surface and to improve the weldability
- Gold foil can be heated on a container, above a gas or alcohol flame, or in an electric furnace at (250–350°C)
- The time of heating depends on the individual material and the degree of surface contamination.

Compaction

The clean and decontaminated gold is packed into the cavity in increments.

Instruments used for Compaction

- A plugger and hand mallet
- A pneumatic vibratory condenser
- An electrically driven condenser.

Points to Note

- The first method requires the greatest time and is the most traumatic
- If the area of the condenser point is too large, there is less pressure applied to the gold for any given force and welding may not be achieved
- If area is too small, the condenser will punch a hole in the metal rather than weld it
- The area of the condenser point should be between 0.3 mm and 1.0 mm
- Force of compaction should be applied perpendicular to the surface of the foil or else shear stresses can get incorporated dislodging the foil.

PROPERTIES

Density

- The density of pure gold is 19.32 g/cm^3
- A gold foil restoration has a density of only about 16 g/cm^3
- This difference is due to the presence of porosity where there is no complete contact between the pieces of foils.

Mechanical Properties

- Properly condensed gold foil is about as hard as the type 1 inlay golds
- The use of foil that has been laminated with platinum gives an even harder restoration
- The strength and hardness of a foil restoration are not sufficient to withstand the direct forces of mastication.

Other Properties

- These materials cause the least gingival irritation of any restorative material
- The corrosion resistance of gold is excellent
- There is very little marginal leakage round a gold foil filling.

RECENT ADVANCES

- E-Z Gold is a new direct filling gold material similar to existing powdered gold formulations. (Late 1980).
  Manipulative characteristics are similar to that of a very stiff amalgam and more sticky (cohesive) than gold foil, hence the name E-Z Gold.
  Composition: It is a mixture of pure gold powder and less than 0.01% organic wax, wrapped in gold foil.
  Advantages: Improved softness and working characteristics when compared to other types of direct gold fillings.[1]
- *Stopfgold*: a new direct filling gold (since 1989)[2]
  Advantages: The final restoration with Stopfgold exhibits greater density than other forms of granular gold with a 50% increase in shear strength when compared to gold foil.
- Nanogold and Resin composites modified with nanogold.
  Few observed properties: Exhibited lower light transmission and have opaque appearance.
  Modified composites exhibited higher microhardness in comparison to non-modified resin composites.
  Diametral Tensile Strength was comparable to nonmodified groups.[3]

REFERENCES

1. Alperstein KS, Yearwood L, Boston D. "Links E-Z Gold: the new Goldent." Oper Dent. 1996;21(1):36-41. Temple University School of Dentistry, Department of Operative Dentistry, Philadelphia, PA 19140, USA.
2. Lambert RL. Stopfgold: a new direct filling gold Oper Dent. 1994;19(1):16-9. University of Colorado Health Sciences Center, School of Dentistry, Department of Restorative Dentistry, Denver 80262.
3. Sokołowski, Jerzy, et al. "Evaluation of resin composites modified with nanogold and nanosilver." Acta of Bioengineering and Biomechanics 16.1 (2014).

33. Define soldering and welding. Describe the precaution that you would take to obtain a good solder joint. Add a note on fluxes.

OR

Define solders. Give examples, composition and uses. Explain the technique of soldering in bridgework prosthesis.

OR

What is soldering? Describe the properties and general requisites of gold alloy solders.

DEFINITIONS

Soldering: Is the joining of metals by the fusion of an intermediary alloy, which has a lower melting point.

Brazing: A term used industrially, is a soldering operation at temperatures above 500°C.

Welding: Is a process in which the parts themselves are joined together, by the application of heat and/or pressure.

SOLDERING

Ideal Properties of Dental Solders

- The fusion temperature must be at least 50–100°C lower than the melting temperature of the alloys to be joined
- The solder should be as strong as the alloys being soldered
- The molten material should flow freely and wet the components well
- Good tarnish and corrosion resistance are necessary
- The color of the solder should be similar to that of the metals being joined.

Gold Solders

Composition

Gold, silver and copper, with lesser quantities of zinc and tin.

Properties

- Gold contributes to the corrosion resistance
- Zinc and tin help to lower the melting range by the formation of eutectic alloys
- Fusion range limits—750–900°C.

Applications

Suitable for most dental gold alloys.

Silver Solders

Composition

These contain silver-copper alloys, zinc and cadmium (lowers the fusion temperature).

Properties

Fusion range limits—600–750°C. Their lower fusion temperature reduces the chances of weld decay.

Uses

Used for base metal alloys and stainless steel.

Fluxes

Functions of a Flux

- To protect the alloy surfaces from oxidation during soldering
- To dissolve metallic oxides as they are formed.

Composition

- Borax or fluorides such as potassium fluoride. This flux is used for the chromium-containing alloys, as it can dissolve the passivating oxide film
- Some fluoride-containing fluxes evolve toxic fluorides when heated. Inhaling such fumes should be avoided.

Practical Points in Soldering

- The metallic parts to be soldered are thoroughly cleaned
- A solder of the correct fusion temperature should be selected
- The reducing zone of the flame is used
- The flame should be removed from the solder soon as it flows
- Immediately after soldering, the work is quenched in water.

Investment Soldering

Procedure

- The parts to be soldered are accurately aligned

- Alignment is achieved by securing the parts with sticky wax
- After embedding the portion to be soldered in investment material, the wax is removed and boiling water and detergent are used to clean the area thoroughly, before soldering is done.

Causes of Soldering Failures

- Improper cleaning of the parts to be soldered
- Improper fluxing
- Poor flow of solder if not sufficiently heated
- Overheating of solder can result in a pitted joint.

WELDING

The most common method of achieving such hot-welding in dentistry is by the application of resistance melting or spot welding.

Procedure

- The pieces to be joined are pressed firmly together between two electrodes
- These electrodes are usually made of copper
- Grooved electrodes are available to give good contact with orthodontic wires
- An electric current is passed through the electrodes and the pieces of metal
- If the parts to be joined are relatively poor conductors of electricity, they will heat up more than the electrodes when the current is passed
- If sufficient heat is generated in the portion of metal in contact with the electrodes and if enough pressure is applied, a welded joint is formed
- A current of 250–750 amperes is usually used, for a time of between 1/25th and l/50th of a second
- Too low a current, or too short a time, results in a weak joint
- Overheating can thin the metal.

This technique is not used

- For gold alloys which are good conductors of electricity
- For butt-joints.

Soldering Methods in Titanium

Though Titanium has ideal properties to be used for dental applications joining titanium has many practical problems.

Conventional dental soldering methods cannot be employed as the dissolved oxygen and hydrogen cause embrittlement in titanium materials.

Techniques used are:

- Laser soldering
- Tungsten inert gas and
- Infrared radiation heating methods

Wang RR. et al, used all the above methods for joining both pure titanium and Ti–6Al–4V alloy. Mechanical tests such as Vickers microhardness and uniaxial tensile testing along with microstructure analysis were done.

Observations were: Samples prepared by the three joining methods had lower tensile elongation.

The changes in microstructure and microhardness values increased in the heat-affected zone for all the specimens tested.[1]

REFERENCE

1. Wang RR, et al. Joining titanium materials with tungsten inert gas welding, laser welding, and infrared brazing. Journal of Prosthetic Dentistry, Volume 74, Issue 5, 521-530.

34. Write in detail about silicate cement, its composition and properties. Write in detail about its dimensional stability and strength.

APPLICATION

Used for filling of anterior teeth.

COMPOSITION

Supplied as powder and liquid.

Powder	Liquid
SiO_2 (Silica)—40%	Phosphoric acid—42%
Al_2O_3 (Alumina)—30% Sodium or calcium phosphate—8%	Aluminium phosphate } Zinc phosphate—18% }
CaF_2—4% Sodium aluminium fluoride—20%	Water—40%

SETTING REACTION

When powder and liquid are mixed, the reaction is that of an acid and base. The surface of powder particle is attacked by acid liquid.

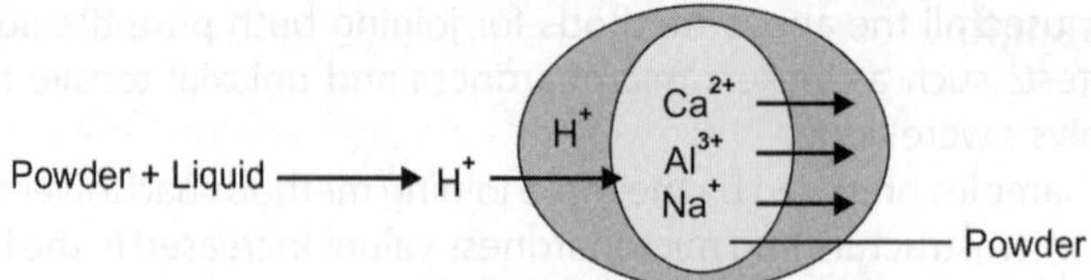

Fig. 12: Setting reaction of silicate cement

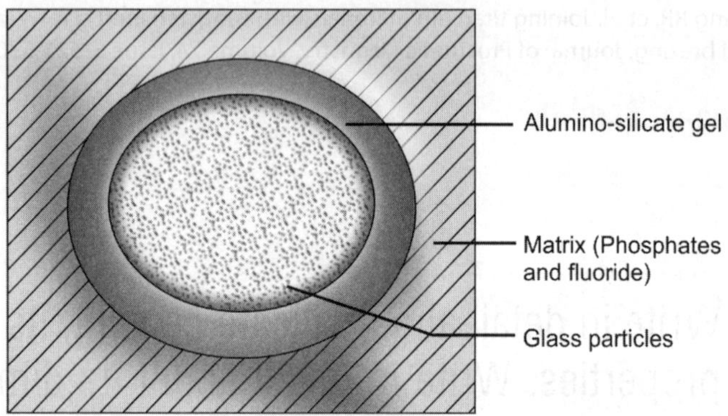

Fig. 13: Set gel structure

Alumino-silicate glass + phosphoric acid → $H^+ + H_2PO_4^-$ (with release of Al^{3+}, Ca^{2+}, Na^+ and F^- ions)

- The liquid dissociates and the H^+ ions migrate into the surface layer of the glass particle. Al^{3+}, Ca^{2+}, Na^+ and F^- ions move from the glass into liquid **(Fig. 12)**.
- The metal ions precipitate to form a gel matrix of phosphates and fluorides
- The matrix binds together the undissolved powder particles to form a composite material as set cement **(Fig. 13)**.

PROPERTIES

It has a pH of 2.8 after 3 minutes or at the time of insertion and pH is 5 after 24 hours.

Thus, it is highly acidic and the pulp needs to be protected by a base to prevent pulpal irritation.

Anticariogenic

The fluoride ions leach out in aqueous medium and react with the enamel to produce a structure that is resistant to acid decalcification.

Acts as antibacterial agent.

Setting Time

3–8 minutes.

Compressive Strength

180 MPa.

Hardness

70 KHN.

Tensile Strength

3.5 MPa.

Very brittle and cannot withstand impact force, hence used in nonstress-bearing areas.

Dimensional Stability

Solubility and Disintegration

- This cement has the maximum solubility—7%
- Solubility increases with low pH (acidic solution)
- Solubility increases with low powder : liquid ratio
- Initial solubility is high as the setting reaction takes a long time for completion
- Disintegration of cement takes place due to moisture contamination before hardening
- Disintegration also takes place if cement dries after setting.

Optical

Due to the unreacted glass, it is translucent. But disintegration causes discoloration.

Adhesion

No adhesion with tooth structure. Mechanical retention has to be given.

PRECAUTIONS

- Plastic or agate spatula should be used to avoid incorporation of wear particles from steel spatula, which can cause color change
- Coating of varnish should be given after completion of the restoration to prevent the oral fluids from coming into contact with it and to prevent excessive drying
- Should not be used in mouth breathers and in patients who consume high alcoholic fluids.

35. Describe the composition, setting reaction, manipulation and uses of zinc polycarboxylate cement.

ZINC POLYCARBOXYLATE CEMENT

Synonyms

Zinc polyacrylate

Formula for Polyacrylic Acid

```
— CH₂ — CH — CH₂ — CH
   |         |
  C=O       C=O
   |         |
   O         O
   |         |
   H         H
```

INTRODUCTION

Zinc polycarboxylate was the first cement system that developed an adhesive bond to tooth structure.

AVAILABILITY

- Powder and liquid in bottles
- Water settable cements
- As precapsulated powder/liquid system.

Commercial Names

Poly F (Dentsply)
Durelon
Carboco (Voco).

COMPOSITION

Supplied as powder and liquid.

Powder	Liquid
ZnO—85% MgO/stannic oxide—10% Stannous fluoride—4–5% Bismuth oxide, Aluminum oxide Color pigments	Aqueous solution of polyacrylic acid or copolymer of acrylic acid—30–40% Itaconic acid—10–45% Tartaric acid—5%

Powder

- Zinc oxide—Basic ingredient
- Magnesium oxide—Principal modifier, also aids in sintering
- Stannous fluorides—Increase strength, modify setting time and impart anticariogenic property.

Liquid

- Aqueous solution of polyacrylic acid
- Copolymer of acrylic acid with other unsaturated carboxylic acid, i.e. itaconic, maleic or tricarboxylic acid.

Role of Carboxylate Functional Group

- Matrix formation
- Bonding to tooth structure.

Bonding to Tooth Structure

The polyacrylic acid reacts with Ca-ions via carboxyl groups on surface of enamel or dentin. Thus, the bond strength to enamel is greater than that of dentin.

WATER SETTABLE CEMENTS

- Polyacid is freeze dried and added to the cement powder
- Water is used as a liquid when powder is mixed with water, the polyacrylic acid goes into the solution and reaction is same as for conventional cements.

Working and Setting Times

- The working time is 2.5 minutes, much shorter than that of zinc phosphate cement (5 minutes)
- The temperature of cool slab can cause the polyacrylic acid to thicken
- So the powder needs to be refrigerated before mixing
- Setting time ranges from 6–9 minutes
- Setting time can be increased by cooling the glass slab
- It also depends on the method of manufacture of powder and liquid.

Manufacture

Powder mixture is sintered at high temperature to reduce the reactivity and then ground into fine particles.

Setting Reaction

- When powder and liquid are mixed, surface of powder particles are attached by an acid, releasing zinc, magnesium and tin ions
- These ions bind to polymer chain via the carboxyl groups. They also react with carboxyl groups of adjacent polyacid chain to form cross-linked salts.

Structure of Set Cement

Hardened cement consists of an amorphous gel matrix of zinc polyacrylate in which unreacted powder particles are dispersed.

PROPERTIES

Mechanical Properties

Comprehensive strength — 55 MPa
Tensile strength — 6.2 MPa

Factors affecting the Strength of Cement

Increases in powder/liquid ratio

- Increases strength
- Low powder/liquid ratio results in a significantly higher solubility and disintegration in the oral cavity.

Molecular weight of polyacrylic acid

- Affects the strength. A mix from lower viscosity liquid is weaker.

Biological Properties

- Excellent biocompatibility to pulp
- Antibacterial and anticarcinogenic due to fluoride
- PH is 1.7 but rises rapidly when mixed powder to neutral
- Produces minimum irritation to the pulp because of quick neutralization
- Large size of acid molecules from complex products limits its diffusion through the dentinal tubules.

Solubility and Disintegration

- Solubility—0.05% in water. Higher in acids like lactic acid and citric acid.

Biocompatibility

- Pulp response is mild despite the initial acidic nature of polycarboxylate cement.
- pH of liquid is 1.0–1.7 and that of freshly mixed cement in 3.0–4.0
- After 24 hours, pH will be 5.0–6.0.

Adhesion

- Cement bonds chemically with tooth structure
- Carboxyl group in polymer molecules chelates with Ca in tooth structure
- Bond strength—3.4–13.1 MN/m^2
- Film thickness—25–30 μm.

Factors affecting bond

- In ideal conditions, polycarboxylate has better adhesion to a clean dry surface of enamel than other cements

- Presence of saliva reduces bond strength
- Adhesion is better on smooth surface rather than on rough surface
- Does not adhere to gold or porcelain
- Adheres to stainless steel. It is used for orthodontics in cementation of fixed appliances.

Optical and Thermal Properties

- They are very opaque due to large quantities of unreacted zinc oxide
- They are also good thermal insulators.

MANIPULATION

Conditioning

Tooth surface is cleaned by 10% polyacrylic acid solution followed by rinsing with water or 1–3% hydrogen peroxide, after which the tooth is dried and isolated.

Proportioning

1.5 parts of powder to 1 part of liquid by weight.

Procedure

- Powder and liquid are dispensed on a cool glass slab
- Liquid is dispensed to mixing and its viscosity increases
- Powder is incorporated into liquid in bulk (90%) with a stiff cement spatula and remaining powder is added to adjust consistency
- The mix appears quite thick, but cement will flow into a thin film when seated under pressure
  - Mixing time → 30–40 seconds.

Surface Preparation and Retention

- Cement may not bond to noble metal in chemically contaminated cast or pickled condition
- Thus, the contaminated surface on cavity side of casting is abraded with a small stone to improve wettability and mechanical bond at metal-cement interface
- After cleaning, cavity should be isolated to prevent contamination by oral fluids.

Removal of Excess Cement

- Excess cement can be removed when cements become hard
- The outer surface of restoration must be coated carefully with a thin layer of separating medium to prevent excess cement from adhering to its surface.

ADVANTAGES

- Biocompatible
- Less irritant
- Good adhesive

- Anti-cariogenic
- Easy manipulation
- Good thermal insulator.

DISADVANTAGES

- If accurate proportioning is not obtained, the properties are affected
- Working time is less
- Not durable; solubility is more in acid
- Less stiff, difficult to remove flash.

36. Classify composite restorative resins. Write about the composition, properties and clinical performance of hybrid composites and their uses. Add a note on the light-activated composite resins.

COMPOSITE RESTORATIVE MATERIALS

- Composite material may be defined as a compound of two or more distinctly different materials with properties that are superior or intermediate to those of the individual constituents
- Development of modern dental composites started in the late 1950s and early 1960s with the work of Dr Ray Bowen.

CLASSIFICATION

Based on the filler particle size and quantity of major filler particles (Weight or volume percent).

Category	Particle size μm	Percentage of filler	
		Volume %	Wt %
Traditional or conventional or macrofilled composites	8–12	60–65	70–80
Small particle filled composites	1–5	65–77	80–90
Microfilled composites	0.04–0.4	20–55	35–60
Hybrid composites	0.6–1.0	60–65	75–80

Depending on the Polymerization

- Self-cured or chemically cured
- Ultraviolet light cured
- Visible light cured
- Heat cured
- Dual cured
- Laser cured.

Based on Filler Particle Size

- Mega fill—0.5–2 mm
- Macrofill—10–100 μm
- Midifill—1–10 μm
- Minifill—0.1–1 μm
- Micro fill—0.01–0.1 μm
- Nano fill—0.005–0.01 μm

COMPOSITION

- A continuous phase (Resin Matrix phase)
- Diluents
- A dispersed phase of filler particles
- Coupling agents
- Initiator-Activator
- Inhibitors
- Optical modifiers.

Resin Matrix Phase

- The organic polymer matrix is either an aromatic or a urethane diacrylate oligomer
- Oligomers are viscous liquids, the viscosity of which is reduced to a useful clinical level by the addition of a diluent monomer
- The two common oligomers used are dimethacrylate (BIS-GMA), (Bis phenol—A—glycidyl methacrylate) and UDMA (Urethane Dimethacrylate).

Diluents

- The high molecular weight monomers especially BIS-GMA are extremely viscous at room temperature
- Hence, diluents are added to reduce the viscosity (e.g. TEGDMA (Triethylene glycol dimethacrylate) to produce pastes of clinically useful consistencies
- Addition of TEGDMA or other low molecular weight dimethacrylate increases the polymerization shrinkage.

Disadvantages of BIS-GMA

- Highly viscous liquid
- Oxygen or air inhibits polymerization
- High water sorption

- Difficulty in synthesizing the material
- To overcome these problems, alternative monomers are used, such as:
  - Monofunctional methyl methacrylate (MMA)
  - Difunctional ethylene glycol dimethacrylate (EDMA) or TEGDMA.

Fillers

Filler Particles Increase

- Strength
- Hardness
- Rigidity
- Modulus of elasticity.

Filler Particles Decrease

- Coefficient of thermal expansion
- Polymerization shrinkage.

The fillers are

Quartz

- Chemically made, but difficult to grind into fine particles
- Were used in early composites, which were difficult to polish and abraded opposing tooth structure.

Silica

- Pure silica
- Fused silica
- Colloidal silica
  - Pyrogenic
  - Precipitated form
- Alumino-silicate
- Borosilicate glasses

Pyrogenic and precipitated forms of colloidal silica are commonly used.

Coupling Agents

- Used to bind filler particles to resin matrix
- They allow the more flexible polymer matrix to transfer stresses to the stiffer filler particles. They provide hydrolytic stability by preventing water from penetrating along the filler-resin interface.

For example, organic silane such as—γ-methacryloxy propyl trimethoxy silane.

Initiator

- Benzoyl peroxide
- For chemically activated resins.

Activator

- Tertiary amine (N, N-dimethyl-p-toluidine)
- For chemically activated resins.

Optical Modifiers

- To match the appearance of teeth, composites must have visual coloration and translucency that can simulate tooth structure
- Shading is obtained by adding different pigments, often metal oxides, in minute amounts.
  - TiO_2 (0.001–0.008 wt%).
  - Al_2O_3

USES

- Anterior esthetic restorative material
- Posterior restorative material in select conditions
- For cementation, (Dual cured resins)
- To veneer metal crowns and bridges
- Pit and fissure sealant
- Core build-up of teeth.

LIGHT-ACTIVATED RESINS

Visible Light-activated Resins

- Visible light activation is initiated by energy transfer to the di-ketone (camphoroquinone) which forms an excited triplet state
- The excited triplet attract the accelerator (DMAEMA) molecules and form exciplexes (i.e. excited complexes) that convert both the camphoroquinone and the DMAEMA molecules to free radicals that initiate addition polymerization.

Activator

- Blue light with a peak wavelength of 470 nm.

Photo Initiator

- Camphoroquinone.

Accelerator

- Organic amine (Diethyl amino ethyl methacrylate)
- Available as a single paste system.

To Provide Radio-opacity

- Filler materials contain heavy metals such as Barium, Strontium and Zirconium and recently Yttrium fluoride and Ytterbium fluoride
- To ensure optimum esthetics, the translucency of the filler must be similar to tooth structure. Mostly glasses have a refractive index of 1.5, which is comparable to dentin (1.52) and enamel (1.62).

U-V Light-curing System

U-V light-activated resins have been replaced by the visible light curing systems.

Initiator

- Benzoyl peroxide.

Activator

- Benzoin methyl ether.

Inhibitors

- Butylated hydroxytoluene—0.01 wt%
- Hydroquinone
- Inhibitors react with the free radicals as soon as they are formed
- Inhibit chain propagation by terminating the ability of free radicals to initiate polymerization.

Dual Cured

- This combines cold curing and visible light curing components in the same material
- They consist of two light curable pastes, one of which contains benzoyl peroxide and a tertiary amine added to the other
- When the two parts are mixed and exposed to light, both light curing and cold curing are achieved with the same material.

37. Describe the composition, properties and clinical performance of composite resins classified based on filler particles.

Add a note on newer developments in composites.

CLASSIFICATION BASED ON FILLER PARTICLES

- Conventional/traditional composites
- Microfilled composites
  - Sintered prepolymerized microfilled complexes
  - Spherical polymer-based microfilled complexes
  - Agglomerated microfilled complexes
- Small particle composites
- Hybrid composites.

CONVENTIONAL/TRADITIONAL COMPOSITES

- Commonly used filler is ground quartz having an average particle size of 8–12 μm.
- Filler loading is 70–80% wt or 60–70% volume.

Properties

These have improved properties compared to unfilled restorative resins.

- *Compressive strength*: 250–300 MPa (4–5 times greater than acrylic resins)
- *Tensile Strength*: 50–65 MPa (Twice that of unfilled resins)
- *Elastic modulus*: 8–15 GPa (4–6 times greater)
- *Hardness*: 55 KHN (considerably greater)
- *Water Sorption*: 0.5–0.7 mg/cm^2 (less than unfilled resins)
- *Coefficient of Thermal expansion*: 25–30 × 10^{-6}/°C. (High filler to resin ratio reduces the expansion coefficient significantly)
- *Esthetic*: Polishing results in roughening of the surface because of selective abrasion of the soft resin matrix surrounding the hard filler particles. Composites stain over a period
- *Radiopacity*: Composites using quartz as filler are radiolucent.

Clinical Performance

- Difficulty in polishing
- Tendency to discolor. The rough surfaces tend to retain stains
- Coefficient of thermal expansion is three times that of tooth structure. Hence has a higher chance of developing secondary caries due to micro-leakage associated with percolation
- Not hard enough; hence undergoes occlusal surface wear. Not indicated as posterior restorative material.

MICROFILLED COMPOSITES

Types of Microfilled Composites

- Sintered prepolymerized microfilled complexes
- Spherical polymer-based microfilled complexes
- Agglomerated microfilled complexes.

Sintered Prepolymerized Microfilled Complexes

- These are made by incorporating 60–70 wt% silica into a resin matrix
- This is then heat-cured and milled into particles of 1–200 μm
- They contain high percentage of inorganic silica.

Spherical Polymer-based Microfilled Composites

- Manufactured by incorporating pyrogenic silica into partially cured polymer spheres 20–30 μm
- This small size distribution permits an extremely dense packing.

Agglomerated Microfiller Composites

- They consist of artificially agglomerated microfillers in the range of 1–25 µm
- These particles are purely inorganic.

Properties

Microfilled composites have physical and mechanical properties that are inferior to conventional composites.

This is because approximately 50% volume is made up of resins.

- Compressive strength — 250–350 MPa
- Tensile strength — 30–50 MPa, lowest among the composites
- Modules of elasticity — 3–6 GPa, lowest among the composites
- Hardness — 25–30 KHN
- Coefficient of thermal expansion — 50 to 10 × 10^{-6}/c, highest among the composites
- Water sorption — 1.4–1.7 mg/cm^2, highest among the composites
- Esthetics — The inorganic fillers are smaller than the abrasive particle used for finishing the restoration. The silica filler is also removed along with the resin in which it is embedded at the same rate and results in a smooth surface finish
- Filler particle size — 0.02–0.04 µm, which is 200 to 300 times smaller than the average quartz particle in conventional composites
- The disadvantage with using colloidal silica was that, because of its large surface area, it could not be adequately wetted by the resin matrix
- Adding small amounts of microfillers resulted in undue thickening of the resin matrix.

Clinical Performance

- Microfilled composites can be polished to the highest lustre and smoothest surface of all composites
- Primary indication is for esthetic restorations; but in nonstress-bearing areas
- Good choice for restoring Class V cervical lesions due to their low modulus of elasticity allows them to flex during tooth flexure.

SMALL PARTICLE COMPOSITES

They were introduced to approach the surface smoothness afforded by microfilled composites and yet retain or improve upon the physical and mechanical properties of conventional composites.

Composition

- Fillers used are glasses containing heavy metals.
- Average filler size ranges from 1 µm and 5 µm and they have a broad size distribution, which facilitates higher filler loading
- Filler content—65–77 vol%, 80–90 wt% (more than conventional composites).

Properties

The best physical and mechanical properties are seen with this type of composites, due to its high filler content.

• Compressive strength	350–400 MPa—highest among the composites
• Tensile strength	75–90 MPa—Double that of microfilled and 50% greater than conventional
• Modulus of elasticity	15–20 GPa—highest
• Hardness	50–60 KHN—similar to conventional; but has improved wear resistance
• Coefficient of thermal expansion	19–26 × 10^{-6}/°C—lowest; but twice that of tooth structure
• Water sorption	0.5–0.6 mg/cm^2—similar to conventional
• Esthetics	Better surface smoothness than conventional
• Polymerization shrinkage	Comparable to or less than conventional
• Radiopacity	Radiopaque due to the use of glasses containing heavy metals as fillers.

Clinical Performance

- Due to their improved strength and abrasion resistance, they are suggested for use in Class IV and Class II restorations
- They are not as good as the microfilled in this regard.

HYBRID COMPOSITES

They were developed in an effort to obtain even better surface smoothness than that provided by small particles composites and maintaining the properties of the latter.

Composition

The organic matrix is reinforced with microfillers to decrease the differences in properties between inorganic macrofillers and unfilled organic matrix.

Two Kinds of Filler Particles are Employed

- Colloidal Silver—10–20 wt% of the total filler content
- Ground particles of glass containing heavy metals.

There is a blend of submicron (0.04 μm) and small particle (1–4 μm) fillers with an average size range of 0.6–1 μm.

Properties

Their physical and mechanical properties range between conventional and small particle composites and are generally superior to microfilled composites.

• Compressive strength	300–350 MPa—slightly less than small particle
• Tensile strength	70–90 MPa—comparable to that of small particle
• Modulus of elasticity	7–12 GPa—between conventional and microfilled
• Hardness	50–60 KHN—similar to small particle

- Coefficient of thermal expansion — $30–40 \times 10^{-6}/°C$—less than microfilled
- Water sorption — 0.5–0.7 mg/cm^2—similar to conventional
- Esthetics — Surface smoothness and esthetics comparable with microfilled composites
- Radio-opacity — The presence of glasses containing heavy metals makes it radiopaque.

Clinical Performance

- They are widely used for anterior restorations due to their good esthetics
- Combination of medium and small filler particles improves the physical and mechanical properties
- They can be used in stress-bearing areas as Cl-IV and Cl-II.

RECENT ADVANCES IN COMPOSITES

The disadvantages of older composites are
- High polymerization shrinkage
- Lack of ability to condense
- Lack of wear resistance.

Recently introduced composite materials have compensated some of these disadvantages.

High Viscosity Composites (Condensable/Packable)

- These composites contain a wide range of filler particles (0.04 μ–20 μ) and have 60–70% filler by volume
- These materials can be compacted, e.g. solitaire, surefil.

Flowable Composites

- They are 'painted on' in small increments, thereby building the restoration
- They have a low filler loading and the particle sizes are small (less than 50% by volume) This has a very low modulus of elasticity, which allows it to flex and flow
- It can also absorb polymerization stresses, e.g. revolution.

Uses

- Class V cavities
- Pit and fissure sealant
- Base for classes—I, II and III.

Smart Composites

- They can release fluoride ions, hydroxyl ions and calcium when the PH in the restoration is less than 5.5
- This was said to neutralize acid and counteract decalcification, e.g. Ariston PHC (PH Control).

PRIMM (Polymeric Rigid Inorganic Matrix Material)

- This has a resin and a ceramic component
- It consists of a continuous network of ceramic fibers (Al_2O_3 + SiO_2) of diameter 2μ, which are fused together at various sites to produce a continuous network of small chambers into which BISGMA/UDMA flow.

Advantages

- Low polymerization shrinkage
- Are packable
- Depth of polymerization—6 mm (light conducting through ceramic fibers).

Nanocomposites

- They have size below the wavelength of visible light
- These do not scatter/absorb light
- These small particles fill spaces between larger filler particles and allow increased filler loading (95% by weight). This reduces polymerization shrinkage
- They also provide a means for incorporating radiopacity without interfering in the esthetics.

Nanomaterials for Restorative Dentistry

Types

- Nanocomposites
- Nanoionomers
- Endodontic sealers and tooth regeneration.

Nano was coined by the noble laureate Sir Richard Feynman in 1959.

Nano varieties are supposed to decrease polymerization shrinkage, increase wear resistance, micro hardness and achieve good esthetic patient satisfaction.

Nanocomposites[1]

Types of Nanocomposites

Nanofills and nanohybrids are the common types.

- *Nanofills*: Small particle size 1 to 100 nm.
- *Nanohybrids*: Larger particles ranging from 0.4 μm to 5 μm. (E.g. NANOSIT™ Nordiska Dental, Angelholm, Sweden) is a nanohybrid composite. (7 nm to ≤ 2000 nm).
- *Nanofillers*: Ranges from 5 nm to 20 nm as in 3M ESPE (Filtek™ Supreme Plus, 3M ESPE, St. Paul, MN, USA).
- *Nanocomposites*: Main purposes of using nanomeric particles are to reduce the particle size and thereby the wavelength of visible light (400 nm to 800 nm) leading to highly translucent materials with high surface area to volume ratio.

Types of nanometric particles used are:

- Nano-agglomerated particles of silica or zirconia, surface coated with coupling agent to enhance bonding. (Drawback was poor rheological properties)

- Nanoclusters was developed to overcome the drawback of nanoagglomerates—Nanoclusters were synthesized by lightly sintering nanomeric oxides. (Like a bunch of grapes with an average size range of 0.6 μm), e.g. Filtek™ Supreme Plus (3M ESPE).
- Coupling agents (such as gamma-methacryloxypropyltrimethoxysilane (MTPS) are used to achieve a strong covalent bond between the organic matrix and inorganic fillers.
- One side of the coupling agent bond with hydroxyl groups of silica particles and other is copolymerized with polymer matrix.
- Other agents in minor amounts which are added are accelerators, pigments and initiator is camphoquinone (CQ).

Other types:

1. The addition of using monovinyl methacrylate monomers into dental resin by Decker reported enhanced polymerization kinetics and improved mechanical properties.
   They were made up of urethanes, carbonates or cyclic carbonates. They were also referred to as ultra-rapid monomethacrylates.
2. Recently options of adding acidic functional groups in monomers are also under trial.[2]
3. Carbon nanotubes have superior and exceptional mechanical properties as well as unique bioactivity[3]
   Drawback was hydrophobicity and chemical inertness leading to their limited applications.

REFERENCES

1. Ozak ST, Ozkan P. Nanotechnology and dentistry. Eur J Dent. 2013;7:145-51.
2. Cramer, NB, Stansbury JW, Bowman CN. Recent advances and developments in composite dental restorative materials. J. Dent. Res. 2011;90:402-16.
3. Kealley C, Elcombe M, van Riessen A, Ben-Nissan B. Development of carbon nanotube-reinforced hydroxyapatite bioceramics. Phys. B Condens. Matter 2006;385:496-498.

38. Classify dentin-bonding agents. What are adhesive materials? Write a note on composition. Enumerate the uses and advantages of direct bonding materials.

INTRODUCTION

- One of the most effective ways of improving mechanical bonding and the marginal seal of resin-based restorative materials is by the use of acid-etch technique
- Acid etching of enamel provides good mechanical bonding

- Dentin contains higher volume percent of organic components 30 volume % and 20 volume % of fluid
- Its tubular nature allows fluid to the surface, hence, adversely affects adhesion
- The presence of smear layer on the surface of cut dentin interferes in bonding
- Fusayama introduced the *total etch concept* in 1978. This involved the simultaneous etching of Enamel and Dentin with 37% phosphoric acid.

BONDING

Dental adhesives can be defined as an agent or series of substances which mediate a bond to the dental hard tissue without relying on the interlocking effect or retention of the prepared cavity.

Dentin-bonding System consists of Three Components

1. Dentin conditioner
2. Dentin primer
3. Dentin adhesive.

Dentin Conditioner

After the preparation of tooth, a smear layer is formed. Smear layer inhibits proper bonding, hence dentin-conditioning needs to be done.

Conditioning can be done by using:

- Acids, e.g. H_3PO_4(37%), HNO_3-25%
- Chelators
- Lasers
- Microabrasion.

Dentin Primer

This is an adhesion promoter in a solvent such as water, ethanol or acetone.

Dentin Adhesive/Bonding Agent

Contains both hydrophilic and hydrophobic groups that interact with the moist dentinal surface as well as to the restorative resin.

MECHANISM OF BONDING

- Acid etching/conditioning leaves a layer of dentin anchored collagen fibers on the surface of demineralized dentin
- Into this, the hydrophilic resins (Dentin Primer) infiltrate forming a hybrid layer consisting of resin-infiltrated dentin
- The adhesive then bonds to the primer leaving the hydrophobic groups exposed to create a favorable surface for the restorative resins.

CLASSIFICATION

I Generation

- Based on NPG-GMA (N-phenyl glycine glycidyl methacrylate)
- Mediates water resistant chemical bonds of resin to dentinal calcium
- Bond strength—low (2 MPa).

II Generation

- Phosphate bonding systems
- There is ionic interaction between chlorophosphate group and calcium
- This is not strong enough to resist the hydrolysis resulting from saliva exposure or moisture from dentin itself
- Bond strength—4–6 MPa.

III Generation

- Based on oxalate bonding system
- Here dentin conditioning was done to modify and remove the smear layer
- Dentin primers were used, e.g. Hydrophilic resin monomers (HEMA) (Multistep Adhesive System)
- Bond strength—10 MPa.

IV Generation

- Introduction of Total Etch Concept by Fusayama. (1979–Etching, both enamel and dentin)
- Based on 4-META
- Concept of wet/moist dentinal bonding was introduced
- Intertubular and dentinal tubules were used for bonding
- Bond strength—18 MPa.

V Generation

- Two different types of adhesive material:
  - One-bottle systems (containing primer and adhesive)
  - Self-etching Primer (conditioner and primer)
- Monofillers are present
- The self-etching primers eliminate the need to wash out the acidic gel.

VI Generation

- One-step bonding system
- No etching is required
- Device consists of two chambers:
  - First and uppermost contains methacrylated phosphoric esters, initiators and stabilizers
  - Second chamber contains a fluoride-complex, water and stabilizer

- The system is activated by squeezing the upper chamber first and then the second chamber, forcing the material into the pocket, which contains the application device
- This is rubbed on to the tooth surface.

Advantages

- No acid etching
- No washing/air dispersing
- No light curing of bonding agent.

Most of the presently used bonding systems belong to the IV, V or the latest VI generation. Improvements in the bonding system reduce number of steps and time.

39. What are the ideal requirements of restorative dental cements? Classify them. Write in detail about $ZnPO_4$ cement including the control of setting time and technical considerations.

REQUIREMENTS OF CEMENTS

Chemical and Biological

- Should be nontoxic, nonpoisonous, nonirritant and chemically inert
- Should be biocompatible to the pulp and soft tissues
- Should have anticariogenic property
- Should be insoluble and should not absorb the oral fluids
- Should be chemically bonded with tooth structure
- Should be bacteriostatic and obtundent
- Should be able to facilitate growth of secondary dentin
- Setting action should be controllable.

Physical and Mechanical

- Restorative cements should have adequate value of mechanical properties (surface hardness, compressive strength, tensile strength, proportional limit, modulus of elasticity)
- Should be adhesive to enamel and dentin
- Dimensional change should be minimum during setting

- Some restorative materials have low strengths compared with those of composites and amalgam, but they can be used for low stress areas
- Glass ionomer cements, polyacid modified resin composites, metal modified or resin modified glass ionomers have good strength and, hence, can be used as permanent restorative material.

Thermal

- Softening temperature should be high
- Thermal conductivity should be low
- Coefficient of thermal expansions should match with that of tooth structure, i.e. should be low to prevent dimensional change leading to leakage and percolations, e.g. silicate cements.

Esthetics

- The material should have ability to incorporate color pigments
- The material used for anterior restoration must be translucent.
- The material should not discolor or stain
- Glass ionomer cements, resin modified glass ionomers, etc. can have sufficient translucency and so are useful as anterior restorative materials.

General Properties

- Easily available
- Long storage life
- Easy to manipulate.

CLASSIFICATION

Craig's Classification

Based on Function

Function	Examples
• Final cementation of completed restoration	Zinc phosphate, zinc silico-phosphate, reinforced ZOE, Zn polycarboxylate
• Temporary cementation of completed restoration or cementation of temporary restoration	ZOE, non-eugenol ZnO
• High strength bases	$ZnPO_4$, Reinforced ZOE, Zn polycarboxylate, glass-ionomer
• Temporary fillings	ZOE, reinforced ZOE, Zn polycarboxylate.
• Low strength bases	ZOE, $Ca(OH)_2$
• Liners	$Ca(OH)_2$ in a suspension
• Varnishes	Resin in a solvent.

Based on Special Applications

Application	Examples
Root canal sealant	ZOE, Zn polycarboxylate
Gingival tissue pack	ZOE
Surgical dressing	ZOE, zinc oxide preparation
Cementation of orthodontic bands	$ZnPO_4$, Zn pol-carboxylate
Orthodontic direct bonding	Acrylic resin, composite resin.

ZINC PHOSPHATE CEMENT

- Zinc phosphate is the oldest of the luting cements
- It consists of powder and liquid in two separate bottles.

Types

Type I

- Fine-grained or with small-sized particles
- Used for luting or cementation of cast restoration
- Film thickness—25 μm.

Type II

- Medium grained
- Used for thermal insulating base and temporary filling
- Film thickness—40 μm.

Composition

Supplied as powder and liquid.

Powder	Liquid
Zinc oxide—90% Magnesium oxide—10% Metallic oxides SiO_2—1.5–5% Bi_2O_3—0.1% BaO, CaO—0.1%	Phosphoric acid } 54% Aluminum phosphate } $ZnPO_4$ } 10% Buffers } H_2O—36% Or Aqueous solution of H_3PO_4—50–60% + Buffering agents.

Powder

- The ingredients of the powder are sintered at temperatures between 1000°C and 1400°C into a cake that is subsequently ground into a fine powder
- The acidic content of most liquids is 33 ± 5 wt%.

Setting Reaction

$ZnO_3 + H_3PO_4 \longrightarrow ZnHPO_4 + \text{Heat}$

Zinc oxide + Phosphoric acid → Amorphous zinc phosphate + heat

- The buffering agents reduce the rate of reaction of liquid with powder
- They also stabilize the PH of acid and make the cement smooth, nongranular and workable
- Water controls the ionization of the acid, which influences the acid base reaction
- The set cement consists of a cored structure
- The core consists of unreacted ZnO particles in a matrix of Zn_3PO_4, which binds the core
- The set mass is porous
- In the presence of excess water, a noncohesive crystalline mass called hoplite $[(Zn_3(PO_4)_2].4H_2O)$ develops
- When the powder is mixed with the liquid, phosphoric acid attacks the surface of the particles and releases zinc ions into the liquid
- Aluminum, which already forms a complex with the phosphoric acid, reacts with zinc and yields a zinc alumino-phosphate gel. Thus, the set cement is a cored structure consisting primarily of unreacted zinc oxide particles embedded in a cohesive amorphous matrix of zinc alumino-phosphate.

Working and Setting Times

- Working time is measured as the time from the start of mixing to the maximum time at which the consistency of the mix is low enough to flow readily under pressure to form a thin film
- Setting time is defined as the elapsed time from the start of mixing to the point at which the needle no longer makes a complete circular indentation in the cement.
  Setting time of zinc phosphate is between 2.5 minutes and 8 minutes.

Factors Affecting Setting Time

- *Sintering temperature*: Increase in temperature increases the setting time
- *Particle size*: Decrease in size decreases the setting time
- *Composition of liquid*: Increase in water decreases the setting time (controlled by operator)
- *Powder/Liquid ratio (P/L)*: The recommended P/L ratio is about 1.4 gm of powder to 0.5 mL of liquid. Reducing the P/L ratio produces a thinner mix, which increases the setting time
- *Rate of powder incorporation*: The smaller the increment of powder, the larger will be the setting time
- *Spatulation time*: Increased spatulation time decreases the setting time
- *Mixing temperature*: The cooler the temperature, the more will be the setting time.

Physical Properties

- Compressive strength—104 MPa
- Tensile strength—5.5 MPa
- Modulus of elasticity—13.7 GPa
- Hardness—60 KHN. Hence, highly resistant to elastic deformation and can be used as luting agents.

Consistency and Film Thickness

- Thick/luting consistency—for fixing of inlays crowns and bridges
  Film thickness—25 μm
- Thick/Base consistency—used for base and temporary filling.
  Film thickness—40 μm.

Thermal Properties

- Acts as a good thermal insulating base under metallic restoration.

Biological Properties

- The acidity of zinc phosphate cement is high at the time of prosthesis placement on a prepared tooth
- Two minutes after the start of mixing, the pH of the cement is approximately 2 and later increases rapidly
- At 24 hours, it is only about 5.5
- Solubility—0.06% wt
- Solubility is greater in organic acids like lactic, acetic and citric acids
- Adhesion: It has mechanical adhesion.

Manipulation

- Cement should be mixed on a cool slab to prolong the working and setting times and permit incorporation of maximum amount of powder
- The liquid should not be dispensed until mixing is initiated because water will be lost by evaporation
- The powder should be divided into several increments and mixing should be started with a small amount of powder
- The time required to spatulate each increment is approximately 15 to 20 seconds before adding another increment
- Completion of the mix requires approximately 1.5 to 2 minutes.
- For a fixed partial denture, a slightly decreased viscosity is required and field of operation should be kept dry
- After the prosthesis has been seated, it should be held under pressure until the cement sets
- Excessive cement can be removed after it has set
- A layer of varnish can be applied to the margin to prevent the dissolution of luting agent in oral fluid.

Advantages

- Easy to handle and has a long record of clinical durability.
- High compressive strength and low film thickness.
- Working time can be controlled.
- Permanent luting agent.

Disadvantages

- Set cement is brittle.
- High solubility in organic acids and oral fluids.

- Low pH value at early stages and so produces pulpal irritation.
- Lack of chemical bonding to tooth structure.
- Lack of anticariogenic property.
- Setting reaction is exothermic and rapid.

Uses

- For luting
- As a thermal insulating base
- Cementation of cast restoration and orthodontic appliances
- Temporary restorations.

40. Describe briefly the composition, chemical reaction, manipulation, types, uses and properties of glass ionomer.

SYNONYMS

Alumino-silicate polyacrylic cement (ASPA).
Acid soluble calcium fluoro-alumino-silicate glass.

COMPOSITION

Powder	Liquid
Silica (SiO_2)—29.0% Alumina (Al_2O_3)—16.6% Aluminum fluoride (AlF_3)—5.3% Calcium fluoride (CaF_2)—34.3% Aluminum phosphate ($AlPO_4$)—9.9% Cryolite—5.0%.	Aqueous polyacrylic acid—45–50% Copolymer of itaconic acid and maleic acid—10% Tartaric acid—5%

Functions of the Constituents

Fluoride	Improves the working characteristic, enhances translucency, anticariogenic and increases strength
Silica glass	Controls the setting rate, provides translucency
Copolymeric acid	Irregularly arranged; thus decreases setting
Itaconic acid	Increases the reactivity of liquid
Maleic acid	Decreases viscosity and decreases tendency to gel
Tartaric acid	Increases working time, but shortens setting time.

- Freeze-dried acid powder and glass powder in one bottle and tartaric acid in another bottle is available as the liquid component. This on mixing has longer working time and is also called as Semi-hydrous/Water settable/Anhydrous cement.

SETTING REACTION

- Decomposition of the powder (glass) due to acid attack and release of metal ions (Ca^{2+}, Al^{3+}, Na^{+} and F^{-}).
- Migration of these ions into the aqueous phase of the cement. The outer layer of glass particles is thus depleted of metal ions and degraded to silica gel
- Gelation of the polyacids by the metal ions (Ca^{2+} and polysalts) leading to set
- Initially polyacrylic acid are cross-linked by calcium to form a solid mass
- Within 24 hours, a new phase forms in which aluminum becomes bound in the cement mix
- The set cement consists of an agglomeration of unreacted powder particles surrounded by silica gel in a matrix of hydrated calcium and aluminum polysalts.

Chemistry of Setting

The setting reaction is an acid-base reaction between the acidic polyelectrolyte and the alumino-silicate glass.

- Polyacids attack the glass to release cations and fluoride ions
- These metal fluoride complexes react with the polyanions to form salt gel matrix
- In the first 3 hours, calcium ions react with the polycarboxylate chains
- The trivalent aluminum ions react for at least 48 hours
- The polyacrylic acid chains are cross-linked by the calcium ions that are replaced by aluminum ions within the next 24 hours
- Sodium and fluorine ions do not participate in the cross-linking of the cement
- The cross-linked phase becomes hydrated over time with the same water used for mixing. This process is called Maturation
- The unreacted portion of glass particles are sheathed by a silica gel
- Thus, the set cement consists of an agglomeration of unreacted powder particles surrounded by a silica gel in an amorphous matrix of hydrated calcium and aluminum polysalts **(Fig. 14)**.

The solid black particles represent unreacted glass particles surrounded by the gel (shaded) that form when Al^{+++} ions and Ca^{++} ions are leached from the glass as a result of attack by the polyacrylic acid.

The Ca^{++} and Al^{+++} ions form polysalts with the COO^{-} groups of the polyacrylic acid to form cross-linked structures **(Fig. 15)**.

The carboxyl groups react with calcium in enamel and dentin.

Mechanism of Adhesion

- The Ca^{2+} and Al^{3+} ions from the powder react with the carboxylate groups to cross-link the polymeric acid
- The same carboxylate groups interact strongly with surface Ca^{2+} ions in enamel or dentin to yield chemical adhesion to tooth structure
- The bond strength to enamel is always higher than that to dentin because of the greater inorganic content of the enamel.

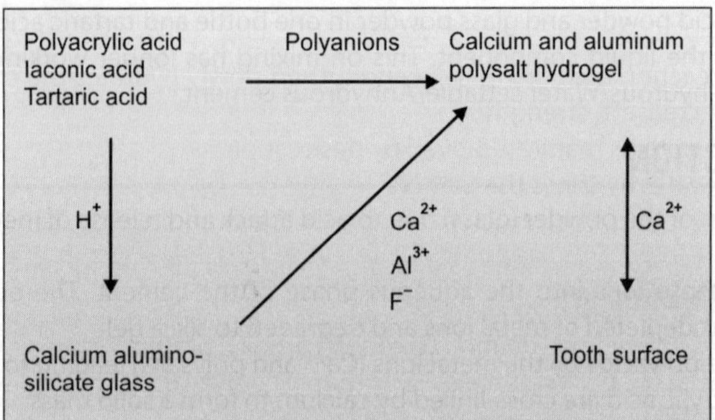

Fig. 14: Setting reaction of glass ionomer

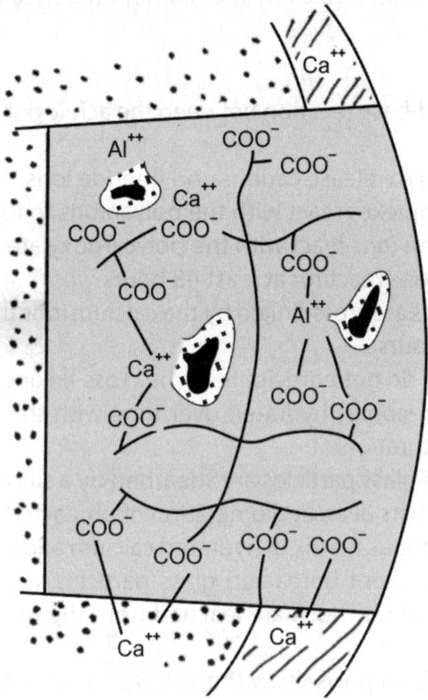

Fig. 15: Structure of glass ionomer cement

Manipulation

- For mixing a wax paper and agate, spatula is used
- Mixing has three stages:
  1. The powder is divided into two halves
  2. The first half is folded into the liquid for 10–15 seconds
  3. The second increment is mixed into the resulting thin paste within the next 15 seconds.
- *For luting, cement powder*: Liquid ratio—1.5:1
- For restorative, cement: Liquid ratio—2.8:1

Role of Water

- Serves as the reaction medium initially and it then slowly hydrates the cross-linked matrix, leading to an increase in strength
- Loosely bound water is readily removed by desiccation
- Tightly bound water hydrates the matrix
- Hydration yields a stable gel structure and builds the strength of the cement.

Bonding to Tooth Structure

- The adhesion to enamel and dentin is through carboxyl group calcium of the tooth
- Chelation takes place between the COO^- group of polyacids and calcium on the apatite of enamel and dentin.

TYPES

Wilson and McLean (1988).

Type I

Luting.

Type II

Restorative material.
Esthetic filling material.
BIS-GMA reinforced filling material.

Type III

Liners/base and fissure sealing material.

PROPERTIES

- High compressive and low tensile strength
- Compressive strength Type I—80–130 MPa, Type II—150 MPa
- Diametrical tensile strength—Type II—6.6 MPa
- It is a biocompatible material and is kind to pulp
- Anticariogenic, due to fluoride release
- Adequate working time and a rapid set at mouth temperature, if protected from moisture contamination
- Strength—Type I—6–8 minutes, Type II—4–5 minutes.
- Low viscosity and film thickness (Film Thickness—250–30 μm)
- Resistance to plastic deformation
- Modulus of elasticity—5.6–9.5 GPa
- Adhesion to tooth structure and restoration
- Translucent
- Radiopaque
- Good resistance to aqueous/acid attack
- Solubility—0.4%.

USES

- Restoration of erosion/abrasion lesions without cavity preparation
- Sealing and filling of occlusal pits and fissure
- Restoration of deciduous teeth
- Repair of defective margins in restoration
- As a base/lining material
- For core build up
- As a luting agent for indirect restorations.

RECENT ADVANCES IN GLASS IONOMERS

Nano Ionomers (Nano Filled Type of Glass Ionomers)

There is no universally accepted cement that fulfills all applications.

Cements used for long-term restorations are:

- Compomer
- Glass ionomers
- Hybrid ionomers
- Zinc phosphate
- Zinc poly-carboxylate
- Resin-based cement.

Glass ionomers: Introduced by Wilson and Kent in the 1970s[1]

Common short coming were:

- Poor esthetic
- Prolonged setting reaction
- Weak bond strength.

To overcome these shortcomings, various changes and techniques such as the addition of cellulose fibers, hydroxyapatite, and nanotechnology was researched.[2]

Nano ionomers

- *Resin modified glass ionomers* were modified with nonoparticles such as nanomers and nanoclusters of fluoroaluminosilicate (FAS) glass, e.g. Ketac™ Nano; 3M ESPE. This improved esthetics and polishablilty but knoop hardness of Ketec nano was low hence cannot be used in high stress bearing areas.
  Equia® system: 15% wt Inorganic silica nanofillers (40 nm size) are dispersed in liquid and reinforce the resulting polymer matrix.
- *Advantages were*: Good wear resistance and reduction in the initial setting time. Maintains polished surface for a longer period of time and is highly esthetic and good as a posterior filling material.[3]
- *Addition of nanoscale hydroxyapatite (HA) and fluoroapatite (FA)*: The addition increased the bond strength with the addition of micro HA (5–10 μm) and Nano-HA (100–150 nm) improved bond strength further and helps filling the demineralizing micro-pores in the tooth structure.
- Ethanol based sol-gel Nano-HA and Nano-FA Eg Fuji II glass ionomers showed better mechanical properties.

- Nano materials are also researched with alumina, alumina/titania, zirconia and yttria stabilized zirconia.

REFERENCES

1. (Guggenberger R, May R, Stefan K, New trends in glass-ionomer chemistry. Biomaterials. 1998;19:479-483).
2. Moshaverinia A, Ansari S, Movasaghi Z, Billington RW, Darr JA, Rehman IU. Modification of conventional glass-ionomer cements with vinylpyrrolidone containing polyacids, nano-hydroxy and fluoroapatite to improve mechanical properties. Dent. Mater. 2008;24:1381-90.
3. Basso M. Teeth restoration using a high-viscosity glass ionomer cement: The Equia® system. J. Minim. Interv. Dent. 2011;4:74-76.

41. Discuss in detail zinc oxide eugenol cement. Add a note on modified zinc oxide eugenol cement.

ZINC OXIDE EUGENOL CEMENT

Introduction

- Zinc oxide eugenol (ZOE) has a pH of 7. So it is the least irritating of all dental materials
- Used in dentistry since 1890s as cavity liners, cementing restorations, bases, root canal sealants, periodontal dressings and temporary and intermediate restorations
- Have low strength and have an abundant (sedative) effect on exposed dentin
- To improve strength many modified zinc oxide eugenol cements have been introduced. For example, EBA—alumina modified and polymer—reinforced zinc oxide—eugenol cements
- Recently, non-eugenol zinc oxide cements have become available for patients sensitive to eugenol.

CLASSIFICATIONS

Type I

Temporary ZOE luting cement.

Type II

Long-term ZOE luting cement.

Type III

Temporary ZOE restorations.

Type IV

Intermediate ZOE restorations.

Type I—Temporary ZOE Luting Cement

- The strength of temporary cement must be sufficiently low to permit removal of the restoration without trauma to the teeth and damage to the restoration.
- It seals the cavity against the ingress of oral fluids at least for a short time; hence, irritation caused by microleakage is minimized.

Type II—Long-term ZOE Luting Cement

- The compressive strength of these cements is acceptable, but overall their strength values are inferior to those of other cements
- They are difficult to manipulate in the oral cavity
- The film thickness of some products tends to be high and the cement excess after setting may be quite difficult to remove
- For these reasons, the use of ZOE cements for long-term applications has been confined primarily to those situations in which tooth sensitivity might be a problem.

Type III—Temporary ZOE Restorations

- Materials used for temporary restorations are expected to last from a few days to a few weeks at most
- They can provide a temporary restorative treatment while the pulp heals or until a more long lasting restoration can be fabricated and cemented.

Type IV—Intermediate ZOE Restorations

Clinical experience with this type of material indicates that it can serve effectively as a restorative material for at least 1 year.

MODE OF SUPPLY

It is dispensed in two forms:

a. Powder and liquid.
b. Two-paste system.

COMMERCIAL NAMES

Unmodified

- Tempac — Type III
- Cavitic — Type IV
- Tempbond — Type I

EBA Alumina Modified

- Opotow alumina EBA — Type II

Polymer Modified

- Fynal — Type II
- IRM — Type III

Non-Eugenol

- Neogenol — Type I
- Freegenol — Type I

COMPOSITION

Powder

Constituent	Percentage	Function
Zinc oxide	69%	Principal ingredient
White rosin	29.3%	To reduce brittleness of set cement
Zinc stearate	1%	Accelerator, plasticizer
Zinc acetate	0.7%	Accelerator, improves strength
Magnesium oxide		Is added in some powders; it reacts with Eugenol

Liquid

Constituent	Percentage	Function
Eugenol	85%	Reacts with zinc oxide
Olive oil	15%	Plasticizer

SETTING REACTION

- In the first reaction, hydrolysis of zinc oxide to its hydroxide takes place. Water is essential for the reactions to proceed

  $$ZnO + H_2O \rightarrow Zn(OH)_2$$

- The reaction proceeds as a typical acid-base reaction to form a chelate

  $$\underset{\text{(Zinc hydroxide)}}{Zn(OH)_2} + \underset{\text{(Eugenol)}}{2HE} \rightarrow \underset{\text{(Zinc eugenolate)}}{ZnE_2 + 2H_2O}$$

- The chelate forms an amorphous gel that tends to crystallize imparting strength to the set mass.

Structure of Set Cement

The set cement consists of particles of zinc oxide embedded in a matrix of particles of zinc eugenolate.

Setting Time

4–10 minutes.

Factors-affecting Setting Time

Manufacture

The most active zinc oxide powders are those formed by decomposing zinc salts such as zinc hydroxide and zinc carbonate by heating at 300°C.

Particle Size

Cements from powders containing smaller zinc oxide particles set faster.

Accelerators

Alcohol, glacial acetic acid and small amount of water accelerate the reactions.

Heat

- High temperature accelerates setting
- Lower temperature (e.g. cooling the glass slab) slows the reaction.

Retarders

The set can be retarded with glycol and glycerine.

Powder-to-Liquid Ratio

The higher the ratio, the faster is the set.

PROPERTIES

Mechanical Properties

Compressive Strength

- They are relatively weak cements
- The strength depends on the use of the materials
- Cements used as temporary restorations and cavity liners will have low strength
- Cements for permanent cementation and intermediate restorations will be stronger
- The compressive strength ranges from 3–4 MPa up to 50–55 MPa.

Tensile Strength

- It varies according to use
- Ranges from 0.32 MPa to 5.8 MPa.

Modulus of Elasticity

- Ranges from 0.22 GPa to 5.4 GPa (0.03–0.79 psi).

Thermal Properties

Thermal Conductivity

- Their thermal insulating properties are excellent and are approximately the same as for human dentin
- The thermal conductivity is 3.98 [cal.Sec^{-1} cm^{-2} (^{0}C/cm)$^{-1}$] $\times 10^{-4}$

Coefficient of Thermal Expansion

35 x 10^{-6}/°C

Solubility and Disintegration

- 0.04% ult
- The solubility of the set cement is high, the highest among the dental cements
- They disintegrate in oral fluids
- This breakdown is due to hydrolysis of the zinc hydroxides and eugenol solubility is reduced by increasing the powder/liquid ratio.

Film Thickness

- This property is important for those cements used for cementation of restorations
- The film thickness of zinc-oxide eugenol cement is higher than other cements.

Adhesion

These cements do not adhere to enamel or dentin.

Biological Properties

pH and Effects on Pulp

- They are the least irritating of all dental cements. In terms of pulpal response, they are classified as mild
- pH is 6.6 to 8.0.

Bacteriostatic and Obtundent Properties

They inhibit the growth of bacteria and have an anodyne or soothing effect on the pulp in deep cavities, reducing pain when it is present.

Optical Property

The set cement is opaque.

MANIPULATION

Powder–liquid System

Powder–liquid Ratio

4:1 to 6:1 by wt.

Procedure

- The bottles are shaken gently
- Measured quantity of powder and liquid is dispensed on to a cool glass slab or paper pad
- The bulk of the powder is incorporated into the liquid and spatulated thoroughly in a circular motion with a stiff-bladed stainless steel spatula
- Smaller increments are then added until the mix is complete
- Oil of orange can be used to clean eugenol cements from instruments.

Two Paste System

Equal lengths of each paste are dispensed and mixed until a uniform color is observed.

APPLICATIONS

Base

- Materials having compressive strength of 5.5 to 39 MN/m^2 are used as a cement base and the strength reaches a maximum in about 12 to 15 minutes
- They are normally used under zinc phosphate cement.

Temporary Cementation

The unmodified zinc oxide eugenol cements are used also as luting materials for temporary crowns and for temporary cementation of gold restoration.

Temporary Restorations

- The EBA-alumina modified cements have been tried as temporary restorations based on their physical properties
- They show ease of manipulation and possess improved carvability
- The EBA-alumina modified cements, despite their low solubility in water, disintegrate excessively in mouth.

Permanent Cementation

The EBA-alumina modified zinc oxide eugenol cements have been used successfully for permanent cementation of crowns and bridges.

Endodontic Sealers

- Endodontic zinc oxide eugenol preparations have been used as root canal sealer alone and with gutta percha and silver points
- There are two major groups of products based on zinc-oxide eugenol cements—conventional and therapeutic sealers.

Tissue Management

For Mechanical Displacement of Soft Tissue

When these cements are used as a mechanical tissue pack, a thin consistency is incorporated into cotton fibers that are placed into the gingival sulcus.

For Dressing Soft Tissue after the Surgery has been Performed

- As a surgical dressing, it provides comfort to the patient during eating, obtunds the surgerized tissue, promotes epithelial growth and helps prevent the overgrowth of granulation tissue
- These zinc oxide eugenol surgical cements have long working and setting time
- Usually no accelerator is added to these materials.

MODIFIED ZINC OXIDE EUGENOL CEMENTS

EBA-Alumina Modified Cement

These were introduced in an effort to improve the mechanical properties of zinc-oxide eugenol cement.

Composition

Powder	Liquid
ZnO—60%–70% Aluminum/quartz—20–30% Rosin—5–10% Zinc acetate—0.4%	Ethoxy benzoic acid—62.5% Eugenol—37.5%

Properties

- Better than that of unmodified ZOE
- Compressive strength is 55 MPa
- Tensile strength is 4.1 MPa
- Modulus of elasticity is 2.5 GPa
- Film thickness 25 μm
- Solubility and disintegration in water 0.05% wt.

Manipulation

- Glass slabs are recommended for EBA-alumina modified cements
- After dispensing, the powder is incorporated into the liquid in bulk
- It is kneaded for 30 seconds and then stopped for an additional 60 seconds with broad strokes of the spatula to obtain a creamy consistency
- They have long working hours.

Setting Time

9.5 minutes.

Polymer Reinforced Zinc Oxide Eugenol Cement

The polymer reinforced cement was introduced in an effort to improve the mechanical properties of conventional zinc oxide eugenol cement.

These have been used

- As luting agents
- As bases

- As temporary filling materials
- As cavity liner.

Resin-bonded Cement (KALZINOL)

Composition

Powder	Liquid
ZnO—60%	Eugenol—85%
White resin—5–10%	Olive oil—15%
Natural or synthetic resin—10–40%	Acetic acid—1%
Zinc acetate—0.5%	Thymol

Setting Reaction

The setting reaction is similar to zinc oxide eugenol cements.

Acidic resins, if present, may react with zinc oxide, strengthening the matrix.

Setting Time

6–10 minutes.

Factors Affecting Setting Time

- *Powder liquid ratio*: Lower powder liquid ratio increases the setting time
- Moisture accelerates the setting time.

Properties

- Compressive strength—48 MPa
- Tensile strength—4.1 MPa
- Modulus of elasticity—2.5 GPa
- Film thickness—32 μm
- Solubility and disintegration—0.03% wt
- Improved abrasion resistance and toughness.

Manipulation

- The proper powder/liquid ratio is dispensed on a dry glass slab
- The powder is mixed into the liquid in small portions with vigorous spatulations.

Working Time

These cements have longer working time.

Cements Containing Vanillate Esters

- Recently cements have been developed containing Hexyl vanillate and Ortho Ethoxy Benzoic acid, as a substitute for eugenol

- This liquid is mixed with zincoxide powder
  It has been claimed that these cements have high strength and low solubility.

Special Zinc Oxide Eugenol Products

Antibiotic/Steroid incorporated

Some zinc oxide eugenol materials contain antibiotics such as tetracycline and steroids as anti-inflammatory agents. Their principal use is in pulp capping and root canal therapy.

Radiopaque cement

It contains barium sulfate, which is radiopaque.

42. Compare and contrast the physical, mechanical, biologic and esthetic properties of anterior and posterior restorative materials.

ANTERIOR RESTORATIVE MATERIALS

Physical and Mechanical Properties

Composites

Property	Conventional	Microfilled	Hybrid
Compressive strength	36,000–43,000	50,000	60,000
Tensile strength	7,000	7,500	10,000–13,000
Coefficient of thermal expansion	25×10^{-6}/°C	50×10^{-6}/°C	$30–40 \times 10^{-6}$/°C
Expansion	0.5%	1.4%	0.5%
Water sorption	1.2–1.3%	1.5–2%	1–1.5%
Polymerization shrinkage	50–60	20–30	50–60
KHN	8–15	3–6	7–12

- Hardness is greater for composites than for unfilled acrylic resins.

Conventional composite

- Can cause roughening of the surface because of selective abrasion of the softer resin matrix
- Finishing of restoration produces roughened surface
- Polymerization shrinkage and coefficient of thermal expansion is significantly reduced.

Microfilled composites

- Have greater water sorption, high coefficient of thermal expansion, and decreased elastic modulus
- Has decreased tensile strength
- Has wear resistance and provides a smoother surface finish
- In stress bearing areas, chipping of these composites can occur.

Hybrid composites

Physical and mechanical properties are superior to those of microfilled composites, so used in stress-bearing areas.

Acrylic Resins

- Compressive strength is less—69 MPa
- Low tensile strength 24 MPa
- Low modulus of elasticity 2.4 GPa
- Proportional limit is low
- Low hardness and abrasion resistance
- It is the softest of all restorative materials
- Hardness—15 KHN
- Coefficient of thermal expansion is very high—$92.8 \times 10^{-6} mm^2/°C$. It is 8 times greater than enamel and dentin
- Alteration in mouth temperature causes expansion or contraction of resin leading to percolation of oral fluids at the margins leading to discoloration and secondary caries.

Glass Ionomer

- Light cured universal restorative material can be used as anterior restorative material and Fuji 2 as cervical restorations
- Light cured once have coefficient of thermal expansion similar to dentin
- Good fracture strength
- Good radiopacity, polishability and wear resistance
- Fuji 2 has fluoride-releasing property.

Biological Properties

Composites

Composite resins affect the pulp in two aspects.

- Inherent chemical toxicity of material
- Pulpal involvement due to micro leakage.
- Monomer from improperly cured/uncured composites enters the dentinal tubules and causes pulpal inflammation
- So, a layer of $Ca(OH)_2$ or GIC is applied as a protection to pulpal wall before the insertion of resin paste.

Acrylic Resins

- It has low thermal conductivity

- Polymerization shrinkage is high. It causes a gap between the cavity margins and restoration leading to discoloration and secondary caries
- Insoluble in water and oral fluids, yet can absorb water and swell. Water sorption is 1.7 mg/cm^2
- Monomer can penetrate the dentinal tubules and cause pulpal irritation. A $Ca(OH)_2$ or glass ionomer lining should be applied for pulp protection.

Glass Ionomer

Good radiopacity and good biocompatibility with tooth tissue.

Esthetic Properties

Composites

Highly acceptable esthetics.

Conventional

Polishing results in rough surface. It resulted in a tendency to stain over a period.

Microfilled

- Increased resin content and presence of microfillers is responsible for increased surface smoothness
- Microfilled composites are the resin of choice for esthetic restoration of anterior teeth in nonstress-bearing situations.

Hybrid

Surface smoothness and esthetics make it a material for anterior restoration.

Acrylic Resins

- Excellent matching with tooth color
- But it tends to discolor and stain with use.

Glass Ionomer

- Light cured GIC has good esthetic, enamel-like translucency
- Fuji 2 can be used as an anterior restorative material if in cervical region as it is not as esthetic as composites.

POSTERIOR RESTORATIVE MATERIALS

Physical and Mechanical Properties

Amalgam

Creep

- Time dependent strain or deformation is produced by a stress
- Creep phenomenon causes an amalgam restoration to extend out of the cavity preparation leading to marginal breakdown
- Creep value for low copper alloy is high (6.3%)

- High copper amalgam has low creep value
- Over trituration of alloys increases creep of dental amalgam and under trituration lowers it
- Dental amalgam has components with melting point that is slightly above room temperature and the creep produced may be very destructive to the restoration.

Tarnish and corrosion results from

- High residual mercury
- Surface texture–small scratches and exposed voids
- Contact of dissimilar metals
- Patients on high sulfur diet
- Moisture contamination during condensation
- Type of alloy–Low copper amalgam has increased susceptibility of corrosion (increased γ_2 content).

Corrosion can be reduced by

- Smoothening and polishing the restoration
- Correct mercury and alloy ratio and proper manipulation
- Avoid dissimilar metals including mixing of high and low copper amalgam.

Strength

- Compressive strength 145 MPa within 1 hour
- Tensile strength 48–70 MPa
- Compressive strength of amalgam should be at least 310 MPa
- High tensile strength resists fracture by premature biting forces.

Hardness

- ADA stipulates a minimum of 80 MPa at 1 hour.

Elastic modulus

About 62,000 M_N/M^2.

Dimensional change

If zinc-containing alloys are contaminated by moisture during trituration or condensation, a large (delayed) expansion can occur.

Composite Resins for Posterior Restorations

- All types of composites are used
- Material shrinks away from margins leading to gap formation
- Wear faster than amalgam. Wear is greater in contact areas. Larger restorations wear faster than smaller ones.

Glass Ionomer Cement

Compressive strength

120–200 MPa—Lesser than silicates.

Tensile strength

8–30.5 MPa—Greater than silicates.

Hardness

48 KHN—Wear resistance is less compared to composites.

Fracture roughness

Inferior compared to composites.

Bond strength

1–3 MN/m^{2-}—Lower than zinc polycarboxylate.

Modulus of elasticity

2,900,000 Psi.

Film thickness

18–25 μm.

Zinc Oxide Eugenol

Compressive strength

- 3–55 MPa
- It depends on the use of cement
- Relatively weak cement.

Tensile strength

0.32–5.8 MPa.

Modulus of elasticity

0.03–0.79 Psi

Film thickness

- 25 μm
- Higher than any other cements.

Setting time

6–8 minutes.

Adhesion

Does not adhere to enamel and dentin. So, they are not used for final cementation of dental restoration.

Silicate Cements

Silicate is the strongest of all dental cements.

Compressive strength

180 MPa.

Tensile strength

3.5 MPa.

They are stronger in compression and weak in tension.

Hardness

70 KHN.

Coefficient of thermal expansion

- Lower than any other restorative material
- Solubility is about 0.7%. It has high solubility.

Adhesion

No adhesive bond between silicates and enamel. It mechanically adheres to tooth structure. Slightly contract on setting.

Biologic Properties

Amalgam

- Microleakage is prevented in amalgam restoration by its own corrosion materials over a period; hence, amalgam is a self-sealing restoration
- Both low and high copper amalgams are capable of sealing against microleakage but the accumulation of corrosion products is slower with high copper alloys
- Excessive cavity cutting is required because of its poor edge strength
- As silver is a good thermal conductor, a base is required under these restorations
- Oral lichen planus has been reported with silver amalgam.

Composite Resins for Posterior Restorations

Biologic properties are the same as that for anterior composite.

Glass Ionomers

Anticariogenic

- Type II Glass-ionomers release fluoride more than silicate cements
- They have good adhesive effect; hence, reduce infiltration of oral fluids at cement-tooth interface.

Zinc Oxide Eugenol

- Excellent thermal insulating properties. It is in the range of cork and asbestos. It is about $3.95 \times 10^{-6}/°C$
- Solubility is the highest among other dental cements. They disintegrate in oral fluids
- They are least irritating of all dental cements. It is mild irritant, pH is 6.6 to 8
- It has bacteriostatic and obtundent effect. They inhibit growth of bacteria and have an anodyne or soothing effect in pulp in deep cavities, reducing pain, if present.

Biocompatibility

- *Type I*: More hazardous because of increased acidity and slower set
- *Type II*: Elicits greater pulpal reaction than ZnOE but less than zinc phosphate cement.

Silicate Cements

- Disintegrate in oral fluids due to high solubility
- Severe irritant to pulp. Acts as standard for comparing pulpal response to other materials
- Pulp protection is done with ZnOE/Ca $(OH)_2$ or varnish
- Reduced incidence of secondary caries
- Reduced incidence of contact caries due to fluoride release.

Esthetic Properties

Amalgam

Even the properly polished silver amalgam restorations are not esthetically acceptable.

Composite Resins for Posterior Restorations

They are highly esthetic.

Glass Ionomer

Not as esthetic as composites.

Zinc Oxide Eugenol

- Inferior to silicates and composites
- 90% radiopacity
- Lack radiolucency
- Have a rough surface texture.

Silicate Cements

- They are translucent and resemble porcelain in appearance
- Initial esthetic is excellent but becomes stained over a period
- Refractive index is similar to enamel and dentin
- Surface of silicate is difficult to polish
- If the restoration is allowed to dry, the surface becomes powdery and opaque, hence contraindicated in mouth breathers.

43. Write in detail about the various cavity varnishes, liners and bases used in dentistry.

MATERIALS DEVELOPED FOR PULP PROTECTION

These include:
- Varnishes
- Calcium hydroxide cement
- Zinc oxide-based cement
- Glass ionomer cement
- Visible light-cured resins
- Glass ionomer cement resin hybrids.

CAVITY VARNISHES

Composition

Natural Gums

For example, Copals.

Resins or Synthetic Resins

Dissolved in an organic solvent like acetone, chloroforms, or ether.

Mode of Application

- Applied in two or three coatings on the cavity walls using a thin brush
- Single layer application can cause an evaporation of the solvent, which can leave voids.

Mode of Action

- They form a coating on the tooth by evaporation of the solvent
- It is painted onto the cavity and the solvent evaporates to leave a thin layer of resin, which helps to seal the ends of the dentinal tubules
- Varnish does not give adequate thermal protection in deep cavities since it forms only a thin layer.

Function

- They reduce microleakage and prevent penetration of corrosion products of amalgams into the dentinal tubules
- They do not provide insulation.

Contraindications

- They are not indicated under adhesive material like glass ionomer and composites

- Heat is liberated by filling materials while setting (e.g. light activated composites show an increase of 200–400°C for an average-sized cavity) causing injury to pulp
- Under glass-ionomer, they prevent the carboxylic groups from coming in contact with calcium of enamel and dentin
- Under composites, they interfere with the polymerization reaction and may cause softening of the resin.

CAVITY LINERS

Cavity liners are placed on the base of the cavity and on the axial dentinal wall for Class II cavities prior to the filling placement.

Requirements of Cavity Liners

These depend on:
- Depth of cavity, which determines the thickness of residual dentin between the base of the cavity and the dental pulp
- The type of filling material used to restore the tooth
- The degree of set achieved at the time the filling material is placed
- Strength of the set material and its thickness
- Type of cavity
- Pressure exerted during placement of the filling material
- Degree of support from surrounding structures
- Ideally, the lining material should be radiopaque so that they can be observed on radiographs
- The lining chosen must be compatible with the filling. Its constituents should not have any effect on setting characters or properties of filling
- If the lining is not set when amalgam condensation starts, then the material can displace due to high condensation pressures.

Functions

- Acts as a barrier between the filling material and dentin
- Should have sufficient mechanical strength to resist displacement during placement of fillings
- Liners act as thermal, chemical and electrical barriers
- It acts as a thermal insulating barrier to protect the pulp from sudden, intolerable changes in temperature, especially under a metallic filling such as amalgam. The thermal diffusivity of amalgam is about 40 times greater than that of dentin
- Lining materials are also placed to form a protective barrier against chemical irritants present in some filling materials, e.g. phosphoric acid in silicate materials
- When an amalgam restoration opposes a gold restoration, a galvanic cell forms that may accelerate corrosion and cause pain. Varnishes consisting of less polar resin, such as polystyrene may be used for electrical resistance
- Bacteria and endotoxins can be prevented from causing pulpal irritation by coating with varnish.

Other materials that can be used as liners and their functions

- Glass ionomer cement—Anticariogenic
- Zinc oxide eugenol—Obtundent/Soothening effect on pulp
- For Class I cavities, the fracture of a set cement lining is rare as it is supported on all sides by tooth substance **(Fig. 16)**
- For Class II, if the lining displaces upwards during condensing of amalgam, the thickness of the amalgam restoration decreases in that area
- For Class II, the axial wall lining is unsupported and can fracture during the condensing of amalgam; this results in an incompletely filled cavity having voids **(Fig. 17)**.

Correct technique to condense amalgam into the interproximal box. This provides support for lining of axial wall, which can then withstand forces **(Figs 18A and B)**.

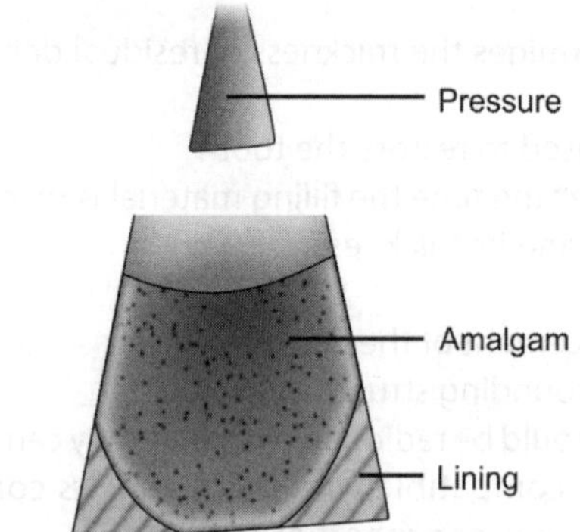

Fig. 16: Class I cavity showing set cement lining

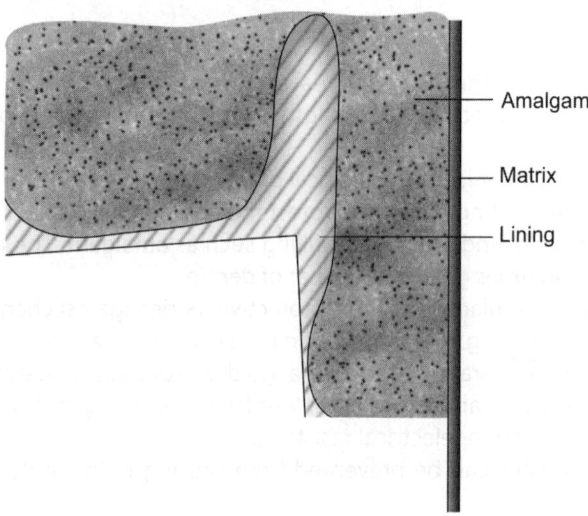

Fig. 17: Class II cavity with lining

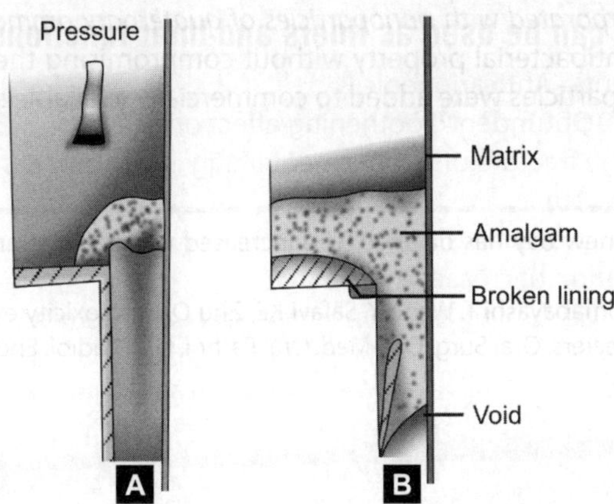

Figs 18A and B: Correct (A) and incorrect (B) condensing techniques

CAVITY BASES

- Cements when used as bases are applied in thick layer (0.75 mm) under restoration to protect the pulp against the thermal injury, galvanic shock and chemical irritation
- Bases need to be of good strength to withstand condensation forces during placement of restoration and should be able to resist fracture under masticatory stress.

Cement	Indication	Precaution
Zinc phosphate	Under amalgam restoration in normal cavities.	1. If used in deep cavities, use a cavity liner on the pulpal floor before its use. 2. In routine use, apply cavity varnish before and after placement of base.
Zinc oxide eugenol	Reinforced ZOE may be used as a base under amalgam restoration.	Not indicated under composites as eugenol interferes with the polymerization.
Zinc polycarboxylate	Can be used under amalgam restoration.	Very biocompatible; hence no varnish required prior to its placement. Varnish can be applied after base placement.
Glass ionomer	Under amalgam and composites.	When placing very close to the pulp, a liner of $Ca(OH)_2$ may be applied.

NANO BASED-ENDODONTIC SEALER

Bioceramic-based Nanomaterials (EndoSequence BC sealer)

- Composed of calcium silicate, calcium phosphate, calcium hydroxide, zirconia and a thickening agent, has been developed. Upon setting, it forms hydroxyapatite with highly alkaline pH of 12.8 providing bioactivity and antimicrobial properties[1]
- *Silicon-based sealer (Gutta-Flow Sealer)*: It is composed of gutta-percha powder and silver nanoparticles. Available in the form of unidose capsule which can be mixed and injected.[2] Advantages are that it is dimensionally stable and sets within half an hour with good sealing ability and antibacterial activity.

- *Existing sealers incorporated with nanoparticles of quaternary ammonium polyethyleneimine (QPEI)*: Increasing antibacterial property without compromising the mechanical properties. 0–2 wt% QPEI nanoparticles were added to commercially available sealers.

REFERENCES

1. Koch K, Brave D. A new day has dawned: The increased use of bioceramics in endodontics. Dent. 2009;10:39-43.
2. Zoufan K, Jiang J, Komabayashi T, Wang Y, Safavi KE, Zhu Q. Cytotoxicity evaluation of Gutta flow and endoSequence BC sealers. Oral Surg. Oral Med. Oral Pathol. Oral Radiol. Endodontol. 2011;112:657-61.

44. Classify gold alloys with their composition. Describe the various heat treatment procedures for these alloys to alter their physical properties. Add a note on white alloys with their uses.

PURE GOLD

Pure gold is soft and ductile, hence, it is alloyed with elements as copper, silver, platinum, palladium, nickel and zinc. These alloys can be used for inlays, crowns, bridges and partial dentures.

CLASSIFICATION OF GOLD ALLOYS

Depending on the Application

Type I Alloys

For inlays in low stress situations. These alloys are highly ductile and can be burnished easily. They are less fracture prone.

Type II Alloys

For most inlays. Inlays with thin sections should be avoided as deformation can occur.

Type III Alloys

Used for all inlays, onlays, full coverage crowns and short-span bridges, cast posts and cores because of their greater strength. They are difficult to burnish and can fracture when compared to Types II and I.

Type IV alloys

Used for cast posts, cores, long-span bridges, in partial denture construction and clasp arms. The low elastic modulus and high yield strength of the gold alloy provide a high degree of flexibility to clasp arms.

Depending on the Content of Gold

- High gold alloys
- Medium gold alloys
- Low gold alloys.
- The carat is expressed as the number of 24th part of gold in the alloy: 24-carat gold is pure gold, 18-carat gold contains 75% gold
- The fineness rating is the parts per thousand of gold; 24 carat gold is 1000 fine and 18 carat gold is 750 fine.

High-gold Alloys

The gold content must not be less than 75%. The noble metal content is gold, silver, platinum and palladium.

Composition of high gold alloys

Silver	Strengthens the alloy and counteracts the reddish tint of the copper.
Copper	Imparts strength, particularly of the Types III and IV gold alloys and reduces the melting temperature. Maximum is 16%, amounts above this can cause the alloy to tarnish.
Platinum	Increases both the strength and the melting temperature.
Palladium	Its effects are the same as that for platinum, but are cheaper.
Zinc	Acts as a scavenger during casting, preventing oxidation and improves the castability.
Trace elements	Indium and ruthenium (<0.5%) may be present. These have very high melting temperature and act as nucleating sites during solidification, thus helping to produce a fine grain size.

Medium-gold Alloys

- Medium-gold alloys, with the gold content varying from 40–60%
- These medium gold alloys were introduced in the early 1970s
- The palladium and silver contents were increased to compensate for the reduced gold content, while the copper content is in the range of 10–15%
- Palladium is added to counteract the tendency of silver to tarnish
- Palladium, silver and copper readily form substitutional solid solutions, with the gold producing a single-phase structure throughout the entire compositional range. Copper in the alloy causes order hardening, just as with the Types III and IV gold alloys.

Low-gold Alloys

Gold	15–20%
Silver	40–60%
Palladium	up to 40%

- Due to the reduced gold content, these alloys are white in appearance
- For better esthetics, copper-free, low-gold alloys with high levels of indium can be used. These have a two-phase structure, one consisting of an FCC matrix and the other a BCC phase due to the high indium content
- The matrix phase is essentially an Ag-Au solid solution with minor additions of palladium, indium and zinc. The BCC phase consists of Pd-In with substantial amounts of gold, silver and zinc, giving the alloy its yellow color.

HEAT TREATMENT

Heat treatment increases yield strength of the gold alloy by forming a solid solution, the addition of copper in what is known as **order hardening**.

Stage 1

The alloy is usually quenched after casting.

Stage 2

- Homogenization is carried out since coring occurs with alloys containing platinum. The alloy is heated to 700°C for 10 minutes, then quenched
- The alloy is reheated to 400°C and holding it at that temperature for approximately 30 minutes. This allows the copper atoms to arrange themselves in little ordered clusters
- This ordered structure prevents slippage of the atomic layers, which has the effect of raising the yield stress and the hardness of the alloy
- There must be at least 11% copper in the gold alloy for order hardening to occur, so it cannot occur in Type I and Type II gold alloys
- The addition of copper, combined with the hardening heat treatment can result in a tenfold increase in the yield strength
- Hardening heat treatment causes a reduction in the ductility of the alloy. Excessive bending may give rise to brittle fracture. The heat treated alloy can be benched cool or quenched immediately on casting. This technique is commonly known as self-hardening.

Stage 3

If any cold working is done to the alloy, for example, adjustment of clasps, a stress relief anneal is carried out.

Stage 4

Heat hardening is achieved by heating and maintaining the alloy at an elevated temperature for a sufficient time for diffusion of atoms to occur, to permit order and precipitation hardening.

This is achieved by one of the following:

- Cooling the alloy slowly from 700°C

- Cooling the alloy from 450 to 250°C over 30 minutes, followed by quenching
- Maintaining the alloy at between 350°C and 450°C for around 15 minutes, followed by quenching.
  The effects of this heat treatment on the mechanical properties of these alloys are improved.

WHITE GOLD ALLOYS

Silver-palladium Alloy

Composition

- Silver
- Palladium (at least 5%)
- Gold
- Copper
- Indium
- Zinc.

Function of Components

- The palladium improves the resistance to corrosion and helps to prevent tarnish
- These alloys were introduced in the 1960s as an alternative to the high-gold alloys and are commonly called 'white golds'
- The properties are generally inferior when compared to a carefully controlled hardening heat treatment.

Disadvantage

They are difficult to cast than gold alloys, owing to their density and to the dissolution of oxygen by molten alloys, resulting in porosity in castings.

Other alloys are:

- Copper (brass) with indium and nickel
- Silver-indium with palladium
- Aluminum-bronze.

Applications

- Low stress-bearing inlays
- Used for crowns, short-span bridges and post and cores
- This may be associated with the high casting temperatures for these alloys which is the second most notable feature of these materials.

Disadvantages

- Alloys have a tendency to work harden rapidly, which precludes excessive adjustment and any burnishing
- Although they are highly biocompatible, tarnishing does occur with these alloys.

45. Compare and contrast the general properties of Co-Cr-Mo with a Type-IV dental casting gold alloy. Make particular reference to composition, strength and rigidity. What are the ideal requirements of these alloys used in dentistry?

Comparison with Gold Alloys

- The proportional limit of cobalt-chromium alloys is less than that of the hardened gold alloys
- The ultimate tensile strength of cobalt-chromium alloys is slightly lower than that of Type IV gold alloys
- The cobalt-chromium alloys have a modulus of elasticity about twice that of gold alloys. Hence, sections of cobalt-chromium alloys of about half the thickness of gold alloys can be used to achieve the same degree of rigidity
- The cobalt-chromium alloys are more brittle (lower percentage elongation) than Type IV gold alloys
- Cobalt-chromium alloys have higher melting range and greater hardness than Type IV gold alloys
- The casting shrinkage of cobalt-chromium alloys is greater than that of the gold-containing materials but the investment materials used for base metal alloys compensate for this contraction. For gold alloys—Gypsum-bonded investment and for base-metals—Phosphate-bonded investments.
- The density of cobalt-chromium is about half that of gold. Hence, lighter dentures can be made with Co-Cr.

Composition and Ingredient Functions

Composition

Cobalt	55–65%
Chromium	30%
Molybdenum	4–5%
In some cases, titanium	5%

Functions of Ingredients

- The cobalt and chromium form a solid solution for up to 30% chromium, which is the limit of solubility of chromium in cobalt
- If chromium content is more, the corrosion resistance of the alloy is better. Hence, the amount of chromium is increased avoiding the brittle second phase
- Molybdenum is a grain refiner, which provides more sites for crystal nucleation during solidification. It also produces a hardening effect
- Carbon increases the strength and hardness of the alloy

- Excess carbon can cause brittleness
- Nickel allergic patients can use nickel-free Co-Cr alloys. The mechanical grinding and polishing process cause the release of beryllium, which is a known carcinogen.

IDEAL REQUIREMENTS OF CASTING ALLOYS

- Should be nonallergenic and should not contain toxic components during grinding and polishing procedures and in oral environment
- Should possess good corrosion and tarnish resistance
- Should have adequate yield stress to withstand large forces in situ
- Should be ductile enough to be burnished
- Should possess adequate strength and hardness
- Should have adequate density and good fluidity when molten, hence easy to cast
- Should not be expensive in terms of material and labor costs.

46. Discuss the materials (alloy, resin cement) which may be used in resin-bonded bridge restoration. What are the various special pretreatments of the enamel and alloy contact surfaces required before bonding?

RESIN-BONDED BRIDGES

Definition

- Resin-bonded bridges are fixed partial dentures, which are cemented onto the abutments using special resins
- First described by Rochette in 1973 (Mandibular anterior teeth).

Classification

- Rochette Bridge
- Maryland Bridge
- Virginia Bridge
- Cast mesh fixed partial dentures.

Rochette Bridge (1973)

- Has a wing-like retainer with six perforations to provide mechanical undercuts for resin cement **(Fig. 19)**

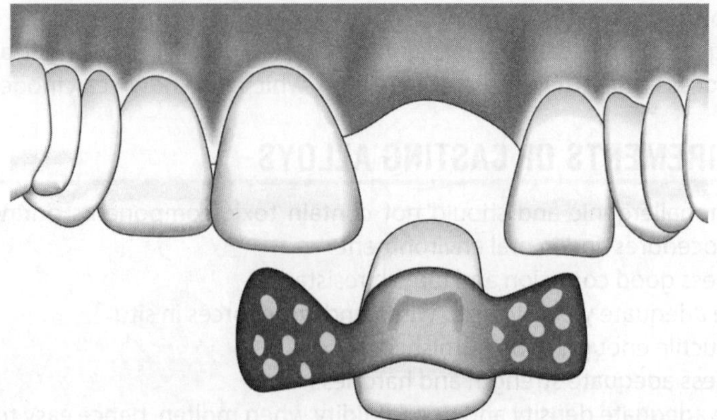

Fig. 19: Rochette bridge

- Etched retainers are coated with pyrolized silane and bonded with resin cements.

Design

- Has six perforations on metal castings, bonded with cold-cure acrylic resin
- Used to splint mobile lower incisors. Later one of the incisors was extracted and a pontic was attached to the splint.

Disadvantages

The composite resin used to lute the restoration failed and the attachment weakened over a period of time.

Variation

Nonperforated retainers can be used.

Maryland Bridges

(Livaditis and Thompson from University of Maryland School of Dentistry)

- A nonperforated retainer was etched for mechanical retention to form microporosities and was bonded by resin cement **(Fig. 20)**
- In 1980s, the metal used as wings on the abutment teeth was electro-etched
- Electro-etching provided for strong luting with composite luting resins
- It bonds the entire area of the retainer to the etched enamel and protects the underlying resin.

Modified Design

The wings resting on the abutments were roughened and treated to form an oxidized layer so that chemically adhesive composite luting resins adhere chemically and mechanically to the retainer surfaces.

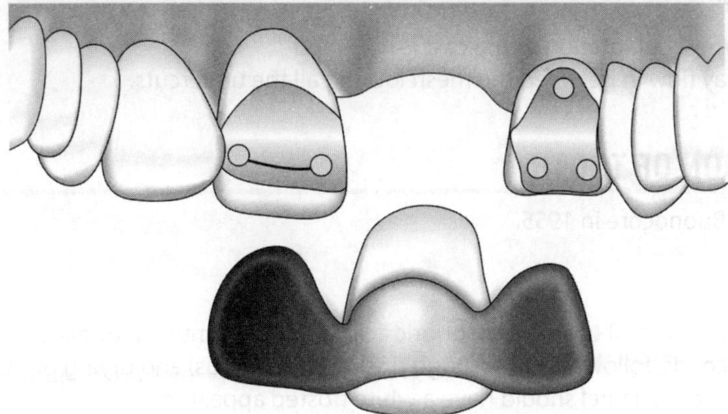

Fig. 20: Maryland bridge

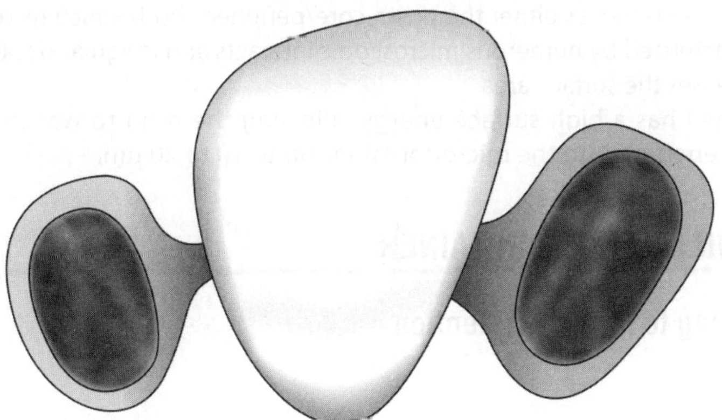

Fig. 21: Cast mesh fixed partial denture

Advantages

- Minimal enamel preparation does not require local anesthetics
- Conservative tooth preparation
- Less chances of pulpal irritation.

Disadvantages

- High debonding rate for the retainers
- Color changes as metal retainers can be seen through (overcome to some degree by using opaque composite luting resins).

Cast Mesh Fixed Partial Denture

A nylon mesh is placed on the tissue surface of the retainer wax pattern before fabricating the wax pattern **(Fig. 21)**.

Disadvantages

- The nylon mesh adaptation to the cast is not good
- The wax may flow in between the mesh locking all the undercuts.

PREPARATION OF TOOTH

Developed by Buonocore in 1955.

Procedure

- A solution or gel of 30 to 50% phosphoric acid (37%—optimum) is applied to the enamel for 15 to 30 seconds, followed by thorough rinsing (15 seconds) and drying of that area
- After drying, the enamel should have a white frosted appearance.

Mode of Action

- The acid solution removes either the prism core/periphery/both which results in an enamel surface characterized by numerous microscopic interacts and irregular peaks
- Etching increases the surface area
- Etched enamel has a high surface energy, allowing the resin to wet the tooth surface better and penetrate into the microporosities up to 10 to 20 μm.

PREPARATION OF METAL RETAINER

Types of Bonding to Provide Retention

- Mechanical
- Chemical.

Mechanical Bonding

Macroscopic Retention

By mechanical locks as in Rochette's (six perforations in metal), mesh and water-soluble salt crystal.

Microscopic Retention

By electrolytic etching (Maryland Bridge).

Chemical Bonding

Chemical Bonding of Resin

Chemical etching
Tin-plating.

Mechanical Etching Techniques

Electrochemical Etching

Results in microscopic porosity.

Non-Beryllium nickel chromium alloys

- Retainer is immersed in 35% nitric acid under a current of 250 milliamps per square centimeter for 5 minutes
- Retainer is cleaned by immersing in 18% HCl in an ultrasonic cleaner for 10 minutes.

Beryllium containing nickel chromium alloys

- Retainer is immersed in 10% H_2SO_4 under a current of 300 milliamps per square centimeter
- Retainer is cleaned by immersing in 18% HCl in an ultrasonic cleaner for 10 minutes.

Another technique (McLaughlin technique)

- Retainer is etched with a mixture of HCl and H_2SO_4 in a beaker
- The beaker with the retainer is directly placed in an ultrasonic cleanser for 99 seconds under an electrical field.

Nonelectrochemical

Roughening by aluminum oxide-air abrasion.

Chemical Bonding of Resin

Chemical Etching

A gel consisting of nitric and hydrochloric acids is applied to the internal surface of the metal framework for approximately 25 minutes.

Tin-plating

Precious alloys can be plated with tin and used as retainers to increase adhesiveness of resins, thereby increasing bond strengths.

ALLOYS USED

Ni-Cr or Co-Cr alloys.

RESIN LUTING AGENTS USED

The composite luting resins, chemically cured systems with less filler content to ensure a low film thickness.

RECENT ADVANCES IN MATERIALS FOR RESIN BONDED BRIDGES

- *All ceramic resin bonded fixed dental prosthesis*: It was introduced in 1990s and also by then the double retainer concept was replaced slowly by single retainer concept due to multiple retainer failures[1]
- Glass infiltrated alumina ceramic was first used as double retainer this caused fracture between the connector area and hence in 1997 a single retainer was introduced[2]

- *Lithium disilicate resin bridges*: Monolithic lithium disilicate resin bonded bridges was strong and can be fabricated by milling or pressing. Clinical trials have shown no chipping or fracture after three year follow up by Dr. Dennis Fasbinder[3]
- Layered lithium disilicate can be used for anterior segments for better esthetics (Utilizing lithium disilicate as a core and then layering porcelain onto the facial and occlusal surfaces).

REFERENCES

1. MJ. Shaw, WM. Tay Clinical performance of resin-bonded cast metal bridges (Rochette bridges). A preliminary report. Br Dent J. 1982;152(11):378-80.
2. Kern M, Glaser R. Cantilevered all-ceramic, resin-bonded fixed... 1997]. Bassett JL. Pract Periodontics Aesthet Dent. 1997;9(4):455-61; quiz 462.
3. Ritter RG, Rego NA. Material considerations for using lithium disilicate as a thin veneer option. J Cosmet Dent. 2009;25(3):111-7.

47. Describe in detail the various materials used for implants.

MATERIALS

- Metals
- Stainless steel
- Cobalt-Chromium-Molybdenum Alloy
- Titanium and Titanium-Aluminum-Vanadium alloy
- Metals with surface coatings
- Ceramics
- Polymers and composites
- Gold, palladium, tantalum and platinum.

METALS

- Metals and alloys such as stainless steel and a cobalt-chromium alloy are used for dental implants
- These materials have good physical properties, good corrosion resistance and biocompatibility
- Common materials used for implants presently are pure titanium or titanium alloys. These materials are highly biocompatible.

Stainless Steel

Composition (Surgical Austenitic Steel)

Iron-carbon	0.05%	Alloy
Chromium	18%	Aids in corrosion resistance
Nickel	8%	Stabilizes the austenitic structure

- These alloys can be used as wrought or heat-treated
- They possess high strength and ductility, hence are resistant to brittle fracture.

Disadvantages

- Subject to pitting corrosion (If the surface oxide is retained, corrosion is prevented).
- A noble or base metal alloy, when in constant contact with a stainless steel implant, can cause galvanic circuit.

Cobalt-Chromium-Molybdenum Alloy

Composition

Cobalt	63%
Chromium	30%
Molybdenum	5%
Carbon, manganese and nickel	Traces

The molybdenum serves to stabilize the structure and carbon acts as a hardener.

Properties

- Have good resistance to corrosion and a high modulus
- Less ductility
- Excellent biocompatibility
- Low cost and long-term clinical success, both stainless steel and cobalt-chromium alloys have been used extensively
- Used as cast or cast-and-annealed and, hence, fabrication of custom designs is possible, as in subperiosteal frames.

Titanium and Titanium-Aluminum-Vanadium Alloy

Commercially Pure Titanium (cpTi)

- Titanium is a highly reactive metal which oxidizes (passivates) on contact with air or normal tissue fluids
- Passivation makes it highly biocompatible
- An oxide layer 10A thick is formed on the cut surface of pure titanium within a millisecond
- Titanium can also be passivated by placing in a bath of nitric acid.

Composition of pure titanium

- *Oxygen*: (0.5% maximum)
- *Nitrogen, carbon and hydrogen*: Minor traces.

Composition of Titanium Alloy

- *Titanium*: 90 wt%
- *Aluminum*: 6 wt%
- *Vanadium*: 4 wt%

Properties

- Titanium has a density of approximately 4.5 g/cm^3, which is 40% lighter than steel
- Possesses a high strength—weight ratio
- Titanium has a modulus of elasticity 5 to 10 times higher than that of bone, and one-half that of stainless steel or cobalt-chromium alloys
- The mechanical properties of the titanium alloy are better than pure titanium
- Titanium is biologically a compatible metal with high corrosion resistance
- Titanium oxide surface releases titanium ions at a low rate into blood and saliva
- The compatibility depends on the composition, the fabrication and preparation of the implant surface
- The high dielectric properties of titanium oxide make it more biocompatible as the surface becomes more reactive to biomolecules.

Metal with Surface Coatings

Surface Coatings

- Plasma spray
- Coating of calcium phosphate ceramic
- Coating the implant with tricalcium phosphate or hydroxyapatite.

Significance

- Calcium and phosphorus form a bioactive surface that promotes bone growth and induces a direct bond between the implant and the hard tissue *(Bioactive materials are inorganic materials that develop an adherent, bonded interface with bone).*
- Spraying on titanium alloy increases the ductility and tensile strength of metal substructure
- The coating on implants and its durability depends on the ceramic-metal bond during function, as well as the characteristics and uniformity of the coating
- A plasma-sprayed surface provides a rough surface for bone ingrowth to ensure anchorage in the jaw
- Sprayed implants can be either screw-shaped or nonthreaded cylinders.

Ceramics

- They are brittle and susceptible to flexural fracture
- They have excellent biocompatibility and inert behavior
- They do not actively participate in the process of bone deposition.

Types

- Bioactive—Hydroxyapatite, bioglass
- Non reactive ceramics—which include alumina and sapphire.

Bioactive Ceramics

Are ceramics or glasses that are rich in calcium and phosphate.

Hydroxyapatite

- $(Ca_{10}(PO_4)_6(OH)_2)$
- Similar to that of bone and teeth
- Used for augmenting alveolar ridges or filling bony defects.

Availability

- As a block or granular form
- The material can be synthesized as dense or porous form
- The porous forms have porosity of 100 to 300 µm in size, which is adequate for bone in growth.

Disadvantages

- Granular form is difficult to keep it localized at the site of implantation
- Can be used only in areas of very-low-stress applications, as its strength and ductility are low
- Newer materials as hydroxyapatite as a coating for titanium substructures utilises strength of titanium and bioactivity of hydroxyapatite.

Bioglass

- Is a bioactive dense ceramic material
- (CaO, Na_2O, P_2O_5 and SiO_2).

Mechanism of bone formation

- When pH in the region of implant changes, the Bioglass surface releases sodium, calcium and phosphate ions into local tissue. The Bioglass is replaced by hydrogen ions from the local tissue fluids
- At the surface, a silica-rich gel forms
- After some time, the calcium and phosphate ions migrate to the silica gel surface from within both the Bioglass and the tissue fluids, to form a calcium-phosphorus layer
- When the concentration of phosphorus increases, the osteoblasts begin to proliferate, producing collagen fibrils that are anchored by the calcium-phosphorus crystals
- This strong bonding layer has been shown to be 100 to 200 A thick
- The bond is so strong that when tested to failure, fracture occurs within the bone or Bioglass material, leaving the interface intact.

Nonreactive Ceramics

Aluminum oxide (Al_2O_3)

- Is a nonreactive ceramic implant material, made from aluminum oxide (Al_2O_3), either as a polycrystalline form or as a single crystal (sapphire)
- It is biocompatible but not bioactive (as it does not promote the formation of bone).

Polymers and Composites

Availability

Porous and solid forms for tissue attachment and replacement augmentation and as coatings for force transfer to soft and hard tissues.

Uses

Used principally for internal force distribution as connectors for osseointegrated implants.

Other Implant Materials

- Were made of gold, palladium, tantalum, platinum and alloys of these metals
- More recently, zirconium and tungsten have been evaluated.

Advances in Implant Biomaterials

1. *Biomodification of titanium implant*: This is done by coating calcium and phosphate-based materials by various techniques such as plasma spraying, laser, etc.
   Advantages: High biocompatibility and osteoconduction. For example, hydroxyapatite (HA) coated metallic implants.
   Disadvantage: Delamination or dissolution of coating. But laser (Nd: YAG)/ablative coating technique increased hardness, corrosion resistance, and had thicker oxide layer.
   Sputter deposition especially radiofrequency magnetron sputtering aids in achieving deposition of thin films of calcium phosphate coatings on titanium implants. Various studies proved these coatings to be more retentive.[1]
   Antibiotic coatings: Gentamycin along with the layer of HA can be coated onto the implant surface. Tetracycline-HCl treatment decontaminates and detoxifies implant surfaces. It inhibits collagenase activity, increases cell proliferation and bone healing.
2. *Ceramic biomaterials*: Bioinert ceramics oxide, ceramic coatings on metals possess high biocompatibility but studies show poor survival rates and hence not very commonly used. Recently zirconium dioxide [Yttrium Stabilized Tetragonal Zirconium Polycrystal (Y-TZP)].
   Advantages of zirconia: Good strength and toughness, stability highly esthetic as ivory in color. Accumulates less plaque than titanium. Studies showed good bone to implant contact area less bleeding on probing with zirconia implants compared to titanium.[2]
3. *Calcium phosphate materials* (CaPs), such as TCP (tricalcium phosphate), glass ceramics, hydroxyapatite can be coated with biomimetic growth factors, BMPs, osteogenic drugs which is observed to increase osteoconductivity.[3]
4. *Carbon and carbon silicone compounds*: In vitro study has shown better cell attachment on carbon-coated zirconia than uncoated disc.[4]
5. *Synthetic biomaterials*: Biodegradable polymers such as Polyvinyl alcohol, polylactides cyanoacrylates forms have been combined with biodegradable CaPO4 eg IMZ implants have a polymethylene intramobile element .
6. *Nanostructured ceramic materials like polymer nanocomposites (PNC)*: This is at research level now.
7. *Other nano-coated materials*: Nano-coating of HA-CaP crystals applied to the surface of the implant. Another type of pico meter thin TiO_2 coating improves the bioreactivity of microrough implant surfaces.

REFERENCES

1. McCafferty MM, Burke GA, Meenan BJ. Mesenchymal stem cell response to conformal sputter deposited calcium phosphate thin films on nanostructured titanium surfaces. J Biomed Mater Res A 2013 Nov 1. doi: 10.1002/jbm.a.35018. [Epub ahead of print].
2. Van Brakel R, Cune MS, van Winkelhoff AJ, de Putter C, Verhoeven JW, van der Reijden W. Early bacterial colonization and soft tissue health around zirconia and titanium abutments: An In vivo study in man. Clin Oral Impl Res. 2011;22:571-7.
3. Liu Y, Huse RO, de Groot K, Buser D, Hunziker EB. Delivery mode and efficacy of BMP-2 in association with implants. J Dent Res. 2007;86:84-9.
4. Kou W, Akasaka T, Watari F, Sjögren G. An in vitro evaluation of the biological effects of carbon nanotube-coated dental zirconia. ISRN Dent 2013 August 20;2013:296727. doi: 10.1155/2013/296727.

Short Notes

1. American Dental Association Acceptance Program.

- The American Dental Association (ADA) on dental materials and devices was established in 1966 and is presently known as the Council on Scientific Affairs
- Till 1965, National Institute of Standards and Technology (NIST) was formulating standards/ specifications for dental materials.

ROLE OF AMERICAN DENTAL ASSOCIATION

- American Dental Association (ADA) measures the physical and chemical properties of dental materials, helps in development of new materials, instruments and test methods
- It also evaluates the development and certification of products certified by ADA.

SIGNIFICANCE OF AMERICAN DENTAL ASSOCIATION

- The ADA Council operates under the direction of the American National Standards Institute
- All products are to maintain regulations
- ADA specifies and standardizes the quality and properties of particular dental materials
- The specifications laid out for each material by the Acceptance Program of the Council are evaluated by ADA and are tested for these specification requirements
- When a product satisfies the ADA specifications, the manufacturer can label the product as 'ADA Accepted'
- The Council on Scientific Affairs evaluates drugs and therapeutic agents and dental X-ray film used in dentistry
- Once a specification has been approved by the ASC MD156, it is submitted to the American National Standards Institute. On acceptance, the Council on Scientific Affairs accepts the ADA specification
- New specifications are continually being developed to apply to new program areas
- Existing specifications are periodically revised to incorporate changes in product formulations
- Each material is specified by a specification number as the ADA Specification
- *Example:* No. 1 for dental amalgam.

OTHER IMPORTANT COUNCILS

Bureau of Standards

- It is now known as the National Institute of Standards and Technology (NIST)
- It was set-up for the evaluation and selection of dental amalgams under the leadership of Wilmer Souder in 1920 and later it was supported by the Weinstein Research Laboratories

- In 1928, the Dental Research Fellowship at the National Bureau of Standards was assumed by the American Dental Association (ADA)
- Wilmer Souder, George C Paffenbarger and William T Sweeney were the pioneer researchers.

Federal Regulations and Standards

- On May 28, 1976, legislation was signed into law that gave the US Food and Drug Administration (FDA) the authority to protect the public from hazardous or ineffective medical (and dental) devices
- This newer legislation, named the Medical Device Amendments of 1976, requires that all medical and dental devices be classified and regulated, that are intended for human use.

ACCORDING TO THE FEDERAL REGISTER

Device

It is any instrument, apparatus, implement, machine, contrivance, implant, or in vitro reagent used in the diagnosis, cure, mitigation, treatment, or prevention of disease in man and which does not achieve any of its principal intended purposes through chemical action within or on the body, of man or other animals and which is not dependent upon being metabolized for the achievement of any of its principal intended purposes.

The Dental Products Panel identifies devices into one of the three classification groups based on relative risk factors.

Class I

Devices are considered to be of low risk, but they need to have the registration of the manufacturer's products and record-keeping requirements.

Class II

- When risk factors are involved, the device is placed into this class
- Class II products require to meet performance standards established by the FDA or CE mark of conformity.

2. Adhesion and Bonding.

ADHESION

Definition

When unlike molecules are attracted to each other or brought into intimate contact, it is called adhesion.

Adhesive

It is the material or film added to produce the adhesion.

Adherend

It is the material to which it is applied.

Example: The retention of artificial dentures—due to adhesion between the denture and saliva and between the saliva and soft tissue.

FACTORS IN ADHESION

Surface Energy

The increase in energy per unit area of surface is referred to as the surface energy or surface tension.

Factors Affecting Surface Energy

- The outer surface of solid has greater energy (atoms have unequal attraction) than its inner surface. The greater the surface energy, the greater is the capacity for adhesion
- The atoms in solids form bonds to other atoms that are in close proximity and reduce the surface energy of the solid. This attraction across the interface between unlike molecules is called adhesion
- Surface impurities (as adsorbed gas or an oxide) reduce surface energy and adhesion.

Wetting

- It is a phenomenon in which the liquid must flow easily over the entire surface and adhere to the solid
- When two polished glass plates are placed one on top of the other and pressed together with a film placed between the two plates, water molecules are attracted to the glass plate
- The attraction is less when the surface molecules of the attracting substances are separated by distances greater than 0.7 nm.

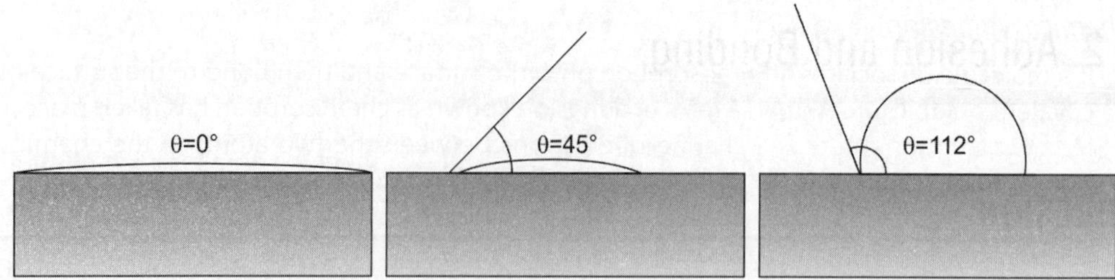

Fig. 22: Contact angle of wetting

Factors Affecting Wetting

- Impurities on the surface of the solid
- An oxide film on a metallic surface
- The surface energy of some substances is so low that few, if any, liquids wet their surfaces
- Close packing of the structural organic groups and the presence of halogens may prevent wetting. Teflon (polytetrafluoroethylene), a commercial synthetic resin, prevents the adhesion of films to its surface
- It is the angle formed when the adhesive wets the surface of an adherent
- The contact angle is the angle formed by the adhesive with the adherent at their interface
- If the wetting is complete, the liquid adhesive will spread completely over the surface of the solid and no angle ($\theta = 0°$) will be formed **(Fig. 22)**.

TYPES OF ADHESION

- Mechanical
- Physical
- Chemical
- Combination of all the above.

Mechanical Adhesion

It is caused by penetration of the adhesive into microscopic or submicroscopic irregularities.

Example: Composite with bonding agent on tooth after etching. The acid produces minute pores in the enamel surface into which the resin flows.

Physical and Chemical Adhesion

Physical and chemical adhesion involve a molecular attraction between the adhesive and the substrate, whereas mechanical adhesion does not require molecular interaction at the interface.

Physical Adhesion

- When two surfaces are in close proximity, secondary forces of attraction arise through dipole-dipole interactions between polar molecules
- This is a weaker bond than ionic or covalent bonds
- This type of bonding is rapid with no activation energy and is reversible as there is no chemical bonding
- Physical adsorption fails when thermal energy is applied.

Chemical Adhesion

- If a molecule dissociates after adsorption onto the surface and then bond to the surface by covalent or ionic forces, then a form of adhesion known as chemisorption has taken place
- In chemisorption, there is a sharing of electrons between the two atoms in the chemical bond
- *Example:* Formation of covalent bonds, in the bonding of reactive isocyanates to polymeric surfaces containing hydroxyl and amino groups.

TYPES OF BONDS

Primary Bonds

If adhesion is by primary bonding, it is termed chemisorption and the bond is *intramolecular*. Chemisorption is limited to the mono-layer of adhesive present on the adherend.

Secondary Bonds

If adhesion is by secondary or Van der Waal's forces, it is weak and is *intermolecular*.

Bond Strength

The strength of the adhesive bond depends on:

- Stress concentrations in the adhesive or at the interface weaken the bond
- The adhesive must be a thin film thickness, greater thickness of adhesive causes shrinkage during setting process, resulting in debonding.

Bond strength is increased by:

Adhesion promoters

- These are the bonding agents which help to wet the two surfaces in contact to form stronger bonds. Examples are bonding of glass filler particles and resin in composite resin
- Adhesion promoters act as intermediary substance that aids in bonding both of the materials in question
- Primers modify the characteristics of the surface of one or the two materials so that a bond can be created.

Coupling agents

- The surface of glass is ionic in nature and can adsorb water, forming a bonded surface layer
- If a coupling agent is applied to the glass, the bonded water layer will be displaced
- Hence, the function of a coupling agent is to displace the adsorbed water and provide a strong chemical bond between the oxide groups on the glass surface and the polymer molecules of the resin.

3. Color, Color Perception, Color Matching and Bezold-Brücke Effect.

COLOR

Color is an individual perception which is subjective, nonquantifiable and time-dependent.

PRIMARY COLORS

- Red
- Green
- Blue.

SECONDARY COLORS

The secondary additive colors are associated with pairs of receptors being stimulated.

- Cyan
- Magenta
- Yellow.

COLOR PERCEPTION

Young-Helmholtz Theory of Color Vision

Proposes that the mechanism of color perception is the stimulation by visible light of certain type of receptors in the fovea.

Receptors

Three types of spectral sensitivity are as follows:

1. 460 nm (blue)
2. 530 nm (green)
3. 580 nm (red).

   Color perception is due to the stimulation of these receptors, in varying proportions.

   The chromatic stimulus is measured in terms of the wavelength and intensity of visible light.

FACTORS AFFECTING VISION

- The intensity of light
- The source of light
- Color blindness.

Process in Color Perception

Subtractive

It is a process in which the illuminated object may remove, or *subtract*, certain wavelengths depending on relative intensities of the emitted and absorbed light.

Diffuse reflection

It is a true selective absorption of the incident light.

Specular reflection

It is a reflection occurring from a polished surface.

Achromatic

- Achromatic colors are black, white and gray
- These colors help to grade the saturation (chroma) and luminosity (value) of color perception
- Partial absorption and reflection over the complete visible range result in the grays.

COLOR MATCHING

Color matching is the comparison of color perceptions to match the restorative materials to tooth material in a suitable chromatic environment by an individual of normal color vision.

Factors in Color Matching

- The patient should be instructed not to wear chromatic clothing (ideally black, gray or white shirt, blouse, etc). Lip make-up should be absent
- An achromatic, ideally black, rubber dam to mask the gingiva and adjacent teeth and use an achromatic apron to mask any colored clothing on the patient. The reference tooth should be kept moist with water during the comparison
- A first comparison should be made in daylight and second under a diffused dental operating light (quartz halogen)
- The shade guide and tooth should not reflect onto each other, the shade guide should not be held too close
- If the shade guide is presented with tooth anatomy, compare the middle third of the guide with the corresponding section of the tooth
- The comparison should be made as quickly as possible
- If a convenient source of UV-light is available (e.g. a low-pressure mercury discharge tube)
- Dentition should be viewed in daylight, fluorescent light and incandescent light sources (such as the sun, tungsten filaments, etc.).

Color Temperature

The color of a visible light source may be described as a color temperature (in Kelvin)–the temperature to which a perfect radiator would have to be heated to emit light of the spectral distribution.

Daylight sun	5,000–20,000K
Dental operating light (quartz halogen) tungsten filament	3,600–6,500K
Fluorescent daylight tubes	4,800K
Incandescent bulb (100 w) tungsten filament	2,800K

Daylight

- An intense blue summer sky will contain a greater UV component
- As the tooth material is fluorescent, a color match will need to be done in daylight, especially when the UV-component is present.

Color Reference

Shade Guides

- For example, the Vita Lumin^{TM} Vacuum Shade Guide
- It relates to dental porcelain and comprises 16 specimens divided into 4 groups
- Each group is based on the hue Y (yellow) and, within each group, the specimens are ordered in terms of decreasing value and increasing chroma.

Color Atlas

- As the Munsell color system
- Shade selection is difficult as ranges of shades are difficult to obtain from shade guide
- Spectrophotometric analysis of commercial shade guides shows the absence of large regions of hue, value and chroma when compared with the color space determined from measurements of human teeth.

BEZOLD-BRÜCKE EFFECT

When the light is dim, the rods of the human eye are more dominant than the cones and color reception is lost. When the brightness becomes too intense, color appears to change.

4. Metamerism and Fluorescence.

METAMERISM

Objects that appear to be color matched under one type of light may appear different under another light source. This phenomenon is called *metamerism*.

Points to Check in Color Matching

- Color matching should be done under two or more different light sources
- Daylight, incandescent and fluorescent lamps are common sources of light that have different spectral distributions
- Because of the trichromatic nature of color vision, the same color perception may result from different combinations of these three stimuli.

FLUORESCENCE

- Natural tooth structure absorbs light at wavelengths between 300 and 400 nm referred to as *near-ultraviolet radiation*
- These wavelengths are present in natural sunlight, photoflash lamps and in decorative lighting
- The energy that the tooth absorbs is converted into light with longer wavelengths, in which case the tooth actually becomes a light source. This phenomenon is called *fluorescence*
- Fluorescence contributes to the brightness and vital appearance of a human tooth.

Importance

Natural teeth look white under a fluorescent light, but some crowns, bridges or fillings look dark next to the fluorescing natural tooth. Hence, it is important to color match under different light sources.

OPACITY

- Opaque material is one that does not transmit light, but instead absorbs light or reflects or scatters from the surface
- The color of the object will depend on which wavelengths of light are reflected and which are absorbed.

Translucent Material

Allows some light to pass through it, absorbs some of the remainder and scatters and reflects the rest from its surface. An object viewed through such a material will have a distorted appearance.

Transparent Material

Allows the passage of light in such a way that little distortion takes place, meaning thereby that an object can be seen quite clearly through it.

5. Three Dimensions of Color.

COLOR

- Light is a mixture of different wavelengths which combine to produce a distinctive color
- The eye is most sensitive to light in the green-yellow range and is least sensitive at the reds and blues
- The cone-shaped cells switch off when exposed to excessive light of a given wavelength.

The color of an object depends on physical factors as:

- Materials appear different when viewed under different light sources. The color of the surroundings alter the light source
- Objects which reflect light appear white, as it reflects all colors. If it is black, it absorbs all colors. If it is colored, that color is reflected and all others are absorbed by the material
- A translucent material appears lighter in color than an opaque object
- A substance which appears to have a high gloss reflects a large amount of light at the surface
- Fluorescence is defined as the ability to absorb the light of one wavelength and emit light of a different wavelength or color
- For example, natural teeth absorb ultraviolet radiation (400 nm wavelength) and emit light of 400-450 nm wavelength.

THREE DIMENSIONS (3D) OF COLOR

- The three dimensions of color by measurement are *hue, value* and *chroma* according to Munsell terminology
- Hue can be seen as pure color while value and chroma depend on addition of black and white in varying proportions.

Hue

- Describes the dominant color of an object, (as red, green or blue) and refers to the dominant wavelengths present in the spectral distribution
- In the Munsell system, a *hue* is referenced by a number from 1 to 5 and a letter (single or multiple) combination
- The possible colors are violet, indigo, blue, green, yellow, orange and red
- The three primary colors, from which all other colors are produced, are red, green and blue.

Value

- Value is the lightness or darkness of a color, which can be measured independently of the hue
- In Munsell system, it increases toward the top (whiter) and decreases toward the bottom (darker or more black) **(Fig. 23)**

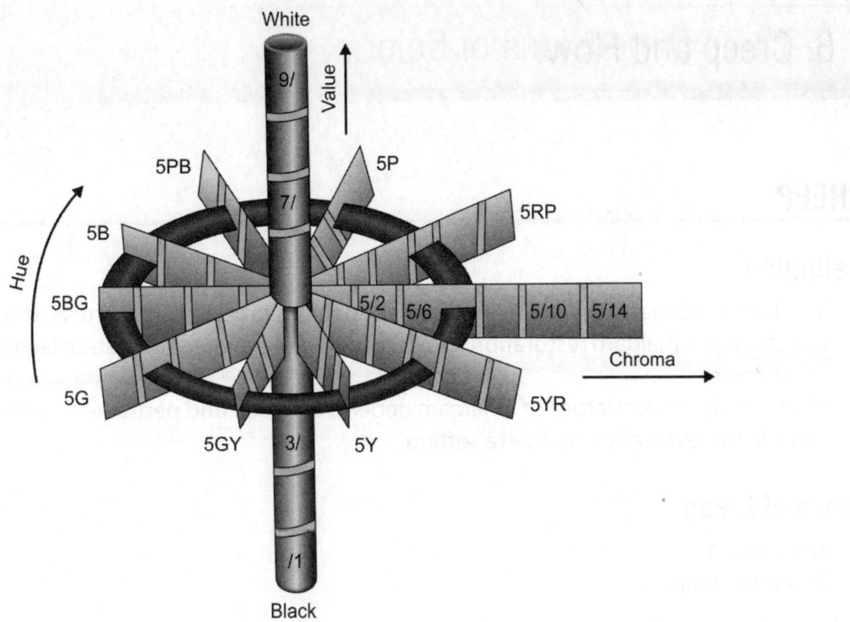

Fig. 23: The Munsell color system

- Forms the vertical axis of the cylindrical system
- The minimum value is referenced as 1 (= black) and the maximum 9 (= white)
- Ranges from black to white for diffusive or reflective objects and from black to clear for translucent objects.

Value Depends on Other Factors

- The incident light
- The surface finish of the object
- The background of the material.

Chroma

- *Chroma* represents degree of saturation of a particular hue
- In Munsell index, chroma varies radially
- The higher the chroma, the more intense is the color. Chroma is associated with hue and value
- In Munsell index, chroma forms the radial axis with a minimum chroma of 1 to a maximum of 12
- For example, a high value and low chroma will produce a pale color while a low value and low chroma produces bright color
- Hue and chroma are properties of the object.

6. Creep and Flow.

CREEP

Definition

- It is the time-dependent strain or deformation that is produced by a stress. The creep process can cause an amalgam restoration to extend out of the cavity preparation leading to marginal breakdown
- The viscoelastic properties of amalgam depend on creep and permanent deformation under static loads, even after complete setting.

Types of Creep

- Static creep
- Dynamic creep.

Static

It is a time-dependent deformation produced in a completely set solid subjected to a constant stress.

Dynamic

It is produced when the applied stress is fluctuating, such as in fatigue type test.

Importance

Dental amalgam has components with melting points that are slightly above room temperature and the creep produced can be very destructive to the restoration.

Creep related to Amalgam

- The phase (Ag, Hg_3) has a primary influence on low-copper amalgam creep rates. Creep rates increase with higher volume fractions and decrease with lower grain sizes
- The presence of γ phase is associated with higher creep rates
- Single composition high copper amalgams have very low creep rates, due to the absence of γ_2 phase and due to the presence of ($Cu_6 Sn_5$) rods which acts as barrier to deformation of the γ_1 phase.

Factors Reducing Creep

- Mercury/Alloy ratio should be kept to a minimum to ensure low creep and high compressive strengths
- Condensing pressure should be maximum for lathe cut or admixed alloys
- Increasing the triturating time increases creep of dental amalgam and decreasing the triturating time lowers creep rates in amalgam.

Creep Value

- According to ADA Specification Number 1, creep should be below 3%
- *Low copper:* 8–8.8%
- *High copper:* 0.4–0.1%
- *Low copper cut alloy:* 6.3% which is the highest value
- High-copper amalgam has low creep value but it increases the brittleness of the amalgam and decreases the relief of stresses at contact areas under load; hence, a high-modulus base is required under a high Cu-amalgam to minimize the development of tensile stresses.

Creep Related to Acrylic Denture Base Resins

- Denture resins are viscoelastic
- When subjected to a constant load, they show primary and secondary creep following the initial instantaneous elastic strain
- The secondary creep rate increases with increase in temperature, stress, residual monomer, plasticizers and cross-linking agent
- The creep rate for self-curing resins increases with stress more rapidly than for heat cure resins.

Creep Related to Noble Metal Alloys for Metal Ceramics

- When a constant stress is applied for a long time, materials can deform permanently even though the stress on the material is below its elastic limit. This time-dependent deformation of materials is known as creep
- At temperatures 40 to 50% less than the absolute melting point, creep is negligible
- Some flow or creep of gold alloy occurs when it approaches 980°C to 1800°C
- When heated to 980°C, ideally a second phase is precipitated, which can produce a strengthening of the alloy
- Creep is evident at high temperatures in excess of half the melting temperature on the absolute scale.

Creep Related to Metals/Alloys

Mechanism of Creep in Metals/Alloys

- Dislocation creep
- Secondary creep
- Diffusional creep or grain boundary sliding (GBS).

Dislocation creep

This takes place through the motion of dislocations within the grains of the metal, or alloy.

Secondary creep

After the dislocation creep slows down over a period of time, due to work hardening, secondary creep occurs. If the grain size is less, the magnitude of creep decreases. Secondary creep occurs at grain boundaries.

Diffusional creep or grain boundary sliding (GBS)

- This occurs by diffusion of atoms at the grain boundaries in metals and alloys that has not undergone work hardening

- Diffusional creep proceeds at constant rate until failure occurs
- Creep tends to increase with decreasing grain size.

Four stages of elongation are present in creep

1. Initial elongation due to the application of the load
2. Transient or primary creep
3. Secondary creep
4. Tertiary creep.

FLOW

Definition

It is the rheologic (or flow) behavior of solid materials.

Rheological Properties

- The science of the study of flow and deformation of matter is termed 'rheology'
- Flow and deformation can be plastic, elastic or viscoelastic.

Factors Affecting Flow

- The ability of the material to flow depends on the viscosity
- When flow decreases, the material begins to solidify (Initial and final setting time)
- The setting of materials initially involves a change in viscosity with time and then the development of an elastic modulus as setting occurs
- The working time is the period during which the material can be manipulated, with no thickening taking place
- The setting time is the time when the material has become rigid.

7. Stress and Strain.

STRESS

Definition

Stress is the internal reaction to the external force and is equal in intensity and opposite in direction to the applied external force.

The stress is calculated as the force per unit area.

$$\text{Stress} = \frac{\text{Force}}{\text{Area}}$$

The unit of stress reported in units of mega-Newton's per square meter (MN/m^2).

Types of Stress

- Tension
- Compression
- Shear
- Complex.

Tension

- Occurs when a body is subjected to two sets of forces that are directed away from each other in the same straight line
- In tension the molecules within the body must resist being pulled apart
- A tensile stress causes a material to stretch or elongate
- A tensile stress is accompanied by tensile strain
- The tensile stress is defined as the tensile force per unit area perpendicular to the force direction (Expressed in pounds per square inch/mega Pascal unit).

Compression

- Results when the body is subjected to two sets of forces in the same straight line and directed toward each other
- When compression is applied, molecules within resist being forced more closely together
- If a body is placed under a load that tends to shorten it, the internal resistance to such a load is called a compression
- Compressive stress is associated with a compressive strain.

Shear

- It is the result of two sets of forces being directed parallel to each other
- When shear stress is applied, one portion of the body must resist sliding past another. Shear resistance represents the elasticity of solid bodies
- Shear stress tends to resist the sliding of one portion of a body over another
- Shear stress is also produced by a twisting or torsional action on a material
- Shear stress is calculated by dividing the force by the area parallel to the force direction.

Complex

- In dental restoration, forces applied are a combination of compressive, tensile and shear stresses
- *In a three-unit bridge:* The occlusal surface of the bridge is subjected to compression and tension and the gingival portion of the pontic is under tensile stress
- The soldered joints are under both tensile and shear stress.

Flexural (bending) stress

Flexural stress is produced by bending forces in dental appliances.

Stress Analysis and Design of Dental Structures

- Brittle coatings
- Strain gauges
- Two- and three-dimensional photoelasticity
- Finite element analysis.

Two-dimensional Photoelasticity

- When a stress is applied to a model material, it becomes anisotropic
- A light is passed through a polarizer and then to the stressed material. This light passing through the stress material changes direction depending on the amount of stress present in each area
- The plane polarized light is converted to circularly polarized light by a quarter-wave plate. This splits the light into two components which changes directions depending on the state of stress in the model
- After the light emerges from the model, it passes through a second quarter-wave plate and an analyzer placed perpendicular to the polarizer
- The interference pattern is recorded photographically, which is the isochromatic fringe pattern.

Pattern reading

- Dark line isochromatic fringes indicate that principle stresses are constant
- Magnitude of stresses can be determined by identification of the order of the isochromatic fringes.

Finite-element Stress Analysis

- Here finite numbers of discrete structural elements are interconnected at finite number of points (nodal points)
- These finite elements are formed when the original structure is divided into a number of shaped sections with actual properties of the original materials.

The stresses and displacements are calculated when:

- The total number of nodal points and elements are present
- A numbering system is required for identifying each nodal point and element
- The elastic modulus and Poisson's ratio for the materials associated with each element can be assessed
- The coordinates of each nodal point
- The type of boundary constraints
- The evaluation of the forces applied to the external nodes.

STRAIN

Definition

- Strain, is the change in length occurring per unit length of the body, when a stress is applied. Strain has no unit of measurement

$$\text{Strain} = \frac{\text{Deformation}}{\text{Original length}}$$

- A body undergoes deformation when a force is applied to it
- The deformation resulting from a tension (pulling force) is an elongation of a body, whereas a compression causes shortening of the body.

Types

Elastic Strain

Reversible.

Plastic Strain

It represents a permanent deformation of the material that never recovers when the force is removed.

8. Young's Modulus.

SYNONYMS

Elastic modulus, Young's modulus or modulus of elasticity.

DEFINITION

- Elastic modulus/Young's modulus describes the relative stiffness or rigidity of a material, within the elastic range
- Elastic modulus is measured by the slope of the elastic region of the stress-strain graph
- If the tensile stress or compressive stress below the proportional limit is divided by its tensile strain or compressive strain, a constant of proportionality is obtained that is known as the Young's modulus (designated by the letter E).

SIGNIFICANCE OF ELASTIC MODULUS

- It represents the elastic qualities of a material
- The interatomic intermolecular arrangement of a material alters the elastic property
- The more the attraction force within the material, the greater is the elastic modulus and rigidity
- Elastic modulus can be measured by application of stress in tension or compression
- Elastomeric impression materials and resins have low values for elastic modulus but metals and alloys have high values

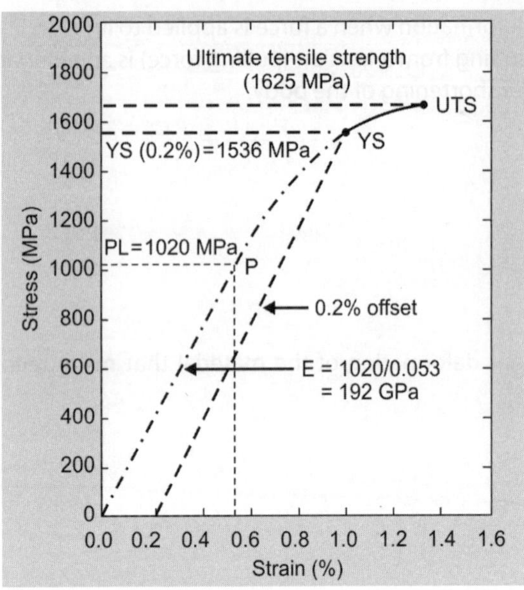

Fig. 24: Stress-strain graph indicating young's modulus

- Elastic and plastic strain occur during burnishing of an open metal margin, when a dental abrasive stone is used to close the marginal gap.

The slope of the straight-line region is the elastic range of the stress-strain graph, which indicates the *rigidity* or *stiffness* of a material.

- The elastic modulus of a material is a constant which is unaffected by the amount of elastic or plastic stress. Hence, it is independent of the ductility of a material and it is not a measure of its strength
- Elastic modulus is tested by means of a tensile test
- Elastic modulus is the ratio of the elastic stress to the elastic strain. Hence, the lower the strain for a given stress, the greater is the value of the modulus
- If one wire was difficult to bend than another of the same shape and size, then it indicates that the wire requiring higher stress to produce deformation possesses a high modulus of elasticity
- Elastic deformation is fully recovered when the force is removed or when the wire fractures
- If the induced stress is within the proportional limit, then the wire returns to its original shape as the force is decreased to zero **(Fig. 24)**.

Evaluation of the stress-strain graph indicates that enamel is stiffer and more brittle and dentin is more flexible and tougher **(Fig. 25)**.

CALCULATION FOR YOUNG'S MODULUS

Modulus of elasticity is given in units of force per unit area [Giga Newtons per square meter (GN/m^2), or gigapascals (GPa)].

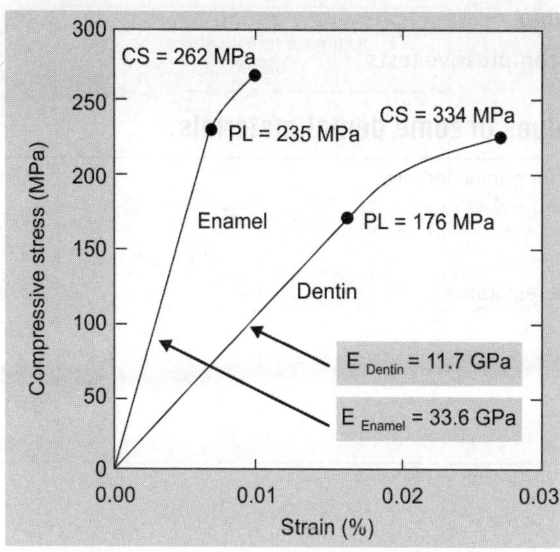

Fig. 25: Stress-strain plot for enamel and dentin

The elastic modulus of a tensile test specimen is calculated as follows:

$$\text{Elastic modulus} = \frac{\text{Stress}}{\text{Strain}} \text{ MN/m}^2 \text{ or lb/inch}^2$$

$$E = \frac{\text{Stress } (P/A)}{\text{Strain } (A_l/A_0)}$$

E = Elastic modulus
P = Applied force or load
A = Cross-sectional area of the material under stress
A_l = Increase in length
A_0 = Original length

MEASUREMENT OF YOUNG'S MODULUS

Methods

- Dynamic
- Static.

Dynamic Young's Modulus

- In dynamic method of measurement, Young's Modulus can be measured by ultrasonic longitudinal and transverse wave transducers and appropriate receivers.
- If velocity and density of the material are known, the elastic modulus and Poisson's ratio can be determined. The values are often found to be higher than the values obtained by static measurements.

Static Young's Modulus

Tested by tensile and compressive tests.

Elastic modulus values of some dental materials

Cobalt chromium alloy for partial denture	218 GN/m^2
Type IV gold alloy	99.3 GN/m^2
Feldspathic porcelain	69.0 GN/m^2
Zinc phosphate cement restorative	22.4 GN/m^2
Composite resin	16.6 GN/m^2
Acrylic resin	2.65 GN/m^2
Enamel	84.1 GN/m^2
Dentin	18.3 GN/m^2

9. Elastic Limit/Proportional Limit.

DEFINITION

Elastic Limit

- The maximum stress a material can withstand before it becomes plastically deformed
- Above *proportional* or *elastic limit* plastic deformation occurs.

Proportional Limit

The stress above which stress is no longer proportional to strain.

Explanation

- The elastic limit of a material is defined as the greatest stress to which a material can be subjected such that it returns to its original dimensions when the force is released
- When a wire is stressed and if the load is removed, the wire will return to its original length
- If the same load is increased progressively and then released at one point, the wire does not return to its original length after it is unloaded.

Hooke's Law

- In which the elastic stress must be directly proportional to the elastic strain; that is, the initial region of the stress-strain plot must be a straight line
- When a material obeys Hooke's law, the elastic stress will be proportional to elastic strain. Within the proportional and elastic limit, the material behaves elastically and it springs back to its initial shape and size when the force is removed
- Beyond proportional and elastic limit, the line becomes nonlinear and stress is no longer proportional to strain.

In a stress-strain plot the first part of the stress-strain plot is a straight-line portion, after which the straight line curves. The stress value at P, the point above which the curve deviates from a straight line, is known as the *proportional limit.*

Factors Related to Proportional Limit

- Proportional limit is the greatest elastic stress and it represents the maximum stress above which stress is no longer proportional to the strain
- Above the proportional limit, before fracture, the removal of the applied force will reduce the stress to zero, but strain does not decrease to zero
- Beyond proportional limit, the material does not return to its original dimension when the force is removed. It remains bent, stretched or compressed **(Fig. 26)**.

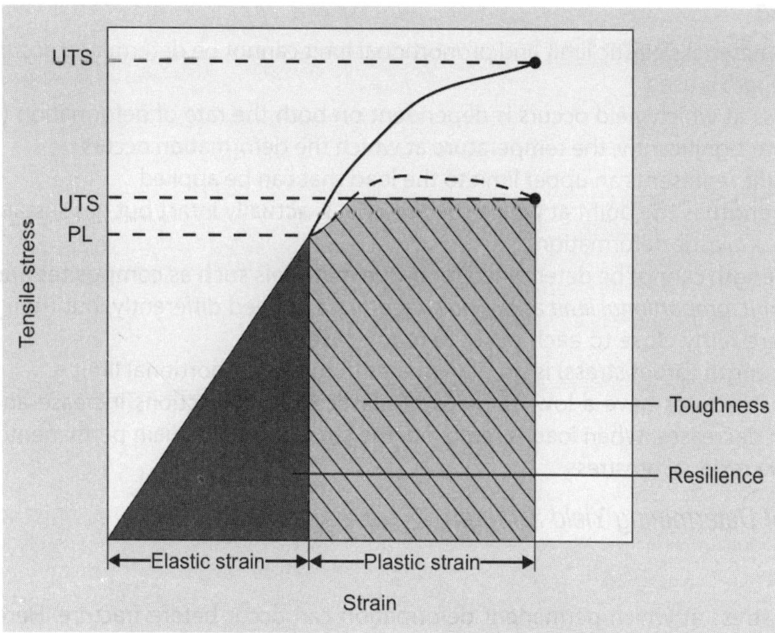

Fig. 26: Stress-strain plot indicating proportional limit

10. Importance of Yield Strength of a Restorative Material.

YIELD STRENGTH (PROOF STRESS)

Definition

It is the stress beyond which permanent strain or plastic deformation occurs. Yield point is the maximum stress which can be applied to a material without causing more than a permissible permanent deformation.

Yield Strength and Deformation

- Before the yield point, the material will deform elastically and will return to its original shape when the applied stress is removed
- Once the yield point is passed, the deformation will be permanent and nonreversible
- This permissible deformation is 0.1 to 0.2% (referred to as percent offset) of the gauge length. Hence, the stress to achieve 0.1% deformation could be 0.1% proof stress.

Significance

- When a material's elastic limit and proportional limit cannot be determined accurately, then *yield strength* is used
- The stress at which yield occurs is dependent on both the rate of deformation (strain rate) and, more significantly, the temperature at which the deformation occurs
- Yield point represents an upper limit to the load that can be applied
- Yield strength is the point at which the material is actually intact but has sustained a small amount of plastic deformation
- Yield strength cannot be determined for brittle materials such as composites and ceramics
- *Elastic limit, proportional limit* and *yield strength* are defined differently, but their values (of stress) are fairly close to each other in many cases
- Yield strength (proof stress) is usually greater than the proportional limit
- Yielded structures have a low modulus of elasticity, so deflections increase and buckling strength decreases. When load is removed, the structure will remain permanently bent and may have residual prestress.

Methods of Determining Yield Strength

Elastic limit

The lowest stress at which permanent deformation can occur before fracture. Here testing is done by load-unload procedure.

Proportional limit

The point at which the stress-strain curve becomes nonlinear. In most metallic materials, the elastic limit and proportional limit are the same.

Offset yield point (proof stress)

As there is no clear demarcation between the elastic and plastic regions, the yield point is often defined as the stress at some arbitrary plastic strain (typically 0.2%). This is determined by the intersection of a line offset from the linear region by the required strain **(Fig. 27)**.

In some materials, there is no linear region and so a certain value of plastic strain is defined.

Theories Related to Yield Criterion

Maximum principal stress theory

Yield occurs when the largest principal stress exceeds the uni-axial tensile yield strength.

Maximum principal strain theory

Yield occurs when the maximum principal strain reaches the strain corresponding to the yield point during a simple tensile test.

Maximum shear stress theory

(*Tresca criterion by Henri Tresca*)

This assumes that yield occurs when the shear stress exceeds the shear yield strength.

Total strain energy theory

Yield occurs when the strain energy per unit volume is greater than the strain energy at the elastic limit in simple tension.

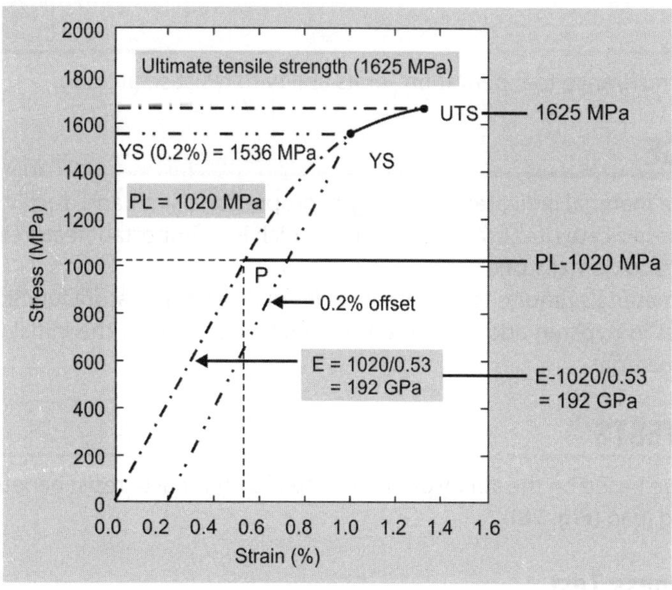

Fig. 27: Yield strength of orthodontic wire subjected to tension

Yield Strength of Few Dental Materials

Gold alloys

Type I .... 400–420 MN/m^2
Type II .... 550–575 MN/m^2
Type III .... 475–525 MN/m^2
Type IV .... 400–525 MN/m^2

Stainless steel .... 248 MN/m^2

Partial denture metals

Nickel chromium .... 690 MN/m^2
Cobalt chromium .... 572 MN/m^2

Gold .... 621 MN/m^2

11. Hardness Tests.

DEFINITION

Hardness is the 'resistance to indentation', or its ability to resist scratching.

SIGNIFICANCE

- Hardness of a material indicates the strength, proportional limit and ductility of the material
- Hardness also indicates its abrasive resistance which is an important feature for die materials, investments and dental stone
- Restorative materials require to be hard in order to resist masticatory function
- Hardness test in gypsum and investment material also indicate the initial and final setting time of the material.

HARDNESS TESTS

Hardness tests are based on the ability of the surface of a material to resist penetration by a point under a specified load **(Fig. 28)**.

Types of Hardness Test

- Brinell
- Rockwell

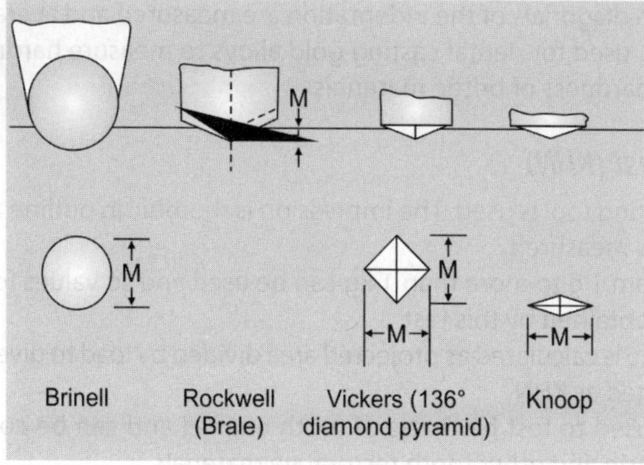

Fig. 28: Various hardness tests

- Vickers
- Knoop
- Barcol
- Shore.

Brinell Hardness Test (BHN)

It is one of the oldest tests employed for determining the hardness of metals.

Procedure

- A hard steel ball is pressed under a specified load into the polished surface of a material
- The hardness is calculated by load divided by the area of the projected surface of the indentation and the measure is abbreviated as BHN
- If the indentation is small, larger is the number and harder is the material
- BHN is related to the proportional limit and the ultimate tensile strength of dental gold alloys.

Rockwell Hardness Test (RHN)

A steel ball or a conical diamond point is used for indentation.

Procedure

- The depth of penetration is measured directly by a dial gauge and the measure is abbreviated as RHN
- Different sizes of indenting points are used for testing different materials
- This test cannot be used for brittle materials.

Vickers Hardness Test (VHN)

- Here a square-based pyramid is used for test and computation is load divided by the projected area of indentation (same as for Brinells)
- The measure is abbreviated as VHN

- The lengths of the diagonals of the indentation are measured and averaged
- The Vickers test is used for dental casting gold alloys to measure hardness of tooth and for determining the hardness of brittle materials.

Knoop Hardness Test (KHN)

- A diamond indenting tool is used. The impression is rhombic in outline and the length of the largest diagonal is measured
- Different loads from 1 g to more than 1 kg can be used and so values for both hard and soft materials can be obtained by this test
- The hardness value is calculated as projected area divided by load to give the Knoop hardness number abbreviated as KHN
- This test can be used to test hardness of tooth enamel and can be compared with that of gold, porcelain, resin and other tooth restorative materials.

Barcol and Shore

Are tests used for determining the hardness of elastic- and rubber-like materials.

Differences Between Tests

- Knoop and Vickers tests use loads less than 9.8 N
- The Rockwell and Brinell tests give average hardness values over much larger areas. Shore and the Barcol tests are used to measure hardness of soft materials as rubbers and plastics. These equipment generally consist of a spring-loaded metal indenter point and a gauge from which the hardness is read directly
- The hardness number is based on the depth of penetration of the indenter point into the material.

12. Brittleness.

DEFINITION

Brittleness is the relative inability of a material to sustain plastic deformation before fracture of a material occurs.

DRAWBACKS OF BRITTLENESS

Brittle material fractures at or near its proportional limit.

Example

Porcelain, luting agents, gypsum products are all brittle.

- Localized high stresses in specific areas develop flaws that later propagate to form cracks causing a failure in the material
- As the stress at the tips of these flaws is higher, it leads to crack initiation and broken bonds
- The stress intensity increases with the length of the flaw in the direction of tensile stress
- Flaws on the surface have higher stresses than the same size flaws in interior regions
- In a ductile material, the flaw tip widens, thereby reducing the localized tensile stress. This is not possible with a brittle material
- Any porosity, roughness and machining damage in brittle materials can also lead to failure
- Any sharp internal angle at the pulpal-axial line angle of a tooth preparation for an amalgam restoration can lead to failure of restoration
- When there is a mismatch in the elastic moduli or thermal coefficients of the two components, bonding failure between the two materials occurs.

PREVENTION OF FAILURE

Factors determining the strength of brittle materials were first stated by AA Griffith.

- Fine polishing of brittle materials to reduce the depth of the flaws such as ceramics, amalgams and composites
- Minimize interior flaws
- The design or preparation should not have any sharp angulations or margins
- Notches should be avoided
- If ceramic is bonded to metal, ceramic should have the lower elastic modulus and metal the higher elastic modulus, so that the stresses can be transferred to the metal
- The above materials must be closely matched in their coefficients of expansion and contraction also
- The cusp tip of an opposing crown or tooth should be well rounded so that occlusal contact areas in the brittle material are large.

TESTING METHODS

A load applied at a point to the surface of a brittle material is called the Hertzian point load.

Griffith's Hypothesis

1. The reduction in strain energy which accompanies the crack.
2. The energy required to create the new surfaces associated with the crack.

When (1) is greater than (2), energy reduction occurs leading to crack progression.

Calculation

When a surface crack, of length *l*, is stressed more, the crack proceeds through the material.

Critical crack length

The crack length that is stable for an applied stress (length *l*).

The tensile strength for a crack of length l, material is given by:

$$\sigma TS = \sqrt{G_c E/\pi l}$$

G_c = amount of energy required to advance the crack by 1 m^2.
E = Young's modulus for the material
l = is crack length.

Thus, the tensile strength of brittle materials is inversely proportional to the square root of the longest crack.

13. Ductility and Malleability.

DEFINITIONS

Ductility

- Ductility is the ability of a material to sustain a large permanent deformation under a tensile load without rupture. A metal that may be drawn readily into a wire is said to be ductile
- When a material is stressed beyond its proportional limit, it becomes permanently deformed. If a material sustains tensile stress without rupture, it is ductile.

Malleability

- The ability of a material to sustain considerable permanent deformation without rupture under compression, as in hammering or rolling into a sheet, is termed malleability
- Not dependent on strength as in ductility.

EXAMPLES OF DUCTILE AND MALLEABLE METALS

- Gold is the most ductile and malleable pure metal (some textbooks refer to tungsten as the most ductile)
- Silver is second and platinum ranks third in ductility
- Silver, aluminum and copper rank second, third and fourth respectively in malleability.

Other Ductile Metals

Iron, nickel, copper, aluminum and zinc.

Other Malleable Metals

Tin, platinum, lead, zinc and iron.

Significance of Ductility and Malleability

- Ductility and malleability are important properties for metals, alloys and few plastics
- The more a metal is ductile, the better is the burnishability
- Metals with good ductility have good margin adaptability, decreasing marginal leakage
- If a metal can be compressed or elongated, it has good ductility and malleability
- Ductility is the maximum plastic deformation a material can withstand when it is stretched at room temperature and this can be assessed by the amount of permanent deformation indicated by the stress-strain curve.

METHODS OF MEASUREMENT OF DUCTILITY (FIG. 29)

1. The percent elongation after fracture
2. A reduction in area in the fractured region ends
3. Cold bend test.

Percent Elongation Test

- The increase in length of a wire or rod after fracture in tension is compared to its length before fracture
- Two marks are placed on the wire or rod at a specified distance and this distance is designated as gauge length (51 mm is standard gauge length)
- The wire or rod is then pulled apart under a tensile load and the fractured ends are fitted together and the gauge length is measured
- The ratio of the increase in length after fracture to the original gauge length is called the percent elongation and represents value of ductility.

Reduction in Area in Fractured Region

- After fracture of a rod or wire, a cone-shaped constriction (referred to as necking) occurs at the fractured end under a tensile load. This indicates the ductility of a material
- The percentage decrease in cross-sectional area of the fractured end in comparison to the original cross-sectional area of the wire or rod is called the reduction in area.

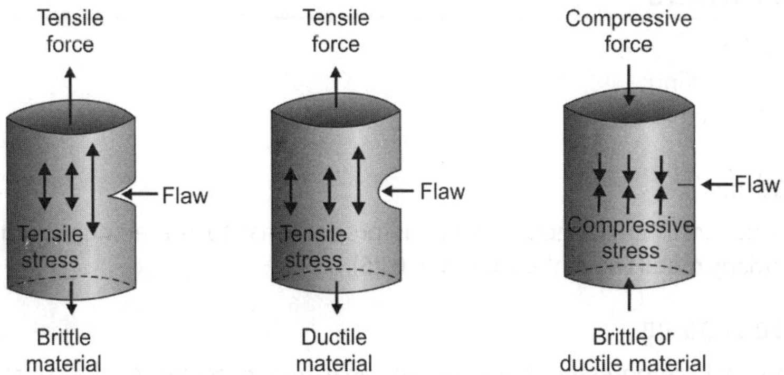

Fig. 29: Influence of tensile and compressive stresses on flaws in brittle and ductile materials

Cold Bend Test

- The material is clamped and bent around a mandrel of a specified radius
- The first bend is made from the vertical to the horizontal and all the rest of the bends are made through 180° angles
- The number of bends required to fracture indicates the ductility of material. The greater the number, the greater is the ductility.

14. Poisson's Ratio.

DEFINITIONS

1. It is the ratio of transverse contraction strain to longitudinal extension strain in the direction of stretching force.
   - Tensile deformation is considered positive and compressive deformation is considered negative
   - The definition of Poisson's ratio contains a minus sign so that normal materials have a positive ratio.

   $\nu = - \varepsilon_{trans} / \varepsilon_{longitudinal}$
2. Poisson's ratio is that ratio in which interatomic bonds realign with deformation.
3. If a cylindrical specimen is subject to a tensile or compressive stress, there is simultaneous axial and lateral strain.
   This ratio of lateral to the axial strain within the elastic range is called Poisson's ratio (ν).

TESTING METHODS

- Tensile loading
- Compressive loading
- Ultrasonic technique.

Tensile Loading

There is a reduction in cross-section which is proportional to the elongation during elastic deformation (Many metals have the value $\nu = 0.25$).

Compressive Loading

- When material is compressed, the cross-sectional area increases. As the stress exceeds the proportional limit, permanent deformation occurs (ν=0.5)

- When there is an increase in length of a material (axial strain), there is also a decrease in cross-sectional area (lateral or transverse strain).

$$\text{Poisson's ratio } (\nu) = \frac{\text{Lateral strain}}{\text{Axial strain}}$$

Significance

Brittle materials show less reduction in cross-section under tensile loading whereas ductile materials show increased reduction in cross-section under tensile loading.

Poisson's Ratio in Viscoelastic Materials

The Poisson's ratio in a viscoelastic material is time dependent in the context of transient tests such as creep and stress relaxation. The transverse strain may be out of phase with the longitudinal strain in a viscoelastic solid.

Examples

- Cork in a bottle
- The cork must be easily inserted and removed, yet it also must withstand the pressure from within the bottle. Rubber, with a Poisson's ratio of 0.5, cannot be used as it expands when compressed into the neck of the bottle and would jam
- Cork, with a Poisson's ratio of nearly zero, is ideal in this application.

Poisson's Ratio of Few Materials

Most materials have Poisson's ratio in the vicinity of 1/3.

Isotropic upper limit	0.5
Amalgam	0.35
Zinc phosphate	0.35
Enamel	0.30
Composite resin	0.24
Acrylic resin	0.35
Lead	0.44
Copper	0.37
Aluminum	0.35
Stainless steel	0.30
Beryllium	0.08
Isotropic lower limit	–1

15. Strength.

DEFINITION

Strength is the maximal stress required to fracture a material.

TYPES RELATED TO DENTAL MATERIALS

- Tensile strength
- Compressive strength
- Shear strength
- Flexure strength
- Fatigue strength
- Impact strength
- Yield strength
- Bond strength
- Tear strength.

TENSILE STRENGTH

Ability of a material to withstand fracture in tension.

Methods of Testing

- Uniaxial tension test
- Diametrical compression test
- Brazilian test
- Indirect tensile test
- Uniaxial and diametrical compression test methods are commonly employed.

Uniaxial Tension Test

This test is determined by subjecting a rod, wire or dumbbell-shaped specimen to tensile loading.

Diametral Compression Test Method

- In compression testing method, a load is placed (a flat plate) against the side of a short cylindrical specimen (disk) **(Fig. 30)**
- The vertical compressive force along the side of the disk produces a tensile stress that is perpendicular to the vertical plane
- Tensile stress is directly proportional to the compressive load applied.
  Tensile stress $S = 2P/(\pi \times D \times T)$
  P = load
  D = diameter
  T = thickness

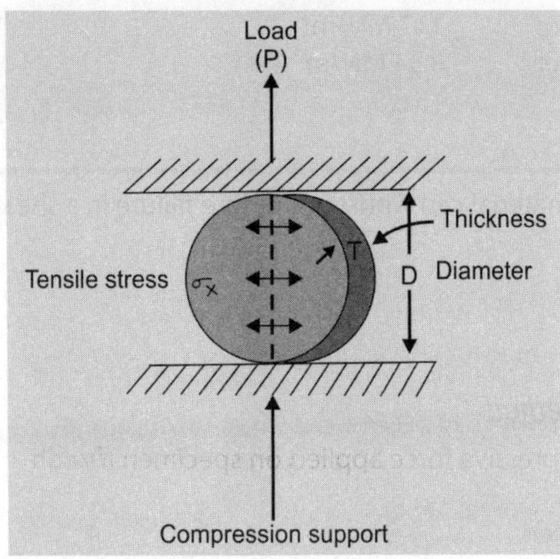

Fig. 30: Diametral compression test

Tensile Strength of Few Important Materials

Amalgam lathe cut	54.7 MN/m^2
Composite	45.5 MN/m^2
Zinc phosphate	8.1 MN/m^2
Calcium hydroxide liner	0.96 MN/m^2

COMPRESSIVE STRENGTH

Ability of a material to withstand permanent deformation under compression.

Testing Method

- Diametral compression testing.

Calculated as

$$\text{Ultimate compressive strength} = \frac{\text{Maximum force (Pounds)}}{\text{Cross-sectional area in square meters (inches)}}$$

Significance

A stress-strain curve can be charted from which other properties as proportional limit and yield strength can be evaluated.

Compressive Strength of Few Materials

Enamel	384 MN/m^2
Amalgam lathe cut	318 MN/m^2
Composite resin	237 MN/m^2

Zinc phosphate cement	117 MN/m^2
Calcium hydroxide liner	8.34 MN/m^2

SHEAR STRENGTH

Is the maximum stress a material can withstand before failure in a shear loading.

Testing Method

- Punch method.

Calculation in Punch Method

- Shear strength = Compressive force applied on specimen (f)/πdh
  D: Diameter of punch
  H: Thickness of specimen
- *Direct shear test:* By shearing a cylindrical specimen with sharp metal knife.

Shear Strength of Few Materials

Aluminous porcelain	165 MN/m^2
Amalgam	188 MN/m^2
Resin	122 MN/m^2
Porcelain	111 MN/m^2
Zinc phosphate	13.1 MN/m^2

FLEXURE STRENGTH

Synonyms

Transverse strength, or modulus of rupture.

Definition

Flexure strength is a strength test of a bar supported at each end, or a thin disk supported along a lower support circle, under a static load.

Testing Methods

- By bending test method
- *Photoelastic method:* To observe isochromatic fringe order.

Bending Test

- When the load is applied, the specimen bends
- The resulting strain causes a decrease in length of the top surface (compressive strain) of a bar specimen or a decrease in diameter of a disk specimen and an increase in the length or diameter of the lower surface (tensile strain)
- There will be a position within the specimen where there is no change, with both stress and strain being zero, known as the *neutral axis.*

Calculation of Flexure Strength

Biaxial Flexure Strength

$$S = \frac{3Wl}{2bd^2}$$

S = Flexural strength
l = Distance between the supports
b = Width of the specimen
d = Depth or thickness of the specimen
W = Maximum load before fracture.

Flexure Strength of Few Materials

Gold foil	292 MN/m^2
Lathe cut amalgam	124 MN/m^2
Composite resin	139 MN/m^2
High strength stone	16.6 MN/m^2

FATIGUE STRENGTH

Definition

- Is the strength of the material that can withstand before premature fracture
- Fatigue failure is a failure occurring below the ultimate tensile strength because microscopic flaws grow slowly over many cycles of stress
- In fatigue failure, crack propagation can lead to unexpected fracture.

Testing

- Fatigue strength is tested by subjecting a material to a cyclic stress of a maximum known value and determining the number of cycles that are required to produce failure
- With this test, a maximum service stress level or an endurance limit is established for each material.

Types

- Static
- Dynamic.

Static Fatigue Failure

Static fatigue is a phenomenon attributed to the interaction of a constant tensile stress with structural flaws over time.

Example: Aqueous solutions degrade dental ceramics by lengthening surface flaws over time in the presence of tensile stress.
(Ceramic orthodontic brackets and activated wires).

Dynamic Fatigue Failure

The delayed fracture of molar ceramic crowns subjected to periodic cyclic forces is due to dynamic fatigue failure.

IMPACT STRENGTH

Definition

Impact strength is defined as the energy required to fracture a material under an impact force.

Testing

- Charpy impact testing
- Izod impact testing.

Charpy Impact Test

- A pendulum is swung to fracture the centre of a specimen supported at both ends
- The energy lost by the pendulum during the fracture of the specimen is calculated by comparing the length of its swing and the impact with its free swing when no impact occurs.
- Described in joules, foot-pounds and inch-pounds.

Izod Impact Tester

- The specimen is clamped vertically at one end
- A blow is delivered at a certain distance above the clamped end
- If the struck object is not permanently deformed, the energy is stored within the specimen in an elastic manner
- A material with a low elastic modulus and a high tensile strength is more resistant to impact forces
- A low elastic modulus and a low tensile strength suggest low-impact resistance.

Tensile strength and elastic modulus values of a few materials

Material	Elastic modulus	Tensile strength
Dental porcelain	40 GPa	50 to 100 MPa
Amalgam	21 GPa	60 MPa
Resin-based composite	17 GPa	30 to 90 MPa
Polymethyl methacrylate	3.5 GPa	60 MPa
Alumina ceramic	350 GPa	120 MPa

Tensile strength of alumina ceramic is 120 MPa, its elastic modulus is 350 GPa, making its impact resistance only fair.

YIELD STRENGTH

Definition

It is the stress at which material exhibits limited deviation from proportionality of stress to strain.

- It is the stress at which material begins to function in plastic manner
- Tested and evaluated by stress-strain curve.

Yield Strength of Few Materials

Nickel chromium	690 MN/m^2
Cobalt chromium	572 MN/m^2
Type IV Gold	621 MN/m^2

BOND STRENGTH

It is the ability of the material to withstand debonding between two materials or between tooth and a material.

Example

- Between porcelain and metal/Composite and enamel
- Bond strength increases after etching enamel, by applying bonding agent and in metal after sand blasting.

Testing Methods

- Placing bond in tension
- Placing bond in shear (push through shear test).

Bond Strength of a Few Materials

Zinc polycarboxylate	3.45 to 13.1 MN/m^2
Glass ionomer	1 to 3 MN/m^2
Ceramic to metal bond strength	117 MN/m^2

TEAR STRENGTH

Definition

It is the resistance to tearing forces.

Testing Method

- Crescent-shaped specimens of 12.7 mm on one side with a 90-degree notch on the other side is made. Cross head speed of 25 cm/min is used to test specimens
- Tear strength is calculated by: maximum load applied/thickness of specimen.

Tear Strength of a Few Dental Materials

Denture liners	2.6 to 45 KN/m
Agar	0.99 KN/m
Alginate	0.47 KN/m
Polysulfide	4.0 KN/m

16. Viscosity.

DEFINITION

- The viscosity of a fluid is a measure of the resistance offered by a fluid to forces producing flow
- When a substance flows under the influence of an external force, the molecules or atoms come into contact with other atoms, during which bonds are broken and remade and this gives rise to a resistance to flow known as viscosity
- Viscosity is shear stress by shear rate
- Viscoelasticity is related to viscosity in which materials require an initial stress application to flow (e.g. waxes, resins and amalgam).

Examples of Viscosity

- As water flows easily, it has a low viscosity
- In polymers, the intermolecular attractions are much stronger and the molecules entangle with one another, hence they possess high viscosities.

METHOD OF DETERMINING VISCOSITY

- It is measured as the time required for a unit amount of liquid to flow through a capillary opening with calibrated diameter and this is compared to a standard material as water
- Stirring a liquid is applying a shear stress and the force of stirring is expressed by the shear rate
- Units of viscosity are Poise or dyne × seconds cm^2 or centipoises (1 poise=100 centipoises).

TYPES OF VISCOSITY (FIG. 31)

- Newtonian
- Dilatant
- Plastic
- Pseudoplastic.

Newtonian

- Newtonian substances have a linear relationship between shear stress and shear rate with single value of viscosity (few impression materials)
- Viscosity of Newtonian is independent of shear rate.

In a flow index, if n = 1, the material is Newtonian, if n is less than 1, it is pseudoplastic, if n is greater than 1, it is dilatants. These are called *power law fluids*.

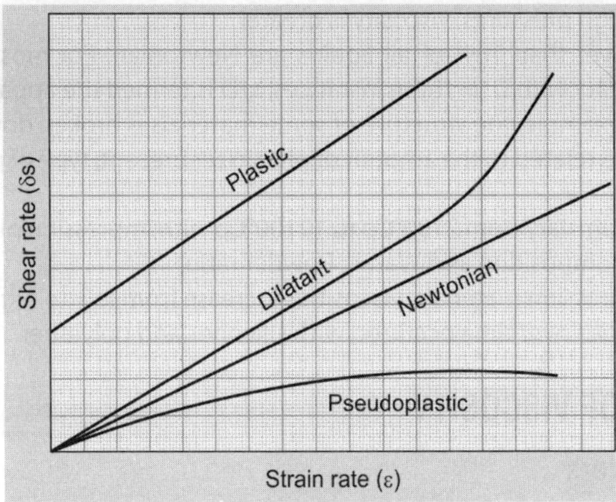

Fig. 31: Types of viscosities

Dilatant

- Dilatant liquids show an increase in viscosity as the shear rate goes up. Hence, the faster the mix, the more difficult it is for the liquid to get mixed
- This liquid flow cannot be defined by a single viscosity.

Pseudoplastic

- In pseudoplastic materials, an increase in shear rate does not increase the shear stress. Hence, pseudoplastic liquid becomes easier to mix at higher shear rates
- For example, silicone impression materials used as syringe material.

Plastic

- Materials, that behave like a rigid body until some minimum value of shear stress is reached, is termed as plastic.
- For example, catsup.

Thixotropy

- Thixotropic materials when mixed, a change in molecular arrangement occurs
- If the material was left long before the second mix, the molecule could recover
- In these, the longer the fluid mixed at a given shear rate, the lower is the shear stress and, hence, the viscosity (e.g. nondrip paint).

FACTORS AFFECTING VISCOSITY

- The nature of the substance
- *The temperature:* The viscosity decreases with increasing temperature
- Time duration

- *Pressure:* At very high pressures, viscosity is greater
- *Shear rate (D):* Fewer than 10% of all liquids are Newtonian. For most fluids, x/D is not a constant but will vary with D. In these instances, x/D is termed the apparent viscosity
- *Shear history:* For example, the structure of some materials is broken down on shearing
- Viscosity in resins is related to the amount of plasticizer present, type of polymer and initiator concentration
- Viscosities in gypsum vary from 2100°Cp to 10100°Cp with impression plaster being 2300°Cp. (Depends on the composition and Water : Powder ratio)
- In elastomeric impression materials, viscosities increase from low to high consistencies
- Increase in viscosities over time occurred with silicones and polyether.

MEASUREMENT OF VISCOSITY

Capillary Viscometers

Used to measure viscosity of Newtonian fluids. Here the fluid is extruded under pressure through a capillary and viscosity is calculated from force of extrusion, volumetric flow rate through the capillary and capillary dimensions.

Falling Body Viscometers

Viscosity can be calculated from the time taken for a sphere to fall or roll through a fluid.

Rotational Viscometers/Coaxial Cylinder Viscometers

The fluid is placed between two coaxial cylinders which are rotated. The shear rate is derived from the speed of rotation and shear stress is obtained from a meter.

Cone-plate Viscometers

Here the fluid is sheared in the gap between a stationary plate and a rotating cone. The shear rate is constant and shear stress is calculated from torque and instrument dimensions. This is used to measure non-Newtonian fluids.

Rotating Spindle Viscometers

A spindle is made to rotate in the fluid and viscous traction is measured.

Parallel Plate Plastometers

Fluid is placed between two discs of the same size and one plate is made to move toward the other. Viscosity is calculated from force applied to move the plate and rate of movement.

Qualitative Instruments

Orifice Viscometers

These consist of a fluid reservoir and an orifice.

Penetrometer

It is a rod with a needle or cone which is dropped on to a sample and depth of penetration is measured.

Oscillating or Reciprocating Rheometer

A plate oscillates in the material and the decrease in amplitude of oscillation is recorded as setting of the material occurs. Can record working and setting times.

Viscoelastic Measurement

Viscoelastic behavior can be assessed by models consisting of springs and dash-pots.

A spring

It is used to record the amount of elastic recovery when a load is applied.

Dashpot

It is a cylinder filled with a Newtonian fluid, with a leak-proof and frictionless piston. The fluid is pressed from one vessel with an opening to a large reservoir by applying force over time (t). This causes a time dependent deformation which stops at time (t), when the load is removed and permanent deformation results.

Combinations of Springs and Dashpots

A Maxwell unit

It is composed of a spring and dashpot in series.

A Voigt unit

It is composed of a spring and a dashpot in parallel.
Viscoelastic properties as creep of dental amalgam, properties of soft lining materials and resins can be assessed by springs and dashpots.

17. Contact Angle.

DEFINITION

- The contact angle is the angle formed by the adhesive with the adherent at their interface
- Contact angle of wetting is the extent to which an adhesive wets the surface of an adherent and is determined by measuring the contact angle between the adhesive and the adherent.

THEORY OF WETTING

- If the molecules of the adhesive are attracted to the molecules of the adherent, the liquid adhesive will spread completely over the surface of the solid and no angle ($\theta=0°$) will be formed.

- Here the forces of adhesion are stronger than the cohesive forces holding the molecules of the adhesive together.

FACTORS AFFECTING WETTING

- Any impurities or contamination of the adherend cause an increase in the contact angle
- Impurities as film of water, an oxide film on a metallic surface can decrease the contact of an adhesive
- Structural organic groups and the presence of halogens may prevent wetting
- Low surface energy solids decrease the wetting as in polytetrafluoroethylene
- If the adhesive is thicker, the wettability is reduced. Thinner adhesive flows and wets better
- If the surface of the solid is not flat, wetting can decrease
- Surface imperfections decrease wetting
- Air pockets decrease the spreading of the adhesive that prevent complete wetting of the entire surface.

Relation of Wetting to Contact Angle

- If the wetting is good, contact angle will be zero
- Contact angle is indicated as θ
- If $\theta = 0°$, wetting is good
- If $\theta = 90°$, wetting is not good **(Fig. 32)**
- When a liquid spreads completely over a surface, the contact angle decreases, the contact angle is an indicator of spreadability or wettability
- The smaller the contact angle between an adhesive and an adherent, the better is the wettability
- Thermal and mechanical stresses on the adhesive joint cause stress concentrations leading to crack propagation and adhesive failure.

Example of Wetting

- When water is coated between two polished glass plates, the surface energy of the glass attracts the molecules of water
- The attraction between glass and water molecules forms a resistance in separation of the two glass plates.

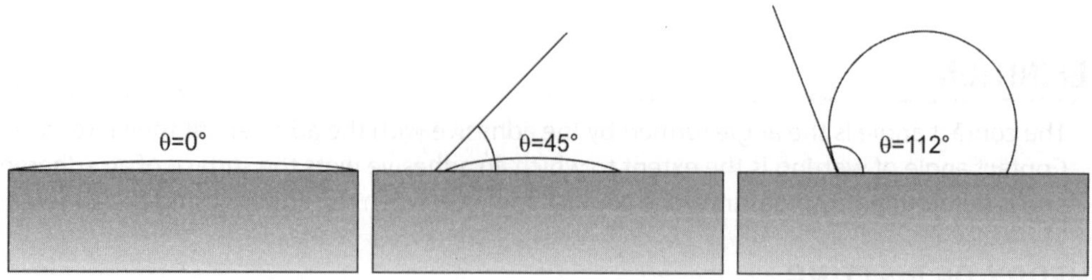

Fig. 32: Contact angle

SIGNIFICANCE OF WETTING/CONTACT ANGLE

- In true wetting, failure occurs cohesively in the solid or in the adhesive itself
- Adhesion of complete denture to tissues where saliva is the adherent
- Metals and oxide films in regard to soldering.

18. Surface Tension/Surface Energy.

DEFINITION

- It is the tension exerted over the surface film of a liquid due to cohesive forces within the liquid and resulting in a tendency for the surface to contract in area
- The increase in energy per unit area of surface is referred to as the surface energy or surface tension
- Surface tension is responsible for wetting and capillary action.

FACTORS IN SURFACE TENSION

Molecular Arrangement

The surface of large molecules is flat but liquid in capillary tube has a curvature.

Molecular Attraction

The attraction of molecules on the outside and inside of the same liquid differs.

Surface Energy

For adhesion to exist, the surfaces must be attracted to one another at their interface.

Cohesive Forces

- The more the cohesive forces between the molecules, the more is the surface tension
- Materials with low surface tensions have better wetting capacity
- Impurities as adsorbed gas or an oxide decrease surface energy and cause decrease in wetting
- The type of crystal plane of a space lattice present at the surface can affect the surface energy
- The greater the surface energy, the greater is the capacity for adhesion.

THEORY BEHIND SURFACE TENSION

- A liquid has molecular attraction in all directions, or in a spherical way in the molecules
- Attraction forces between the molecules on the surface of the liquid are referred to as surface tension
- The cohesive forces within the molecules tend to make the liquid into a spherical droplet representing the lowest energy
- Any media having an interface with two surfaces will possess surface energy
- The energy at the surface of a solid is greater than that of its interior
- In a space lattice, all the atoms are equally attracted to each other with equal interatomic distances and minimum energy
- At the surface of the lattice, the energy is greater as the outermost atoms are not equally attracted in all directions
- The interior atom is balanced due to its surrounding atomic attractions, whereas surface atom has one side that is exposed to outside and is not balanced.

MATERIALS IMPORTANT IN RELATION TO SURFACE TENSION

Mercury

Has high surface tension and forms droplets on amalgam alloy and wets the alloy particles.

Water

Has medium surface tension and forms droplets on silicone and resins but spreads while in contact with metals and porcelain.

Gold Alloys

- When melted, if it has high surface tension, the accuracy of casting is decreased
- Increasing the temperature of molten alloys decreases the surface tension
- Silver, platinum and gold adsorb oxygen readily by adsorption
- Gold attracts oxygen by secondary bonding forces.

Silver

- It forms silver oxide by chemical or primary bonding (termed chemisorption)
- In chemisorption, a chemical bond is formed between the adhesive and the adherent.

19. van der Waals Forces.

Synonyms

Interatomic secondary bonds/Intermolecular weak bonds.

SECONDARY BONDS

- Do not share electrons unlike primary bonds
- Due to the differences in charge among molecules and atomic groups, they form polar forces that attract the molecules.

Examples of Secondary Bonds

Combination of Hydrogen and Secondary Bonding

- No primary bonds exist between water and glass, yet when water freezes to ice crystals, it bonds to an automobile windshield
- Hydrogen bonding occurs in a water molecule in which the oxygen atoms are covalently (share electrons) bonds to two hydrogen atoms.

Mechanism

- The protons of the hydrogen atoms not bonded to the oxygen atoms become positively charged
- On the opposite side of the water molecule, the electrons in the outer orbit of the oxygen have a negative charge
- When such a water molecule comes in contact with another such water molecule, the positive hydrogen portion of one molecule is attracted to the negative oxygen portion of the neighboring molecule, forming hydrogen bridges.

Sorption of Water by Synthetic Dental Resins

This is due to intermolecular reactions.

REASON FOR SECONDARY OR VAN DER WAALS FORCES

- They are formed due to dipole attraction
- Normally, the electrons of the atoms are equally distributed around the nucleus and have an electrostatic field around the atom
- This electron field is fluctuating with positive and negative charges occurring
- A fluctuating dipole attracts other similar dipoles by weak interatomic forces.

FACTORS AFFECTING VAN DER WAALS FORCES

Interatomic Bond Distance

- Is the distance between the center of an atom and that of its neighbor and this depends on the diameter of the atoms involved
- The position at which the repulsion and attraction forces become equal is the equilibrium position of the atoms
- As the forces of attraction increase, the interatomic space decreases.

Bonding Energy

- Energy can be defined as a force integrated over a distance
- Molecules are attracted to each other by the amount of energy present
- Thermal and electrical factors increase the energy.

20. Contact Stomatitis.

Synonyms

Allergic contact stomatitis/Allergic contact dermatitis.

DEFINITION

Allergic contact stomatitis is an adverse reaction to dental materials.

TYPES OF LESIONS

- Local
- Contact-type lesions
- Distant reactions as itching on the palms of the hand or soles of the feet are also seen.

INTENSIVITY OF REACTIONS DEPEND ON

- Composition of the materials and their toxic components
- The amount of degradation products
- The concentration of absorbed and accumulated components.

DEFINITIVE DIAGNOSTIC TEST

Patch Test

- The suspected allergen is applied to the skin. If allergic, a small area of allergic contact dermatitis occurs
- The test generally takes from 48 to 96 hours, although a reaction may appear after 24 hours. This reaction may cause hyperemia, edema, vesicle formation and itching (Slavin and Ducomb, 1989).

ALLERGENS PRESENT IN DENTAL MATERIALS

- Chromium
- Cobalt
- Mercury
- Eugenol
- Monomer
- Colophonium
- Formaldehyde
- Nickel.

Acrylic Resins

- Acrylic resins release minute amounts of formaldehyde as a degradation product of unreacted monomers
- Formaldehyde can cause enhanced tissue reactions if persons are allergic to it
- Residual monomer is present because polymerization of resin-based materials is not complete
- If surface layer of resin is exposed to air, polymerization is incomplete
- Degradation of these materials releases components that cause local and systemic reactions.

This can be reduced by

Heat cured dentures. If chemically cured resins are used, they should be immersed in water for 24 hours before being worn.

Composite Materials

- Composite materials can cause gingival reactions as leachable components enter the permeable gingival epithelium
- The degree of gingival inflammation is less when placed against enamel surfaces.

Gold

- Very rarely some patients develop reaction to gold restorations
- The reactions vary from burning sensations and lichenoid lesions of the oral mucosa
- During patch testing with gold trichloride, few patients developed papular reactions. (Laeijendecker and von Joost, 1994).

Amalgam

- Many patients develop allergic reactions to mercury
- Reactions are seen as oral lichenoid lesions in contact with amalgam restorations.

Symptoms of Methyl Mercury Poisoning

- Weakness
- Fatigue
- Anorexia
- Weight loss
- Insomnia
- Irritability
- Shyness
- Dizziness
- Tremors in the extremities.

The average mercury level in the blood of subjects with amalgams was 0.7 ng/mL.

The lowest level of total blood mercury at which the earliest non-specific symptoms occur is 35 ng/mL. Hence, it was concluded that amalgam restorations are not harmful.

Nickel

- Seen more in female population than in male population (9:1)
- Females are more prone because all gold-plated jewellery is undercoated with a nickel
- Metal parts on clothing are nickel-plated for corrosion resistance
- Incidence of nasal and sinus cancer has been observed among nickel refinery workers (Nickel carbonyl is a known carcinogen).

Others

- Lozenges
- Cough drops
- Mouthwashes
- Dentifrices.

Reactions to these are burning, swelling and ulcerations of the oral tissues.

21. Microleakage.

DEFINITION

Flow of oral fluid bacteria into the microscopic gap between a prepared tooth surface and a restorative material is termed as microleakage.

SCHEMATIC DIAGRAM OF THE MICROLEAKAGE PHENOMENON

- Here the penetration of irritant from the oral cavity has extended along the entire tooth restoration interface, through the dentin and into the pulp
- Gross penetration of acids and micro-organisms leads to caries at the margins of the restoration
- Accumulation of debris in that area causes staining and discoloration
- If the leakage is severe, bacterial growth occurs between the restoration and the cavity wall and even into the dentinal tubules
- The toxic products produce irritation to the pulp leading to postoperative sensitivity following placement of the restoration **(Fig. 33)**
- Microleakage may be the greatest cause for recurrence of caries
- Amalgam restoration minimizes marginal leakage by forming corrosion products, which seal the interfaces between the tooth and the restoration
- The presence of calcium, phosphorus and demineralization of tooth structures adjacent to the amalgam restoration also are corrosion byproducts
- The ability to seal against microleakage is shared by both low and high copper amalgams. It is slower with high copper alloys
- The degree of microleakage at the restoration/tooth interfaces can be monitored by the penetration of tracers staining agents.

Acid Etching

Acid etching of enamel effectively seals interface gaps.

Varnish

Varnish also prevents penetration of corrosion products of amalgam into dentinal tubules, thereby reducing tooth discoloration associated with amalgam restoration. They also reduce tooth sensitivity and reduce infiltration of tissue fluids.

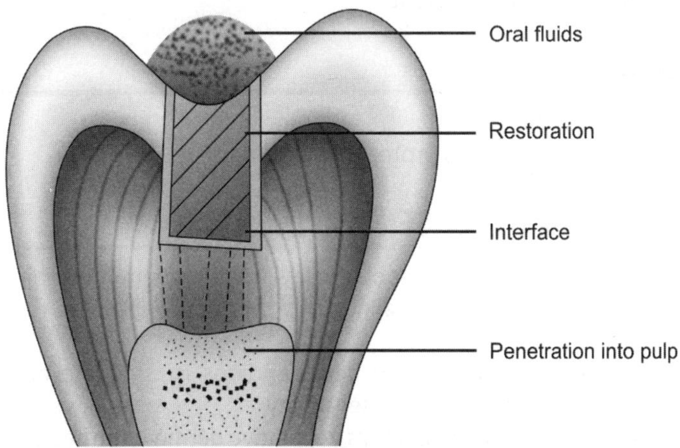

Fig. 33: Microleakage phenomenon

Restorative Materials that Decrease Microleakage

- Glass ionomer
- Polycarboxylate
- Composite.

Only adhesive materials reduce the space between the restoration and prepared cavity. All other restorative materials are more prone to microleakage where fluid debris flows between the restoration and teeth.

22. Dentin Hypersensitivity.

FACTORS INFLUENCING DENTIN HYPERSENSITIVITY

- Age and sex of the patient
- Age of the tooth
- Amount of sclerosis present
- Proximity to the pulp (RDT)
- Presence or absence of CH liners
- Depth of carious lesions
- The thickness of reparative dentin formed.

DENTIN HYPERSENSITIVITY DOES NOT OCCUR

- If sclerosis is present
- If reparative dentin thickness is present.

SYMPTOMS OCCUR

- If insufficient sclerosis is present
- Reparative dentin is not formed to protect the pulp.

REASONS FOR DENTIN HYPERSENSITIVITY

- During a restorative procedure, odontoblastic layer and predentin are injured, which forms outgrowth of dendrites to initiate healing. This process contributes to increased dentin hypersensitivity
- After 21 days, the regeneration of the nerve endings is complete and then dendrites degenerate causing a decrease in dentin sensitivity
- If symptoms disappear within 7 to 12 weeks, reparative dentin is formed to block the tubules and prevent sensitivity.

PROLONGED DENTIN HYPERSENSITIVITY

- When micromechanical bond fails
- When composite resin shrinks during polymerization
- Cohesive failure of the liner or base
- When dentinal tubules are open
- In cusp deformation
- Excessive occlusal loading of Class II posterior resin composites
- Flexing during chewing (because of a low elastic modulus)
- Thermal stimuli can cause thermal contraction of the resin and subsequent microleakage.

TREATING DENTIN HYPERSENSITIVITY

- The existing composite resin needs to be replaced with other conventional restorative material
- Encouraging reparative dentin by sealing the involved tubules
- Varnishes and base help to eliminate sensitivity
- Bonding systems seal dentinal tubules, avoiding postoperative sensitivity
- High resistance to solubility of current luting agents (cements) decreases postoperative sensitivity
- Restorative materials that contract on polymerization or thermal contraction should be avoided to prevent microleakage.

23. Solid Solution.

DEFINITION

When atoms of two metals intermingle randomly in a common space lattice in which the two metals are mutually soluble in the solid state, such alloys are called solid solutions.

Examples

- Most type of gold alloys
- Silver-Palladium system
- Copper in gold, platinum and palladium.

SIGNIFICANCE

- Grains of these alloys are similar to pure metal
- They are homogenous in structure with a single phase

- Most of alloys used in dentistry are solid solution
- In solid solutions, the atom of one of the alloys is distributed randomly through space lattice of the other and remains so after solidification as a single phase.

TERMS RELATED TO SOLID SOLUTION

Solvent

Is that metal which occupies the space lattice (occupies more than one half the total number).

Solute

Is the metal that distributes itself randomly.

TYPES OF SOLID SOLUTION

- Substitutional
- Interstitial
- Ordered.

Substitutional

Here the atoms occupy space lattice positions normally occupied by solvent atoms in the pure metal.

Example

Silver palladium (Pa-solvent and Ag-solute).

Interstitial

- Here solute atoms are present in positions between the solvent atoms
- The solute atoms should be smaller in size and less in concentration than solvent atoms.

Example

Steel (Carbon in iron).

Ordered

When the solute and solvent have affinity toward each other at low temperature, diffusion forms an ordering process.

Example

- Aluminum and copper at high temperature are random or substitutional but at 50% wt of Au and 49.8% wt of Cu
- If cooled below 400°C, Au atoms move to the corner of the cube and Cu atoms to the faces. Here copper atoms are three times more than gold atoms forming a super lattice or ordered structure.

REQUIREMENTS FOR SOLID SOLUBILITY

- Atom size
- Valence
- Chemical affinity
- Lattice type.

Atom size

- If the two atoms in the alloy differ in size by less than 15%, it is favorable for solid solution
- If greater than 15%, then it can cause multiple phases.

Atomic Diameters of a Few Metals

Metal	Diameter in Angstrom units	Type of atom structure
Au	2.882	Face-centered cubic system
Ag	2.888	
Pl	2.775	
Pa	2.750	
Cu	2.556	
Sn	3.016	Body-centered
Zn	2.665	Close-packed
Si	2.351	Diamond cubic

Valence

- Metals of same valence and size form solid solutions
- If valences are different, then higher valence metal will be soluble in lower valence.

Chemical Affinity

- Metals with less affinity are more likely to form solid solutions
- Metals with more affinity will form intermetallic compounds.

Lattice Type

- Metals should be of the same type of crystal lattice
- If size factor is less than 8%, they have a better chance of forming solid solution.

PHYSICAL PROPERTIES OF SOLID SOLUTIONS

- When a solute atom displaces a solvent atom, a strained condition occurs within the lattice and slip is inhibited
- The more the solute metal added to the solvent, the more are the strength and hardness
- This phenomenon increases strength, proportional limit and surface hardness of the alloy but decreases ductility.

Example

Cu 5% in Au: Increases strength and hardness.

24. Composition, Requirements, Types, Properties and Uses of Impression Compounds.

COMPOSITION

- Composed of a mixture of waxes
- Shellac, stearic acid and gutta-percha, which are added to improve plasticity and workability, are referred to as plasticizers
- Thermoplastic resins are used along with natural resins
- The filler which is present is used for strength and to increase the viscosity at temperatures above 37°C and increase the rigidity of the compound at room temperature
- Coloring agent.

REQUIREMENTS OF IMPRESSION COMPOUND

- It should be flowable at oral temperature without hurting soft tissues
- It should be dimensionally stable on hardening
- It should be able to be shaped by trimming and moulding
- It should be economical
- It should possess adequate shelf life.

TYPES

Depending on Softening Temperature

- Low fusing
- Medium fusing
- High fusing.

Low Fusing

Synonym

Tracing sticks.

Availability

Sticks or cones.

Uses

- For border molding (Green sticks)
- For copper band impressions
- Used to stabilize matrix bands.

Properties

Similar to medium fusing except for flow.

Medium Fusing

Availability

Cake form.

Properties

- Are thermoplastic: They soften on heating and harden on cooling
- Softened by immersion in hot water or warming in flame
- Softening in hot water is preferred for uniform heating
- Cannot be used in undercut areas as impression material
- They have low flow and cannot record details as elastic impression materials can
- Repeated use can cause plasticizers to leach out, making the compound brittle.

Use

For impressions of edentulous patient (preliminary impression).

High Fusing

Properties

Fusion Temperature

- It is the temperature at which the softened material remains plastic while the impression is being obtained
- Tray should be held firmly in position until the impression cools below the fusion temperature.

Thermal Conductivity and Contraction

- Thermal conductivity of these materials is low, hence, it needs to be uniformly softened and thoroughly cooled in the tray before the impression is withdrawn from the mouth
- The average linear contraction of impression compounds on cooling from mouth temperature to room temperature of 25°C varies between 0.3% and 0.4%.

Leaching out

Prolonged immersion or overheating in the water bath can produce leaching of the plasticizers, making the compound brittle and grainy.

Flow

- After softening and during the impression, the material should flow easily
- If flow is great, distortion can occur when the impression is withdrawn from the mouth.

Distortion

Relaxation of stresses can result in warpage or distortion of the impression.

To minimize distortion, the impression should be cooled before removal from the mouth and should be immediately poured within the first hour.

Uses

- As special tray material in conjunction with wash impression

- Using this impression as a tray, a thin layer of a second impression material, as ZOE paste, hydrocolloid, or a nonaqueous elastomer is used to make a wash impression (called secondary impression)
- As preliminary impression material

Copper Band Impression/Tube Impression

For a single-tooth preparation, a cylindrical copper band/matrix band is filled with the softened compound.

After cooling the compound, the impression is withdrawn and a cast, or die, is made.

25. Composition of Alginate Impression Material.

ALGINATE

ANSI/ADA Specification No. 18.

COMPOSITION

Potassium alginate	18%	Reacts with calcium ions
Calcium sulfate dihydrate	14%	Reacts with potassium alginate to form insoluble calcium alginate gel
Potassium sulfate/potassium zinc fluoride	10%	Gypsum hardener
Trisodium phosphate	2%	Retarder (increases the working time)
Diatomaceous earth	56%	Filler
Organic glycols	Traces	For dustless alginates
Wintergreen, peppermint	Traces	For flavor
Pigments	Traces	Color
Ammonium salts and chlorhexidine	2%	Disinfectant

COMPONENTS AND THEIR FUNCTIONS

Filler

- Diatomaceous earth increases the strength and stiffness of the alginate gel, produces a smooth texture and ensures a firm gel surface that is not tacky

- It also aids in forming the sol by dispersing the alginate powder particles in the water
- Zinc oxide also acts as a filler and has some influence on the physical properties and setting time of the gel
- The amount of filler present controls the flexibility of the set impression material
- The amount of filler present indicates the hardness or the softness of the material. The injection type is more fluid after mixing and more flexible after setting.

Retarder

- The concentration of sodium phosphate differs depending on regular and fast-set alginates. There are tray and injection types available
- Salts that can be used as retarders are sodium or potassium phosphate, potassium oxalate, or potassium carbonate, trisodium phosphate, sodium tripolyphosphate and tetrasodium pyrophosphate. The latter two are now the most commonly used
- If approximately 15 g of the powder is mixed with 40 ml of water, gelation will occur in about 3 to 4 minutes at room temperature.

Reactor

Calcium sulfate can be used as the reactor. The dihydrate form is generally used, but sometimes the hemihydrate produces an increased shelf life of the powder and gives better dimensional stability of the gel.

Gypsum Hardener

A fluoride, such as potassium titanium fluoride, is added as an accelerator for the setting of the stone to ensure that a hard, dense stone cast surface is produced against the impression.

26. Laminate Technique.

PROCEDURE

This a combination of agar-alginate technique.

The agar impression material is loaded into a syringe. This syringe material is injected around the prepared tooth.

Meanwhile the alginate material is loaded onto a stock tray and impression is made.

The tray containing chilled alginate bonds to the syringe agar.

The alginate gels by a chemical reaction, whereas the agar gels by means of contact with the cool alginate rather than the water circulating through the tray.

As agar is in contact with the prepared teeth, maximum detail is reproduced.

Advantages

- Cost is less because only the syringe material needs to be heated
- Less preparation time
- More accurate detailed reproduction in comparison to alginate impression
- Water cooled trays are not required.

Disadvantages

- The bond between the agar and the alginate is not strong
- The higher viscosity alginate displaces the agar during seating
- The dimensional inaccuracy of the alginate limits the use to single units.

27. Noneugenol Paste.

METHOD OF FORMATION

When zinc oxide reacts with carboxylic acid, saponification produces an insoluble soap.

Reaction

$ZnO + 2RCOOH \rightarrow (RCOO)_2Zn + H_2O$.

- Powdered acids can be dissolved in a liquid-carrying agent, such as ethyl alcohol
- This reaction is not affected by temperature or humidity
- Bactericides and other medicaments can be incorporated without interfering with the reaction.

Other acids that can react with ZOE

- Ortho ethoxybenzoic acid (EBA).

Uses of Eugenol and Noneugenol Paste

Surgical Pastes

- After gingivoplasty, ZOE paste can be placed over the wound to retain the medicament in place and to promote healing
- Surgical pastes are softer and slower setting when compared to impression pastes
- Surgical paste should be capable of being formed into a rope for ease of packing into the gingival wounds and the interproximal spaces

- Surgical paste should be strong enough to resist displacement during mastication, yet not so brittle.

Bite Registration Pastes

- ZOE pastes are used as recording materials in complete dentures and fixed or removable partial denture procedures
- Petrolatum is applied around the patient's oral cavity to prevent the tendency of the paste to adhere to oral tissues
- ZOE impression paste gives an accurate and stable interocclusal relationship as it offers no resistance to closing of the mandible.

Reason for Use of Noneugenol Paste

- ZOE pastes when used as secondary impression material can cause burning sensation when in contact with soft tissues. This is due to the eugenol content
- When it is used as surgical packs, ZOE contains free eugenol which may leach out. Here the Eugenol can cause chronic gastric disturbances
- Many patients find the taste of eugenol disagreeable
- In the above situation, noneugenol pastes are used as substitutes.

28. Electroplating of Impressions.

ELECTROFORMED DIES

Advantages of Electroplated Dies

- High strength
- Hardness
- Abrasion resistance.

Types of Electroplating

- Copper plating
- Silver plating.

Procedure

An elastomeric impression is made which can reproduce a line 4 μm or less in width easily.

Preparation of Impression

- The impression surface required to coat with silver or copper is treated to conduct electricity. This process is referred to as metallizing
- Various metallizing agents such as bronzing powder and aqueous suspensions of silver powder and powdered graphite are burnished on the surface of the impression with a camel-hair brush
- These metallizing agents aid in the deposition of a thin layer of metal, such as silver, on the required area of the impression material. This metal layer represents the finished die

Method of Electroplating

Copper-plated compound dies were used in the early 1930s and silver-plated dies later.

Silver Plating

- The electroplating bath is a solution of silver cyanide or silver nitrate. Cyanide solution is poisonous, hence not commonly used and, if used, precautions need to be taken
- Chemical deposition of silver from a silver nitrate solution gives a greater surface detail reproduction
- In the silver-plating process, the greater the concentration of silver in the bath, the faster the silver is deposited
- The acid content increases the *throwing power*
- Metallized surface of the impression is the cathode in the electroplating bath
- A plate of silver at least twice the size of the area to be plated is used as the anode
- A direct current is applied for approximately 10 hours using 5 to 10 mA/cm^2 of cathode surface
- The impression that contains the electroformed die surface is then filled with dental stone
- These dies have greater surface hardness and resistance to abrasion than one of gypsum
- The model and die are prepared in the normal manner and margins of the die are trimmed with a finishing disk.

Points to Note

- Hydrocolloid impressions are difficult to electroplate
- Silver electroformed dies made from polysulfide rubber impressions are clinically acceptable
- The polysulfide rubber impression is cleaned thoroughly and dried. It is then metallized with a fine silver powder, which results in a superior surface on the electroformed die.

29. Imbibition and Syneresis.

IMBIBITION

If the agar or alginate impression is placed in water or in a humid environment, it will absorb water and this process is called imbibition.

Clinical Significance

The gel swells during imbibition and alters the original dimensions of the impression. Hence, the cast which is made from that will be smaller in dimensions.

Control of Imbibition

- Immediate pouring of cast.
- If there is a period of time before pouring the cast, then the impression should be wrapped in a moist paper towel
- The paper towel should not be too wet or imbibition may occur.

SYNERESIS

If the agar or alginate impression is placed too long in contact with the outside atmosphere, the gel may lose water by evaporation from its surface or by exudation of fluid onto the surface by a process known as *syneresis.*

Clinical Significance

- The gel shrinks during syneresis and alters the original dimensions of the impression. Hence, the cast which is made will alter in dimensions
- The exudate that appears on the surface of the gel during and after syneresis may be either alkaline or acid
- The removal of water or fluid from the micelles of the gel by evaporation or syneresis causes the gel to shrink.

REASON FOR IMBIBITION AND SYNERESIS

- The hydrocolloid gel contains a large percentage of water
- If the water content of the gel is reduced, the gel will shrink and if the gel takes up water, it will expand or swell
- These changes in dimensions can lead to an inaccurate cast.

30. Manipulation of Agar.

MANIPULATION OF AGAR IMPRESSION MATERIALS

Steps in Manipulation

- Advanced preparation of the material
- Preparation immediately before making the impression
- The making of the impression.

Advanced Preparation of the Material

- The hydrocolloid is supplied in two forms, syringe and tray materials. Tubes to fill the water-cooled trays and cartridges for use in the syringes
- The only difference between the syringe and tray material is the color and a greater fluidity of the syringe material
- First the hydrocolloid gel is reverted to the sol state by placing the material in liquefaction bath at 100°C for a minimum of 10 minutes
- After it has been liquefied, the material is stored until it is needed for use.

Preparation Immediately before Making the Impression

Conditioning or Tempering

- A tube of hydrocolloid sol is removed from the storage bath
- The tray is filled
- A gauze pad is placed over the top of the tray material
- The tray is placed in the tempering section (approximately 45°C) of the conditioning unit for 3 to 10 minutes to ensure that all the material has reached a temperature below 55°C which can be tolerated by oral tissues.

Points to follow during Preparation of the Material

- The loaded tray should not be kept in the bath for more than 10 minutes
- A gauze is placed on the material loaded on tray and placed in the storage bath to prevent imbibition
- The gauze is removed and the contaminated surface layer of material is peeled off along with the gauze
- This fresh surface adheres easily to the syringed material injected over the prepared teeth
- The syringe material is taken from the storage bath and applied to the prepared tooth surface.

Impression Making

- The tray is positioned and seated with light pressure and held in place passively
- Gelation is accelerated by circulating cool water, approximately 18° to 21°C through the tray for 3 to 5 minutes

- Waiting an extra minute greatly increases the strength and tear resistance. The impression is removed with a sudden jerk.

Wet Field Technique

The impression areas are flooded with warm water, then the syringe material is introduced quickly in bulk to cover the occlusal and incisal areas. The tray material is then seated over the syringe material.

31. Polysulfide Impression Material.

ADA Specification No. 19.

Composition

Polysulfide impression material consists of a base paste and catalyst paste.

Base Paste Contains

- Polysulfide polymer
- Lithopone or titanium dioxide as filler to provide the required strength
- Dibutyl phthalate as a plasticizer to give appropriate viscosity to the paste
- Sulphur, 0.5%, to enhance the reaction.

Accelerator Paste Contains

- Lead dioxide which gives it a dark-brown color
- Dibutyl phthalate as a plasticizer to give appropriate viscosity to the paste
- Lithopone or titanium dioxide as filler to provide the required strength
- Oleic acid or stearic acid as retarders to control the rate of setting.

Availability

- Light body for wash impression
- Regular body
- Putty
- Monophase.
  Depending on the above, the packing differs.
  Light body and regular body are supplied in tubes and putty in jars.

Factors Affecting the Reaction

- The polymerization reaction of polysulfide polymers is exothermic

- Exothermic reaction depends on the amount of total material and the concentration of initiators
- Moisture and temperature alter the course of reaction
- Hot humid conditions accelerate the setting of polysulfide impression material
- The condensation reaction byproduct is water
- Loss of byproduct from the set material has a significant effect on the dimensional stability of the impression.

Manipulation

- Equal lengths of the two pastes are squeezed onto a pad or glass slab
- Catalyst paste is collected on a stainless steel spatula and then distributed over the base paste spreading over the mixing pad
- The mass is then scraped up with the spatula blade and smoothed until the mixed paste is of uniform color with no streaks of the base or catalyst appearing in the mixture
- Medium-body and heavy-body polysulfide impression pastes are extremely viscous and sticky, making it difficult to mix
- In putty consistencies, the dough of base and catalyst paste are taken in equal amount and kneaded without streaks.

Working and Setting Times

- Working and setting times are measured by an oscillating rheometer
- An increase in temperature accelerates the curing rate decreasing both the setting and working times
- Cooling the glass slab and mixing at low temperature increases the working time
- High oral temperature decreases the setting time of the impression material
- Adding a drop of water accelerates the curing rate
- The curing rate is affected if the base to catalyst paste ratio is altered.

Advantages

- Long working time
- Good accuracy
- High tear resistance
- Less hydrophobic
- Inexpensive and good shelf life.

Disadvantages

- Requires a custom tray
- Must be poured in stone immediately
- Chances for significant distortion
- Odor offends patients
- Messy and stains clothes
- Second pour is less accurate.

Shelf Life

- If stored in the tubes under normal environmental conditions, the shelf life is long
- Storage in a cool environment prolongs shelf life

- Even when stored for 7 days at 60 ± 2°C (140 ± 3.6°F), the material must still meet the test for permanent deformation.

Modifications

- The lead dioxide reactor contributes to some of the disadvantages of polysulfide impression material
- Organic hydroperoxide can be used (e.g. t-butyl hydroperoxide), but these compounds have poor dimensional stability because of the hydroperoxide volatility
- The inorganic hydroxides, such as copper, are used as the cross-linking system in dental polysulfides.

32. Condensation Silicone/Polysilicone Impression Material.

Composition

Supplied as base paste and liquid catalyst.

Base Paste

- A polymer: α-w-hydroxy-terminated polydimethyl siloxane.
- Fillers
- Coloring agents.

Catalyst Liquid

Filler: Colloidal silica or microsized metal oxide.

Availability

Condensation silicone paste materials and putty can be made in a variety of colors. Pastel pinks, blues, greens and purples are common.

Chemistry

- The condensation reaction occurs when the trifunctional and tetrafunctional alkyl silicates (tetraethyl orthosilicate), react in the presence of stannous octoate ($Sn[C_7H_{15}COO]_2$). These reactions take place at room temperature, hence referred to as *room temperature vulcanization* (RTV) silicones
- The filler particle size should be within the range of 5 to 10 μm. The particles are surface treated to provide better compatibility and reinforcement of the silicone rubber.

Disadvantages

- These silicones have low cohesive energy level and a weaker intermolecular interaction
- The filler particles tend to separate from the polymer and the dispensed material appears as two components
- They have large polymerization shrinkage
- Putty material has low polymerization shrinkage because the filler content is more in putty with less polymer present. (Referred to as *law of mixtures*)
- The overall thermal expansion is less than that of the polymer because the filler particle has a smaller coefficient of thermal expansion.

Manipulation

- A length of the base is dispensed from the tube onto a mixing pad and one drop of the liquid catalyst is added for each unit length of base
- They are mixed till a uniform color is obtained indicating a homogenous mix
- The putty material is supplied as a very thick paste and a liquid accelerator. First the liquid accelerator is incorporated into the putty by mixing on a pad, then later kneading with the fingers
- The putty is supplied in a jar and dispensed by using a scoop
- The manufacturer's directions indicate the number of drops of accelerator needed for each scoop
- Two-paste putty systems are also available. This is manipulated by taking equal amount of both base and catalyst paste and kneading the material with the fingers
- Sulphur in the gloves can inhibit the setting of the putty
- Putty is used as the tray material in conjunction with a low-viscosity silicone as in the multiple-mix technique same as for polysulfide.

Advantages

- Adequate working and setting time
- Pleasant odor and no staining
- Adequate tear strength
- Better elastic properties on removal
- Less distortion on removal
- Condensation silicones are compatible with all gypsum products.

Disadvantages

- Adequate accuracy if poured immediately
- Poor dimensional stability
- Potential for significant distortion
- Putty-wash method is technique sensitive
- Slightly more expensive
- Poor to adequate shelf life.

Disinfection of the Impression

By immersing in commercial antimicrobial solutions for less than an hour.

33. Addition Reaction Silicone (Vinyl Polysiloxane).

Synonyms

Polyvinylsiloxane or vinyl polysiloxane.

Brand Names

- Baysilex CD (Miles)
- Examix (GC-Amer)
- Hydrosil (Caulk)
- Imprint (3M).

Composition

It is supplied as base and catalyst paste.

Base Paste Contains

- Vinyl silicone
- Polymethyl hydrogen siloxane
- Siloxane prepolymers
- Hybrid silicone (present if platinum is contained in catalyst paste)
- Filler
- Surfactant (to make it hydrophilic).

Catalyst Paste Contains

- Di-vinyl polydimethyl siloxane
- Siloxane prepolymers
- Platinum salt activator
- Filler
- Retarder
- Platinum or palladium are added to some brands to act as a scavenger for the released hydrogen gas.

Chemistry

- Addition reaction activated by a platinum salt catalyst is terminated with vinyl groups and is cross-linked with hydride groups
- If catalyst to base ratio is precise and if no impurities are present, no reaction byproducts are formed
- If the proportions are not accurate or if impurities (moisture and polymeric) are present, hydrogen gas is formed, which can cause pinpoint voids
- Hydrogen gas can be limited by using impression materials containing platinum or palladium or pouring of the impression can be delayed for an hour.

Manipulation

Light-body and medium-body vinyl polysiloxanes utilize automatic mixing device, can be hand-mixed on a pad also.

Automatic Device

- Aids in greater uniformity in proportioning and mixing, less air entrapment during mixing and less time
- Chances of contamination of the material are minimized
- The tips in the device vary in diameter, in length and number of spiral units
- More spiral units provide better mixing. (As a 13-spiral unit compared to a 11-spiral tip)
- To ensure that the tip is not clogged, a small amount is extruded from the cartridge before mixing tip is attached
- The mixed material should have uniform color
- Due to shear-thinning behavior, they are suitable for automatic dispensing.

Method

- The mixed impression material is ejected directly into the adhesive-coated tray or onto the prepared teeth
- Meanwhile, the medium body can be mixed on a pad with spatula by taking equal lengths of catalyst and base paste and loaded onto the custom tray
- Immediately after syringing the light body material onto the tooth, the medium body loaded onto the tray is positioned and the impression is made
- The putty is supplied as two jars of high-viscosity base and catalyst materials with same viscosities and is manipulated by manual method and formed into a dough. This is used as preliminary impression for edentulous patient or as border molding material
- The monophase can be used as a tray material and syringe material due to its shear thinning property.

Shelf Life

Have a 2-year shelf life. The silicone material tubes or containers must be stored in a cool, dry environment.

Advantages

- Shorter setting time
- Easy to mix—automatic mixing devices
- Adequate tear strength
- Extremely high accuracy
- Undetectable distortion on removal
- Dimensionally stable even after 1 week
- Less distortion on removal
- Good compatibility with gypsum.

Disadvantages

- It is hydrophobic in nature. Presently hydrophilic addition silicones are available in the market that contain a surfactant to wet soft tissue and allow the poured stone to flow better

- These materials need a dry field for accuracy of impression
- Latex gloves contains sulphur that inhibits the setting of the addition silicone impression materials, which, in turn, can cause distortion of the impression
- Expensive.

Recent Advances

- The mixing devices, the gun and holding device, are made smaller, hence are made easier to manipulate. The smaller mixing tubes prevent the excess waste of material and, hence, the cost
- Visible light-curable polyether urethane dimethacrylate was tried which contained light-cure photo initiators, photo accelerators and silicon dioxide filler
- The new hydrophilic polymers as dentin bonding agents can prevent setting problem associated with the above material
- The main problem is to direct the light to all areas of the mouth for proper curing of the material.

34. Describe the Composition, Manipulation, Properties and Uses of Impression Plaster.

IMPRESSION PLASTER

Composition

Powder

Constituent	Function	Percentage
Calcium sulfate β hemihydrate $(CaSO_4)$: H_2O	Main component	
Potassium sulfate	Reduces the expansion	4%
Borax	Reduces the rate of setting	0.4–1%
Starch	To help disintegration of the impression on separation from the plaster/stone model (called soluble plasters).	
Alizarin red	Gives it a pink color so it can be distinguished from the cast.	0.04%
A flavoring agent.		
Gum tragacanth	To improve the cohesive properties of the mixed plaster.	

- The additives may be blended with the plaster powder, or supplied as an aqueous solution to be mixed with plaster
- If as a solution, it contains potassium sulfate, borax and alizarin red in the above percentage. This solution is called 'AE' or 'anti-expansion' solution.

Manipulation

- Calcium sulfate hemihydrate when mixed with water reacts to form a rigid mass of calcium sulfate dihydrate
- The plaster should be mixed with water or an AE solution in the ratio of 100 g to 50–60 mL without air bubbles
- The amount of potassium sulfate is more than found in model plaster, as minimum expansion is only required for impressions.

Proportioning and Mixing

- Impression plaster is mixed in a rubber bowl, with a stiff, wide-bladed spatula
- Variations in the water/powder ratio will affect both the consistency and setting time and the strength of the impression
- Increased amount of water gives a more fluid mix with a longer setting time and a weaker impression
- A suitable quantity of powder is sifted into the required amount of water and left undisturbed for 30 seconds, in which time the powder will be wetted
- The mass is then given the minimum amount of spatulation for a homogenous mass, which usually is 30 seconds or less.

Working Time and Setting Time

- The working time and setting time are 2–3 minutes
- The mixed material is fluid in consistency and the impression technique is called muco-static
- The material is loaded in a special tray, made of acrylic or shellac, or can be used as a wash impression.

Pouring of Impression Plaster

Separating Media

- A separating agent needs to be applied in order to prevent the dental stone poured into the impression from dissolving and penetrating into the porous plaster of the impression
- A separating medium needs to be applied before pouring dental stone into the impression for easy removal of the impression from the cast
- Various separating agents used are alcoholic solutions of varnishes, waxes, ethereal solution of colloid, soap solutions, water glass and liquid paraffin.

Properties

- It is hydrophilic and, hence, adapts readily to the soft tissues, recording their surface detail with great accuracy
- The dimensional stability of impression plaster is very good

- A separating medium as sodium alginate must be used between the model plaster and the impression plaster
- The material is rigid once set and thus unable to record undercuts and hence can be used only in an edentulous patient
- On storage of a plaster impression, the dimensional changes are small, though a small degree of drying shrinkage may occur
- Impression plasters are nontoxic, but are unpleasant for the patient, because they produce a dry sensation in the mouth
- The setting time can be controlled by use of the appropriate quantities of additives
- Plaster is stable on storage, provided it is kept in an airtight container
- If exposed to air during storage, it will absorb water
- This causes crystals of calcium sulfate dihydrate to form on the surface of the hemihydrate crystals which result in shortening of the setting time
- Changes in dimensions occurred after storing the disinfected impressions in air for 24 hours.

Uses

- As an impression material for hyperplastic ridges
- It also can be used as corrective wash, where excessive salivary secretion is present
- Other uses are the mounting of casts on articulators in which impression plaster is mixed with high-strength stone for study models as it sets faster than normal dental stone.

35. Compare and Contrast Between Dental Plaster and Dental Stone.

OR

What is the Difference Between Dental Plaster and Dental Stone? Add a Note on Setting Time and Expansion.

COMPARISON OF DENTAL PLASTER AND DENTAL STONE

Manufacturing

Dental Plaster (β-hemihydrate)

It is also called as 'alabaster'. Plaster, the gypsum, is ground to a fine powder and the material is heated at 120°C in open pans, which results in partial dehydration of the gypsum to yield the hemihydrate.

Dental Stone (α-hemihydrate)

It is also called Hydrocal and is obtained by heating under steam pressure in an autoclave. The hemihydrate produced can recrystallize to yield a more regular crystal form.

Densite Stone

It is also called crystacal. Hemihydrate crystals of a very regular nature can be obtained by adding gypsum to the boiling $CaCl_2$ solution.

Color

Dental Plaster

Cheap and white in color.

Dental Stone

It is more expensive and a dye is added to give it color. Depending on the dye added, the dental stones are available in various colors. Commonest are green and yellow.

Particle Size and Shape

Dental Plaster

Calcined hemihydrate particles are larger, irregular and porous.

Dental Stone

The particles of the autoclaved material are smaller, regular and nonporous.

Water/Powder Ratio

Dental Plaster

Calcined hemihydrate (plaster) 50–60 mL/100 g.

Dental Stone

- Autoclaved hemihydrate (dental stone) 22–35 mL/100 g
- Porous particles as in dental plaster absorb lot of water compared to dental stone
- The greater the quantity of excess water, the more porous (or less dense) is the set material. Thus, the porosity of set plaster is greater than the porosity of set stone.

Mechanical Properties of the Set Material

Strength and hardness depend on the density of the material, thus stone is harder and stronger than plaster.

Applications

- Dental stone is the material of choice for master cast used in construction of dentures, dies for crowns, bridge and inlay work and binders for casting investments

- When strength is not of primary importance, plaster is used as for mounting casts and some orthodontic study casts.

SETTING TIMES AND SETTING EXPANSION

Setting is accompanied by

1. Evolution of heat (exothermic reaction).
2. Development of strength (interpenetration of crystallites).
3. Setting expansion.

Steps in Setting

1. Calcium sulfate hemihydrate dissolves in the water to give (Ca_2 and SO_4) ions. The solubility of hemihydrate is about 0.8%.
2. Induction period is the time between mixing and the formation of the saturated solution, characterized by the ability of the mix to flow.
3. At the end of the induction period, the glossy surface is lost and crystal growth begins.
4. The dissolved calcium sulfate hemihydrate reacts with the water and forms calcium sulfate dihydrate.
5. The solubility of calcium sulfate dihydrate is very low and a supersaturated solution is formed.
6. This supersaturated solution is unstable and calcium sulfate dihydrate crystals precipitate out as stable crystals.
7. Spherulites are rosettes of long, needle-like crystals growing from isolated sites of nucleation.
8. As the stable calcium sulfate dihydrate precipitates out of the solution, more calcium sulfate hemihydrate is dissolved and this continues until all the hemihydrate has dissolved.

Initial set: The setting time is measured by the ability of the setting plaster or stone to withstand a stress. The initial set takes place when the lighter needle *fails to indent* the surface of the setting plaster and during this period, major trimming can be carried out.

Final set: At the final set, the material has become hard and brittle and cannot be cut with a knife.

Hardness testing device: The device consists of a mass of 300 g applied to a flat needle of diameter 1 mm. The material is set when the needle fails to indent the surface by more than 2 mm.

Setting Time

Dental plaster: The setting time is 5–10 minutes.

Dental stone: The setting time can be up to 20 minutes.

Factors in Setting Expansion

- The linear expansion is in the range of 0.3–0.4% for most plasters and 0.35–0.008% for dental stones. This expansion is caused by the outward thrust of the growing crystals of dihydrate
- The expanded set material contains crystals of dihydrate and pores
- The volume of crystals of the set material is less than the initial volume of the hemihydrate, approximately 7%
- If mixed plaster is placed under water at the initial set stage, a greater expansion on setting occurs. This is hygroscopic expansion.

36. Accelerators and Retarders in Gypsum Products.

ACCELERATORS

- Potassium sulfate
- Sodium chloride
- Sodium sulfate
- Calcium sulfate dihydrate.

Potassium Sulfate

- Potassium sulfate (K_2SO_4) reacts with the water and hemihydrate to produce 'syngenite' ($K_2(CaSO_4)$ $2H_2O$) which crystallizes rapidly and increases more crystal growth
- This has the effect of reducing the overall expansion and accelerating the setting reaction. When present as a 2% solution in water, it will reduce the setting time from approximately 10 minutes to 4 minutes.

Sodium Chloride

- Sodium chloride provides additional sites for crystal formation
- The higher density of crystals limits the growth of the crystals and, hence, reduces their ability to push each other apart. This results in a reduction of the apparent expansion.

Calcium Sulfate Dihydrate

- The addition of a small amount of calcium sulfate dihydrate will provide additional sites for nucleation and act as an accelerator.
- It will reduce both the working and the setting times.

Sodium Sulfate

- Can be used as accelerators in low concentrations but act as retarders in high concentrations
- In low concentrations, these materials aid in the dissolution of the plaster powder (decrease induction period), but interfere with the nucleation of gypsum in high concentrations.

RETARDERS

Borax

- The addition of borax ($Na_2B_4O_7$ $10H_2O$) counteracts the increased rate of setting due to the inclusion accelerators
- Borax retards the setting process
- The addition of borax leads to the formation of calcium borate, which deposits on the dihydrate crystals and prevents further growth
- For example, hydrated sodium borate

- When the plaster or stone powder is mixed with an appropriate aqueous solution of borax (0.9%w/w), the powder particles become coated with a thin layer of $Ca_2B_6O_{11}5H_2O$ (*'colemanite'*) which is very insoluble and delays the dissolution of the powder (increased induction period).

Potassium Citrate

- Potassium citrate acts as a retarder and is sometimes added in addition to borax
- By regulating the amount of additives, gypsum products can produce the correct degree of expansion and the correct working and setting times
- The low setting expansion of stone and densite make them ideal for dies and models for metal and ceramic work.

FUNCTION

Combinations of accelerators and retarders, in solution, can control the setting expansion and setting time.

37. Terra Alba.

DEFINITION

- Terra Alba is a pure, white and finely-ground gypsum
- Terra Alba is pulverized gypsum used in making paper, paints and as a nutrient for growing yeast
- Terra in Latin means earth and Alba means white
- Terra Alba is also called food-grade gypsum.

GYPSUM

- Gypsum is calcium sulfate combined with two molecules of water of crystallization
- The other gypsum varieties are alabaster, spar, satin spar and selenite
- Gypsum is a very brilliant white and in tone is bluish
- As the properties are neutral, it can be mixed with most other pigments without affecting them or being affected by them in any way
- Gypsum is soluble in water. At temperature of about 300 degrees F, gypsum loses its water of crystallization and forms a white powder, which has the property of combining with water and setting into a hard mass
- Product is sold as Plaster of Paris.

USES OF TERRA ALBA

As Accelerator

- Terra Alba in the concentration of 0.5%–1.0% in water or slurry water containing terra alba can be used to accelerate setting reaction of gypsum
- Terra Alba 1% acts as an accelerator by providing additional nuclei of crystallization.

As Pigment

- For use as a pigment, it is ground up in the form of a soft white powder
- Particle size is 12 microns and is 98% pure calcium sulfate.

As Food Additive

ACG *Terra Alba* is an economical food additive and pharmaceutical grade calcium sulfate.
As nutrient—in growing yeast.
In making of paper and paints.

38. Space Lattice.

DEFINITION

- Space lattice is the space in which atoms are arranged such that every atom is situated similarly to every other atom
- The type of space lattice is defined by the length of three of the unit cell edges (axes) and the angles between the edges.

Types of Bonds in Space Lattice

- Primary
- Secondary
- Metallic.

Number of Space Lattices Possible

Three types of lattices called P, I and F

1. P—primitive—8 points
2. I—body centered—9 points—one in the middle
3. F—face centered—point on each face.
   There are 230 possible combinations in relation to crystal systems.
   Of these, 14 types of space lattice combinations are possible in various dental materials.

Significance of Space Lattice in Dental Materials

- Most of the dental materials belong to cubic forms
- The atoms are arranged at points of intersection of three sets of parallel planes each set perpendicular to the other planes referred to as crystal planes
- Depending on the space lattice arrangement, the strength of the metal varies
- Even waxes have space lattices, though they are amorphous
- The arrangement within a space lattice always acquires a minimum energy within the structure and causes an equilibrium state to occur
- Most of the space lattices are uniformly spaced and closely arranged to maintain a low internal energy
- Space lattice indicates the stability of a material and, in turn, the strength.

Most common Types of Crystalline Space Lattices

- Simple cubic
- Body-centered cubic
- Face-centered cubic
- Rhobic
- Orthorhombic
- Rhombohedral
- Monoclinic
- Triclinic
- Tetragonal
- Simple hexagonal
- Close-packed hexagonal.

Simple Cubic

In a cubic space lattice, the axes are all of equal length and meet at 90° angle **(Fig. 34)**.

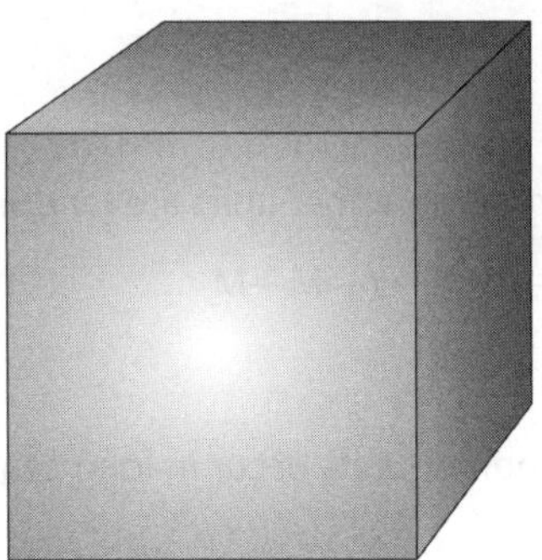

Fig. 34: Simple cubic

Space Lattices in Noncrystalline Form

- Short range order lattice form
- Long range order lattice forms mostly in crystalline forms
- Example of short range lattice form: Glass is a ordered arrangement of units with a number of disordered units present between the ordered structure and are called super-cooled liquids.

39. Explain Copolymerization with the help of Suitable Examples.

COPOLYMERIZATION

Definition

To custom design the physical properties of a polymer, two or more chemically different monomers, each with some desirable property, are combined and this process of formation is known as *copolymerization*. The polymer thus formed is called a *copolymer*.

Importance of Copolymer

- Generally a single large unit (macromolecule) is formed by the polymerization reactions
- In a copolymer, the number and position of the different type units vary among the individual macromolecules
- Different type of monomers can be incorporated into a chain to improve physical properties also the desired properties can be selected by copolymerization
- For example, small amounts of ethyl acrylate can be copolymerized with methyl methacrylate to alter the flexibility of a denture
- Methyl methacrylate and acrylic and methacrylic esters copolymerize readily.

Types of Copolymers

- Random
- Block
- Graft.

Random Copolymerization

In a *random copolymer,* the different monomer units are randomly distributed along the chain:

M—M—M—Y—M—Y—M—M—Y—Y—M—M

Block Polymer

In a block polymer, identical monomer units occur in long sequences along the main polymer chain.

M—M—M-• • M—M—Y—Y—Y • • -Y—Y—Y—M—M—M
where —M-• • M— and —Y • • Y— are identical units.

Graft Polymer

In *graft copolymers,* sequences of one of the monomers are grafted onto a 'backbone' of the second monomer species.

```
M—M—M—M—M—M—M—M—M—M
|   |
Y   Y
```

Block and graft polymers show improved impact strength, adhesive properties of resins and surface characteristics.

40. Types of Polymerization/Addition Polymerization.

TYPES OF POLYMERIZATION

- Addition polymerization
- Condensation polymerization

ADDITION POLYMERIZATION

- In addition reaction, there is no change in composition unlike condensation reaction
- In addition reaction, the monomer and the polymer have the same empirical formulas and the structure of the monomer is repeated many times in the polymer
- The reaction starts from an active centre and one monomer is added at a time and rapidly forms a chain that grows indefinitely, until the monomer content is exhausted.

Requisites for Addition Polymerization

- An unsaturated group is required to form a *double bond*
- Free radicals are required for an addition reaction to progress. (Free radical is an atom or group of atoms having an unpaired electron)
- This free radical and its unpaired electron react with monomer molecule and form a bond between the radical and the monomer molecule, leaving the other electron in an unsaturated electron orbital
- The remaining electron from the unsaturated orbital then acts as a new free radical center
- When the free radical-monomer complex approaches another monomer molecule to form a *dimer,* it also becomes a free radical. This chain process leads to large polymer molecules within a matter of seconds

- The process continues to complete the formation of the desired polymer until the termination reaction occurs
- The reactions are exothermic and heat is evolved
- Most dental resins are polymerized by *addition polymerization.*

Stages in Addition Polymerization

1. Induction
2. Propagation
3. Termination
4. Chain transfer **(Fig. 35)**.

Induction/Initiation/Activation

Free radicals are required to start a reaction. Free radicals are generated by activation of monomer molecules by ultraviolet light, visible light, heat, or energy transfer.

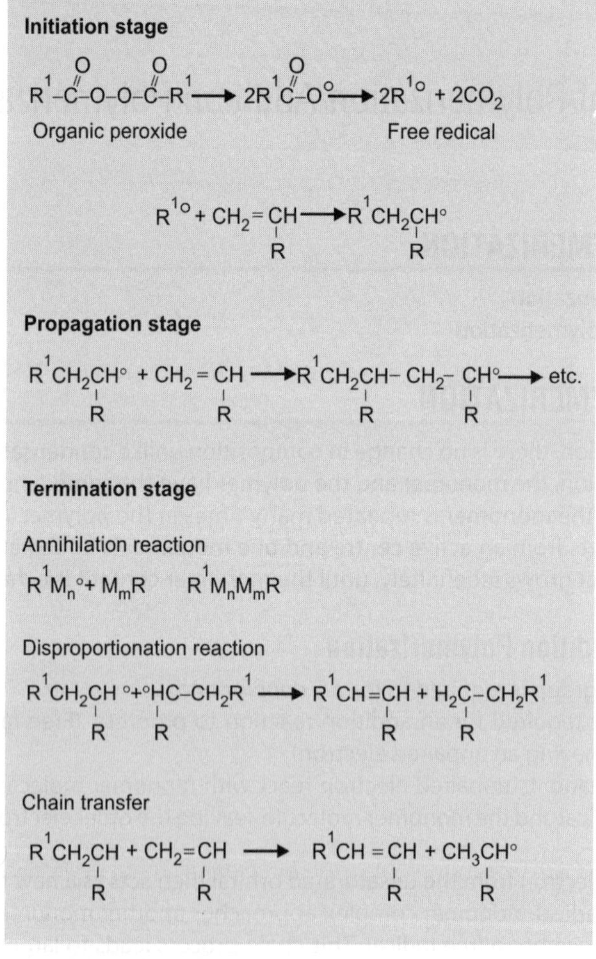

Fig. 35: Stages in addition polymerization

Heat activated

- The free radicals are obtained by heating benzoyl peroxide. The benzoyl peroxide molecule splits into two free radicals to initiate polymerization of methyl methacrylate monomer
- Benzoyl peroxide decomposes between 50° and 100°C
- Impurities in monomer decrease the efficiency of free radical formation
- The higher the temperature, the shorter is the length of the induction period.

Chemically activated

When tertiary amine, the *activator and* benzoyl peroxide, the *initiator* are mixed, the amine catalyzes the split of the benzoyl molecule into two free radicals.

Light activated

Photons activate the initiator to generate free radicals that, in turn, can initiate the polymerization process when UV light is used.

Visible light-cured

Camphoroquinone and dimethylaminoethylmethacrylate, an amine, generate free radicals when irradiated by visible light at a wavelength of about 470 nm.

Propagation

- Once the induction begins, little energy is required for the process to continue
- The chain reactions continue with the evolution of heat, until all of the monomer has been converted to a polymer.

Termination

- Chain reactions terminate either by direct coupling or by the exchange of a hydrogen atom from one growing chain to another
- Finally both molecules combine and become deactivated by an exchange of energy.

Chain Transfer

Chain transfer occurs when the active state is transferred from an activated radical to an inactive molecule. An already terminated chain can be reactivated by chain transfer, which then can continue to grow.

Factors Inhibiting Polymerization

- Any impurity in the monomer can inhibit or retard the polymerization reaction. The presence of such inhibitors alters the length of the initiation period and the degree of polymerization
- Inhibitors such as hydroquinone 0.006% or less are added to monomer to inhibit polymerization of monomer during storage
- The presence of oxygen also causes retardation of the polymerization reaction, because the oxygen reacts with the free radicals
- If resins are manipulated in open containers, the reaction velocity and the degree of polymerization are decreased.

41. Thermoplastic Materials.

DEFINITION

Thermoplastic materials are materials that soften under heat and solidify when they are cooled, with no chemical change taking place.

Example of thermoplastic material:
- Impression compound
- Waxes
- Resins.

IMPRESSION COMPOUND

Types

Depending on Softening Temperature
- Low fusing
- Medium fusing
- High fusing.

Low fusing
- Also known as tracing sticks
- Available as sticks or cones.

Properties
- They soften on heating and harden on cooling
- Softened by immersion in hot water or warming in flame
- Softening in hot water is preferred for uniform heating
- Cannot be used in undercut areas as impression material
- They have low flow and cannot record details as elastic impression materials can
- Repeated use can cause plasticizers to leach out making the compound brittle.

WAXES

Waxes are thermoplastic because they can be softened by heat and solidify without chemical reaction.

Classification according to their use and application
- Pattern wax
- Casting wax
- Base plate wax
- Boxing wax
- Utility wax

- Sticky wax
- Corrective impression wax
- Bite registration wax.

Classification according to their origin

- Natural waxes
  - Mineral
  - Plant
  - Insect
  - Animal
- Synthetic waxes
- Gums
- Fats
- Fatty acids
- Oils
- Natural and synthetic resins.

Properties

Melting Range

- They contain several types of molecules, each having a range of molecular weights and, hence, possess melting ranges rather than melting points
- The melting range for paraffin wax is from 44° to 62°C and for carnauba wax, it is from 50°C to 90°C
- When a mixture of 75% paraffin and 25% carnauba wax was prepared, the melting range increased to 44°C, compared with 18°C for paraffin alone.

Thermal Expansion

- Waxes expand when subjected to a rise in temperature and contract as the temperature decreases
- Dental waxes and their components have the largest coefficient of thermal expansion. The mineral waxes possess higher coefficients of linear thermal expansion than plant waxes. The mineral waxes expand more because they have weak secondary valence forces
- Many waxes exhibit at least two rates of expansion between 72° and 52°C.

THERMOPLASTIC RESINS

- These are synthetic resins which can be moulded by heat and pressure into articles. Thermoplastic resins are fusible and are soluble in organic solvents
- If chemical reaction takes place during molding process, they are called thermosetting resin.

42. What is Meant by Curing Cycle in Acrylic Resin?

DEFINITION

It is the heating process used to control polymerization. When a heat-activated resin is subjected to *polymerization cycle* or *curing cycle*, the reaction is complete and the material sets.

Types of Curing

- Chemically activated and subjecting it to boiling water for one hour
- Heat activated
- Light activated
- Microwave activated.

Techniques for Curing

- One technique involves processing the denture base resin in a constant-temperature water bath at 74°C (165°F) for 8 hours or longer, with no terminal boiling treatment
- The second technique involves processing the resin at 74°C for approximately 2 hours and then increasing the temperature of the water bath to 100°C and processing for 1 hour more.

Factors Affecting Curing/Polymerization

Manipulation Method

- If ideal ratio of polymer to monomer is not present, there is variation in polymerization
- If the material is packed after dough stage or at the stringy stage
- If uniform pressure is not applied for flasking
- A high temperature rise causes the monomer to boil out leading to denture base porosity
- If low temperature is employed, polymerization will not be complete and monomer content will be more and denture distortion chances will increase
- For a proper curing cycle, the resin must be heated more slowly during the polymerization cycle
- If the waxing up was not uniform or uniform pressure was not applied during closure of flask, some portions will be thick compared to others, leading to porosity.
- Rapid cooling can result in warpage of the denture base because of differences in thermal contraction of resin and investing stone
- Slow, even cooling minimizes distortion, hence, should bench cool for 30 minutes and later immersed in cool tap water for 15 minutes.

43. Describe the Physical and Chemical Changes that Take Place during Polymerization of Acrylic.

POROSITIES AND DEFECTS

- Polymerization shrinkage
- Porosity
- Water absorption
- Solubility
- Processing stresses
- Crazing.

Polymerization Shrinkage/Volumetric Shrinkage

When methyl methacrylate monomer is polymerized to form polymethyl methacrylate, the density of the mass changes from 0.94 to 1.19 g/cm. This change in density results in a volumetric shrinkage of 21%. A conventional heat-activated resin mixed at the correct powder-liquid ratio exhibits volumetric shrinkage of approximately 7%.

Linear Shrinkage

- After polymerization of the denture-base resin and removal of the prosthesis from the master cast, the distance between two predetermined reference points in the second molar regions of a completed tooth arrangement is noted. The difference between pre-polymerization and postpolymerization measurements is recorded as linear shrinkage. Acrylic resin denture base exhibits a linear shrinkage of approximately 2%.
- Thermal shrinkage of resin is responsible for the linear shrinkage phenomenon in heat-activated systems
- Complete dentures constructed using chemically activated resins have negligible thermal shrinkage
- Processing shrinkage is measured as 0.26% for chemically activated resin, compared with 0.53% for heat-activated resin.

Porosity

Porosities and Causes of Distortion in Acrylic (Figs 36A to E)

Monomer : Polymer ratio

- If it is too high, not all the polymers will be wetted by monomer and the cured acrylic will be granular
- If too low, there is a shrinkage on polymerization of about 21% by volume for pure monomer. In a correctly proportioned acrylic dough, this is about 1%. If there is too much monomer, there will be greater shrinkage.

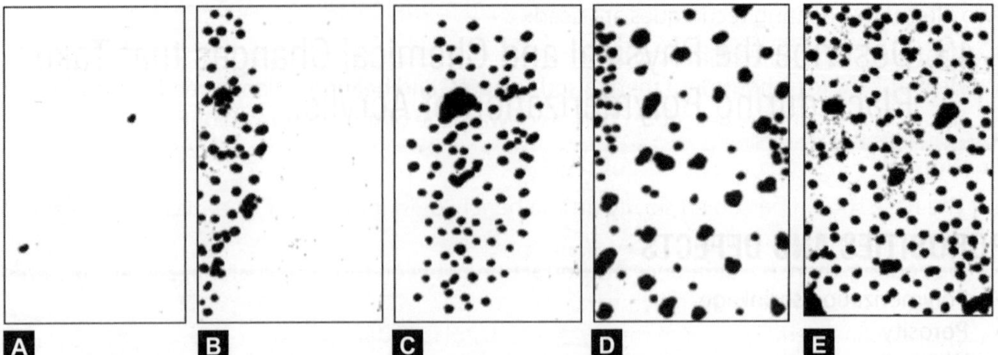

Figs 36A to E: Factors causing porosities in processed denture (A) Properly polymerized—no porosity; (B and C) Rapid heating—relatively small subsurface voids; (D) Insufficient mixing of monomer and polymer, large voids resulting from localized polymerization shrinkage; (E) Insufficient pressure during polymerization—relatively large irregular voids

Manipulation Method

- The acrylic should be packed in dough stage and the correct proportions should be mixed
- If the molecular weight of the polymer is lower, the dough formation is faster
- Plasticizer, when present in some materials, reduces the dough time
- In refrigerated resins, dough formation is delayed.

Avoided by:

- Ensuring homogeneity of the resin mix
- The use of proper polymer-monomer ratios and well-controlled mixing procedures
- Packing the material in dough stage.

Incomplete Wax Elimination

It can cause lack of adherence between teeth and acrylic resin.

Separating Agent

- It is used to prevent monomer penetrating into the mold material and polymerizing there, producing a rough surface with adherent mould material
- It is also used to prevent water from the mold entering into the acrylic resin.

Packing/Curing of Material

- On polymerization, there is contraction which reduces the pressure in the mold. Under-packing can lead to shrinkage porosity
- If the material is undercured, the denture may have a high residual monomer content. It is important that this is avoided
- The rate of temperature rise must not be too high. Monomer boils at 100.3°C causes vaporizing of the monomer, leading to gaseous porosity.

Two alternative heating techniques are used:

- Heat at 72°C for at least 16 hours
- Heat at 72°C for 2 hours and then raised to 100°C and heating is continued for a further two hours. This technique has more chances of warpage of the denture on deflasking.

Cooling

- The flask should be cooled slowly on the bench, or in the oven or water bath. There should never be sudden cooling
- On cooling, there is a difference of contraction between the mold material and acrylic, which causes stresses within the polymer
- Slow cooling permits relief of these stresses by plastic deformation
- Materials cured at higher temperatures will have greater residual stresses and will be more likely to warp.

Deflasking

This has to be done with care to avoid flexing and breaking the denture.

Finishing and polishing

- Final polishing is done with finely ground pumice in water used as a suspension on a wet soft mop
- If dry polishing techniques are used, care must be taken not to overheat the denture.

Storage of denture before delivery

To decrease the chances of dimensional changes, the denture should be stored in water until it is delivered to the patient.

Other types

A final type of porosity is associated with fluid resins. Such porosity appears to be caused by air inclusions incorporated during mixing and pouring procedure. Careful mixing, spruing and venting are required to avoid air inclusions.

Water Absorption

- Polymethyl methacrylate absorbs relatively small amounts of water when placed in an aqueous environment. Water absorption causes a slight expansion of the polymerized mass and water molecules interfere with the entanglement of polymer chains and thereby act as plasticizers
- Polymethyl methacrylate exhibits a water sorption value of 0.69 mg/cm^2
- It has been estimated that for each 1% increase in weight produced by water absorption, acrylic resin expands 0.23% linearly.

Solubility

- Although denture base resins are soluble in a variety of solvents and a small amount of monomer may be leached, they are virtually insoluble in the fluids commonly encountered in the oral cavity
- ADA Specification No. 12 states that the weight loss must not be more than 0.04 mg/cm^2 of specimen surface.

Processing Stresses

These are caused by:
1. Rapid cooling.
2. Improper mixing and handling of the resin.
3. Poorly controlled heating and cooling of the flask assembly.

Total dimensional changes occurring as a result of processing and service are in the range of 0.1 to 0.2 mm (as measured from second molar of right quadrant to second molar of left quadrant in upper denture).

Crazing

- Stress relaxation may produce small surface flaws that adversely affect the esthetic and physical properties of a denture. These microcracks are termed as crazing
- Crazing is seen as small linear cracks that appear to originate at a denture's surface. Crazing in a transparent resin imparts a 'hazy' or 'foggy' appearance. In a tinted resin, crazing imparts a whitish cast
- These surface cracks predispose a denture base to fracture
- Tensile stresses are often responsible for crazing in denture base
- Crazing also may be produced as a result of solvent action as with prolonged contact with ethyl alcohol
- Improved acrylic resin teeth and cross-linked denture base resins have decreased incidence of denture base crazing.

44. Resilient Liners and Tissue Conditioners.

RESILIENT LINERS

When a denture fit is altered, the tissue surfaces must be replaced by *relining* or *rebasing* existing dentures.

Relining

Involves replacement of tissue surface of an existing denture.

Rebasing

Involves replacement of the entire denture base.

Classification

Short-term

- Chemically activated resin (Specification No. 17)
- Light, or microwave energy resins
- Chemically cured soft liners
- Chemically activated silicones
- Polyurethane and polyphosphazine
- Polyvinyl liners.

Long-term

- Heat-cured acrylic soft liners
- Heat-activated silicones.

Method

1. An impression is made using the existing denture as an impression tray.
2. A stone cast is made and the resultant assembly is invested in a denture flask.
3. The flask is opened and prepared for the introduction of resin after the tissue surface is cleaned to enhance bonding between the existing resin and the reline material.
4. The liner is introduced and shaped using a compression-molding technique.
5. For relining, a low polymerization temperature is desirable to minimize distortion of the remaining denture base.
6. A relining jig maintains the correct vertical and horizontal relationships between the cast and the denture.

Uses

Soft liners absorb forces produced by masticatory impact and are referred to as a 'shock absorber'.

Short-term Liners

Chemically Activated Acrylic Soft Liners

Composition

Polymethyl methacrylate or polyethyl methacrylate in powder form are mixed with liquids containing 60% to 80% of a plasticizer (dibutyl phthalate).

(*It does not contain monomer*).

Action of soft liners

- Large plasticizer molecules decrease entanglement of polymer chains permitting slip to occur between chains
- The slipping motion provides the softness and cushioning effect for the underlying tissues.

Chemically Activated Silicones

Supplied as two-component systems that polymerize via condensation reactions.

Long-term Soft Liners

Heat-activated Acrylic Liners

Though considered as long-term, they do not have shelf life as that for silicone liners.

Composition

- Supplied as powder-liquid systems
- Powders consist of acrylic resin polymers and copolymers
- Liquids consist of acrylic monomers and plasticizers.

Disadvantages

- Plasticizers can leach out over a period of time and harden
- If polymethyl methacrylate is replaced by other methacrylates with low softening temperature, such as ethyl, n-propyl and n-butyl, less plasticizer is required and the effect of leaching decreases.

Silicone Rubbers

These do not contain leachable plasticizers and, hence, have long life compared to resin-based liners.

Disadvantages

- Silicone rubbers do not adhere to underlying denture bases
- Silicone liners also gain and lose water and can undergo distortion.

Heat-activated silicones

- Single component systems supplied as pastes or gels
- These materials are applied and contoured using compression-molding techniques
- They can either be applied to polymerized denture base resins, or polymerized in conjunction with freshly mixed resins.

Bonding agents used

- Rubber polymethyl methacrylate cements
- Liquid bonding agents.

TISSUE CONDITIONER

Composition

The material is a three-component system

1. Polyethyl-methacrylate (polymer).
2. Aromatic ester ethyl alcohol mixture of the monomer (liquid).
3. A liquid plasticizer.

These materials, when mixed, form a gel, the ethyl alcohol having great affinity for the polymer.

Uses of Tissue Conditioners

- As adjuncts in conditioning the denture-bearing tissues to a healthy state
- For temporary obturation
- Protection of surgical areas
- Used as stabilizer of base plates or of surgical stents
- In impression-making procedures
- Used as adjuncts in the healing phase of tissue integrated implants.

Adjuncts in Tissue Conditioning

Tissue conditioners are used to condition selected oral structures to bear the stresses of denture prostheses such as:

- In distorted tissues as hypertrophic, irritated, hyperemic and displaced oral mucosa associated with ill-fitting, poorly occluding dentures, bruxism, papillary hyperplasia, depressed areas associated with suction cups and patients with avitaminosis or general debilitating disease
- For preservation of the residual ridge
- To re-establish and maintain proper maxillomandibular jaw relationships.

Temporary Obturators

- Tissue conditioners may be added to an obturator on an existing complete or partial denture by direct or indirect method
- Usually done seven to ten days after surgery
- Tissue conditioner protects the tissues and enhances the healing process as in the cases of resected maxillae
- In obturator patients, it can aid in improving masticatory function, deglutition and speech.

Stabilizers of Base Plates

- In an edentulous cast with undercuts, tissue conditioners can be used to stabilize recording bases and prevent breakage of the cast
- Reduces the error in recording jaw relation records
- Breakage and abrasion of the edentulous cast are prevented with a better finish for the final denture.

Adjunct in the Impression-making

- As a final impression material, when it is difficult to determine the extent of the denture base due to movable oral structures
- They will record the extension in a dynamic form which will help in the making of an impression tray for the final impression.

Technique in the Use of Tissue Conditioner

The dentures to be relined should have:

- Adequate coverage of the denture-bearing area
- A good centric relation

- Adequate occlusal vertical dimension
- No occlusal interferences in eccentric jaw positions.

Preparation of the Denture

- The tissue surface of the denture is relieved of all undercuts and nearly 2 mm of denture material is relieved from all over the tissue surface, sufficient to allow the displaced and traumatized tissue to recover to a normal state
- Retain the borders or flanges and the hard palatal area as vertical stops in seating
- If the denture base is short, extend it by using activated acrylic resin to provide support for the soft material.

Preparation and Placement of Tissue Conditioner in the Mouth

- For conditioning tissues, a ratio of 1¼ parts of polymer to 1 part of monomer is used with the addition of ½ cc of the plasticizer
- Place the material on the denture base and seat without much pressure
- Allow the material to set. A new application of the material is needed every three to four days until the tissues have recovered
- After eight to ten weeks, the resilient liner can be replaced with denture base material.

New Materials

One silicone liner (a silicone copolymer), when cured in conjunction with an acrylic denture base material, contains components capable of bonding to acrylic resins.

45. Maxillofacial Materials.

- Maxillofacial materials are materials used to make maxillofacial prostheses
- Maxillofacial prosthesis reconstructs missing portions of the craniofacial complex
- French surgeon Ambroise Pare categorized various simple prostheses used for the cosmetic and functional replacement of maxillofacial structures.

REQUIREMENTS OF AN IDEAL MATERIAL

- Should be inexpensive.
- Should be biocompatible.
- Possess good strength and should be stable.
- The material should be skin-like in color and texture.

- They should be tear-resistant and should be able to withstand moderate thermal and chemical attack.

No material fulfils all of the above requirements.

Maxillofacial Materials Used

- Waxes
- Resins
- Latexes
- Vinyl plastisols
- Silicone rubbers
- Polyurethane polymers.

Waxes and Resins

These are used in the fabrication of prostheses commonly as they are cheaper compared to silicones.

Latexes

- Latexes are soft, inexpensive materials with skin texture
- They are weak, degenerate rapidly, exhibit color instability and can cause allergic reactions.

Synthetic latex

- Are made from tripolymer of butyl acrylate, methyl methacrylate and methyl methacrylamide
- They are nearly transparent
- Color matching is done by spraying colorants onto the reverse or tissue side of the prosthesis
- The life of synthetic latex prosthesis is short; hence, they are not used presently.

Vinyl Plastisols

- Plastisols are thick liquids consisting of small vinyl particles dispersed in a plasticizer. Colorants are added to these materials to match individual skin tones
- Vinyl plastisols can be heated to impart desired physical characteristics.

Disadvantages

- Vinyl plastisols harden with age because of plasticizer loss
- Ultraviolet light has an adverse effect; hence, the use of vinyl plastisols is limited.

Silicone Rubbers

Types

- Room temperature-vulcanizing silicones
- Heat-vulcanizing.

Room temperature-vulcanizing silicones

- Available as single-paste systems which can be colored by the addition of dyed rayon fibers, dry earth pigments and oil paints
- Prostheses made from room temperature vulcanizing are as strong as the heat-vulcanized silicones
- They are monochromatic.

Heat-vulcanizing silicones

- Supplied as a semi-solid or putty-like material that requires milling
- They are packed under pressure and a 30-minute heat application cycle at 180°C is used to cure them
- Pigments are milled into the material; hence, intrinsic coloring can be done
- Heat-vulcanizing silicones have more strength and color stability than room temperature-vulcanizing silicones.

Disadvantages

- Requirement for a milling machine and a press
- Metal mold is used, which is a lengthy procedure compared to a stone mold
- Stone mold can be used within a denture flask but during deflasking, the material can get damaged.

Polyurethane Polymers

- Polyurethane is a recently used material for maxillofacial prosthetics
- They are available as three components which require accurate proportioning
- The material is placed in a stone or metal mold and allowed to polymerize at room temperature
- Polyurethane prosthesis has a natural feel and appearance, but deteriorates rapidly.

46. Cold Cure Acrylic (ADA-13).

SYNONYMS

- Chemically activated, cold-curing, self-curing, auto polymerizing
- This type has chemical activators within the composition to induce polymerization.

COMPOSITION

Polymer

Emulsion-polymerized beads of PMMA, of average molecular weight 10_5–10_6.

Plasticizer

The polymer beads are more heavily plasticized than the heat-curing materials.

Initiator

Dibenzoyl peroxide—1%.

Pigments

Monomer

Methylmethacrylate.

Cross-linking Agent

Glycol-dimethacrylate 0–10%.

Inhibitor

Hydroquinone.

Tertiary Amine

DMPT—Dimethyl paratoludine.

Stabilizing Agents

Reaction

By chemical activation at room temperature (Cold-curing).

Powder (Polymer + Peroxide) when mixed with monomer + Inhibitor + Amine accelerator → Acrylic resin + heat.

- When polymer and monomer are mixed, tertiary amine reacts with benzoyl peroxide and free radicals are produced initiating polymerization
- The polymerization by cold cure method is not complete and, hence, has residual monomer which can irritate tissues and cause a decrease in strength
- The monomer content can be reduced by placing the tray or appliance on the mold and boiling it in water for one hour or storing it in water for 20 days.

Physical Properties

- Cold-cure resins have less shrinkage and are more accurate in fit than heat-cured acrylic resins
- They imbibe water and become oversized by 0.1% after months of use
- They are easy to make, less time is required and easy to repair
- Warpage and distortion are less in cold-cured resins
- They have low strength when compared to heat-cured resins
- The tertiary amines in cold-cured resins oxidize and alter the color of denture
- Discoloration of resins can be minimized by addition of stabilizing agents that prevent oxidation.

Manipulation Techniques

- For special trays, salt and pepper technique can be used

- For appliances, the correct ratio of monomer and polymer can be mixed and made into a dough which can be shaped to form the base or can be molded using compression techniques
- The working time for chemically activated resins is shorter than for heat-activated materials
- In compression technique, mold preparation and resin packing are the same as for heat-activated denture resins
- For repair, the material can be added to the repair area using a small sable-hair brush or instrument. A slight excess of material is placed at the repair site to compensate for polymerization shrinkage
- After repair work is done, the repaired prosthesis is placed in a pressure chamber and allowed to polymerize and later shaped, finished and polished.

47. Denture Base Materials.

TYPES OF RESINS

- Acrylic resins
- Multifunctional methacrylate and acrylate resins.

Acrylic Resins

Polymethyl Methacrylate

The acrylic resins are derived from ethylene and contain a vinyl group ($H_2C=CH$).

Chemically derived from

Acrylic acid, CH_2—CHCOOH
Methacrylic acid, CH_2—C (CH_3) COOH
Both of these resins polymerize by addition reaction.

Softening temperature

- Ethyl methacrylate—65°C.
- Methyl methacrylate—125°C.
- n-propyl methacrylate—38°C.
- Isopropyl—95°C.
- n-butyl—33°C.
- Isobutyl—70°C.
- Sec-butyl—62°C.
- Tertiary amine—76°C.
- Phenyl—120°C.

Properties

- Polymethyl methacrylate is the hardest resin among the following with the highest softening temperature
- Ethyl methacrylate has low softening point and surface hardness
- n-propyl methacrylate has low softening point and hardness compared to ethyl methacrylate
- The softening temperature of polyisopropyl methacrylate is greater than that of polyethyl methacrylate and the softening temperature of poly-propyl methacrylate is only 38°C
- Polydodecyl methacrylate is a viscous liquid monomer at room temperature
- Isobutylene, may be liquid at temperatures as low as –70°C
- Esterification with an aromatic alcohol increases the softening point.

Polymethyl Methacrylate

- A transparent resin that transmits light in the ultraviolet range to a wavelength of 250 nm
- The Knoop hardness number of polymethyl methacrylate is 18–20 KHN
- Its tensile strength is approximately 60 MPa and its density is 1.19 g/cm^3
- Its modulus of elasticity is approximately 2.4 GPa (2,400 MPa)
- The resin is stable and does not discolor in ultraviolet light
- It is chemically stable to heat and softens at 125°C and it can be molded as a thermoplastic material
- Between 125°C and 200°C, depolymerization takes place
- At 450°C, 90% of the polymer depolymerizes to the monomer
- Polymethyl methacrylate of high molecular weight degrades to a lower polymer at the same time when it converts to the monomer.

Disadvantages

- It has a tendency to absorb water by imbibition
- Due to its high internal energy, molecular diffusion occurs into the resin and polar carboxyl group forms a hydrogen bridge with water. These two factors cause absorption and adsorption termed as *sorption*
- Sorption is reversible if the resin is dried
- Methacrylate resins increase in weight by 0.5 wt% after 1 week in water
- The greater the molecular weight, the lesser is the weight increase
- As polymethyl methacrylate is a linear polymer, it is soluble in chloroform and acetone.

Methyl Methacrylate

- Polymethyl methacrylate alone cannot be used in dental procedures. Only when it is mixed with the liquid monomer methyl methacrylate, acrylic resin is formed
- The monomer partially dissolves the polymer to form a plastic dough. This dough is packed into the mold
- *Melting point*: –48°C
- *Boiling point*: 100.8°C
- *Density*: 0.945 g/mL at 20°C
- *Heat of polymerization*: 12.9 kcal/mol
- It exhibits a high vapor pressure and is an excellent organic solvent

- Methyl methacrylate can be polymerized by ultraviolet light, visible light, or heat and if it is chemically activated, it is polymerized by the use of a chemical initiator.

Factors affecting polymerization

- Temperature
- Method of activation
- Type of initiator
- Initiator concentration
- Purity of chemicals
- A volume shrinkage of 21% occurs during the polymerization of the pure methyl methacrylate monomer.

Multifunctional Methacrylate and Acrylate Resins

Types

- BIS-GMA
- Dipentaerythritol penta-acrylate monophosphate (PENTA-P)
- Hydroxyethyl methacrylate (HEMA).

BIS-GMA

Also known as Bowen's resin.

Composition

- BIS-GMA resin is an aromatic ester of a dimethacrylate, synthesized from epoxy resin (ethylene glycol of bisphenol A) and methyl methacrylate
- To reduce the viscosity, a low-viscosity dimethacrylate such as triethylene glycol dimethacrylate (TEGDMA) is added.

Chemistry

- BIS-GMA has a rigid central structure (two rings) and two OH-groups
- As BIS-GMA is a rigid material, molecule polymerization process is not efficient and only one of the methacrylate groups reacts
- Hence, BIS-GMA molecule forms a branch along the polymer chain. Some of these branches cross-link with adjacent chains
- To reduce the viscosity and increase the degree of conversion, different dimethacrylate resin combinations are tried.

Dipentacrythritol penta-acrylate monophosphate (PENTA-P)

It is a monomer used as dentin bonding agent.

Hydroxy ethyl methacrylate (HEMA)

It is grafted in polyacrylic acid and is used in glass ionomer cement.

Urethane dimethacrylate

It contains any monomer chain containing one or more urethane groups and two methacrylate end groups.

48. Cold Mold Seal.

Cold mold seal is a type of separating agent.

SIGNIFICANCE OF SEPARATING AGENTS

- It prevents the direct contact of resin to gypsum while packing is done
- It prevents water from mold entering the acrylic resin. If water enters the color, rate of polymerization can alter
- Prone to crazing if separating agent is not applied
- Separating agent also prevents monomer penetrating the mold material causing plaster to adhere to acrylic resin.

Types of Separating Agents

- Sodium alginate solution
- Tinfoil
- Cellulose lacquers
- Alginate compounds
- Calcium oleate
- Sodium silicate
- Soft soaps
- Starches.

Cold Mold Seal/Sodium Alginate Solution

This is a water soluble solution. It reacts with calcium of plaster/stone to form insoluble calcium alginate film.

Composition

- Sodium alginate—2%
- Water/alcohol/glycerine
- Sodium phosphate
- Preservatives.

Method of Application

It is applied on plaster and stone surface with fine camel hair brush and the film is allowed to dry and a second coat is applied. The separating agent should be applied to a dry surface.

Points to note

- All impurities from mold surface as waxes, oils need to be removed for the efficiency of the separating agent
- Mold should be warm for a uniform film to be formed. It should not be too cold or too hot
- There should not be any separating agent on the tooth; if present, will hinder the tooth from bonding with denture base resin.

49. Eutectic Alloys.

DEFINITION

Eutectic mixtures occur when the metals are miscible in liquid state but separate in solid state. The two metals precipitate one over another.

Eutectic (lowest melting temperature) alloy systems exhibit complete liquid solubility but limited solid solubility.

Examples of Eutectic Alloy

There are two metals that are partially insoluble in each other in the solid state as silver-copper system (72% Ag and 28% Cu).

ABEGD: Solidus boundary line.

AED: Liquidus boundary line.

Below 780°C: Limited solid solubility composed of the silver-rich alloy and the copper-rich alloy.

E: The liquidus and solidus point where the composition is 71.9% silver, 28.1% copper, known as the *eutectic composition.*

Explanation of the Diagram

- A to B—The silver becomes richer in copper as the temperature decreases
- Copper content increases from 0% to 8.8% at B
- From D to C, the silver atoms increase in the copper space lattice until 8% silver has alloyed with the copper
- Copper is soluble in the silver to an extent of 8.8% when the system is held at the eutectic temperature E
- The solid solution of copper in silver is called the *α-solid solution and* that of silver in copper is called the *β-solid solution*
- Line AB (liquidus) represents the solubility limit of the copper in the silver at the solidus temperatures
- Line BC (solvus) represents the solubility limit of the two metals in the solid state
- If more than 8.8% copper is added to the melt, the eutectic appears on solidification
- The eutectic structure does not appear in alloys of less than 8.8% copper
- Solubility of the copper in the silver becomes less as the temperature decreases below the eutectic solidification temperature
- When this alloy is slowly cooled below 630°C, the solid solution becomes supersaturated with copper and the excess copper is *precipitated.*

Eutectic Reaction

- Liquid $\rightarrow$ α-solid solution + β-solid solution
- Solidus gradually changes to eutectic with decrease in temperature.

Types

Depending on Physical Properties

- There is a difference between composition and physical properties because two different phases are on opposite sides of the eutectic composition
- The mechanical properties of the eutectic alloys do not vary linearly with the composition
- Eutectic alloys are harder and are brittle than the metals used to form alloy
- Eutectic alloys have a melting point and not a melting range
- Alloys with a composition less than that of the eutectic are called *hypoeutectic alloys*. The primary crystals of the hypoeutectic alloys in the copper-silver systems are composed of α-solid solution
- Alloys with a composition greater than the eutectic are known as *hypereutectic alloys*. The primary crystals in the hypereutectic alloys are composed of β-solid solution **(Fig. 37)**

Features of an Eutectic Alloy

- The temperature at which the eutectic occurs is lower than the fusion temperature of either silver or copper (779.4°C)
- There is no solidification range for composition E
- Eutectic alloy solidifies at a constant temperature, similar to a pure metal
- Eutectic alloys are used when a lower fusion temperature is required as in soldering. They are inferior in physical properties to solid solution alloys
- When an eutectic alloy solidifies, constituent metals segregate to form regions of pure parent metals. It forms in layers
- Eutectic alloys have poor corrosion resistance.

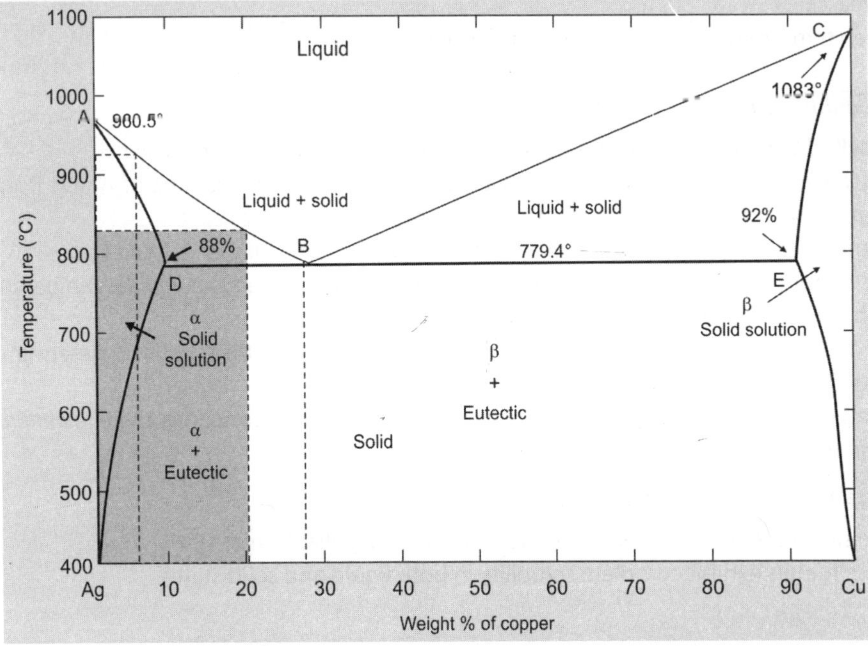

Fig. 37: Silver-copper phase diagram of eutectic alloy

50. Phase Diagrams and Homogenization.

PHASE DIAGRAM

Synonyms

Constitution or equilibrium phase diagram.

Terms Related to Phase Diagrams

Liquidus temperature is the temperature at which the first solid begins to form.

Solidus temperature is the temperature at which the last liquid solidifies.

Examples of Equilibrium Phase

1. Table Salt-water System

- When table salt is dissolved (NaCl) in water, it forms brine
- At a particular temperature, the extent of salt dissolution stops before salt crystals begin to settle out (solubility limit)
- If the solubility limit is exceeded, a two-phase solid-liquid mixture (brine and salt) is formed
- When the temperature of the system is increased, the amount of salt that can be dissolved increases
- When temperature is decreased, *ice* is formed.

2. Palladium Silver Alloy System

- Is melted at high temperatures at all combinations of palladium and silver
- *Pure palladium* and *pure silver* composed of all possible combinations of A and B, ranging from 100% A to 100% B are used to form a equilibrium phase
- A and B are completely soluble at all compositions in both solid and liquid states
- The temperature at which the first solid begins to form (called the *liquidus temperature)* for each composition is determined from the cooling curves
- The temperature at which the last liquid solidifies (called the *solidus*) is determined and plotted
- When the liquidus and solidus points are connected, a smooth curve, the *equilibrium phase diagram* results.

Silver-palladium phase diagram

- Pure silver is represented at 0% palladium and pure palladium at 100%
- These metals exhibit complete solubility in both liquid and solid states.

Interpretation of the Constitution Diagram

- At 1500°C (2732°F), an alloy of composition 65% palladium and 35% silver completely is liquid (line PO)
- At point R—The first solid forms at 1400°C (2552°F) with 65% liquid palladium
- At RM, called the tie line—first alloy solidifies
- A line drawn from (M) to the base line—indicates composition as *77%* palladium
- At S—1370°C (2498°F), the material is partially solid and partially liquid
- At Y—composition of the liquid is 58% palladium
- At W—composition of the solid is about 71% palladium
- At point T (1340°C), the last portion of liquid solidifies
- In Figure 39, point T, the alloy is entirely solid with a composition of 65% palladium
- The larger the temperature range between liquidus and solidus, the greater is the tendency toward coring **(Fig. 38)**.

Explanation

During cooling, the liquidus and solidus points are noted and these points are connected to form a smooth curve that indicates the phase diagram **(Fig. 39)**.

The equilibrium phase diagram indicates:

a. *Liquidus line*: Above this line, the alloy is liquid.

b. *Solidus line*: Below which the alloy is solid.

c. *Between the solidus and liquidus lines*: in which the liquid and solid states are present.

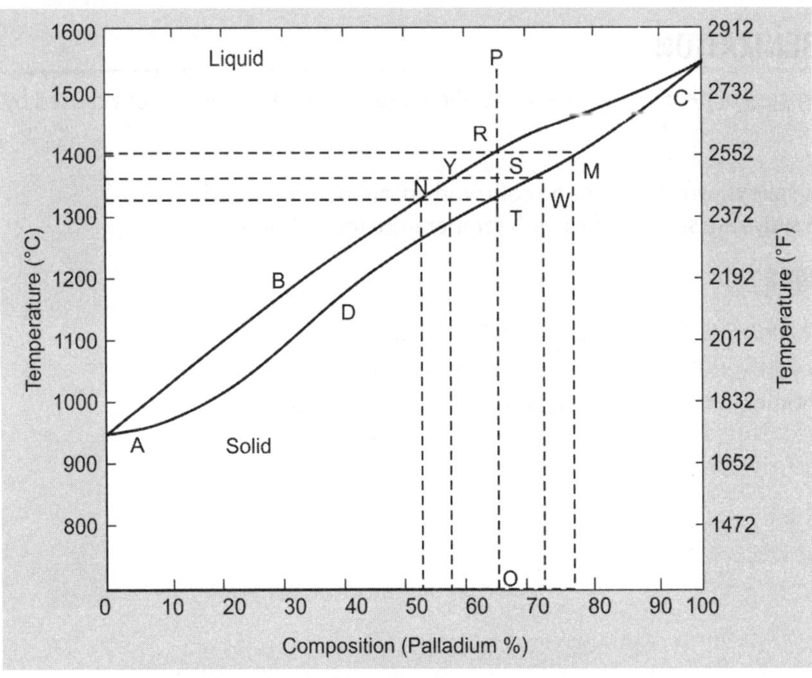

Fig. 38: Silver-Palladium phase diagram

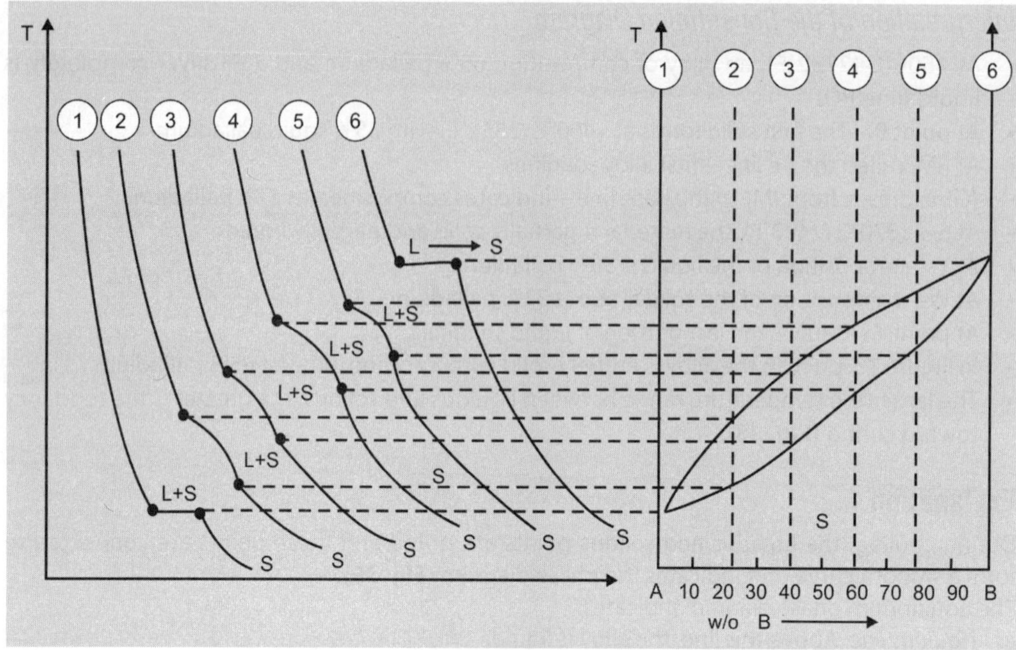

Fig. 39: Cooling curves of six different alloys (equilibrium phase)

HOMOGENIZATION

It is the process of heating a cast alloy to eliminate composition differences caused by coring.

Method

- Casting alloys, which cannot be cold worked, are homogenized
- These alloys are subjected to high temperature for six hours.

Advantages

Coring in Alloys is Relieved by Homogenization

- Homogenized alloys are more resistant to tarnish and corrosion
- After homogenization, the ductility of the alloy increases.

51. Types of Heat Treatments.

TYPES

- Annealing
- Homogenization/Solution or softening heat treatment—To produce a solid solution
- Hardening heat treatment/age hardening: Precipitates a second phase (silver-copper system)
- Self-hardening to form supper lattice, as in gold-copper system.

Annealing

Annealing is a process by which the effects of cold working, such as strain hardening, low ductility and distorted grains are reversed by heating the metal.

Homogenization/Softening Heat Treatment

In this, the alloys are heated to 700°C for 10 minutes and quickly quenched in water. After this treatment, the alloys become more ductile and soft.

Hardening Heat Treatment

- A softened alloy is heated at 450°C for 2 minutes and then uniformly cooled to 250°C in 30 minutes and then quenched in water
- A procedure in which the metal is elevated to a temperature above room temperature and held at that temperature for a length of time
- This procedure can soften or harden an alloy, change its grain size and corrosion resistance. Heat treatment is mostly done for gold alloys.

Quenching

To cool it rapidly from high temperature to room temperature.

Advantages of quenching

- To preserve the stable phase achieved at high temperatures
- To terminate a process immediately only occurring at high temperatures.

Self-hardening to Strengthen Gold Alloys

When copper is added, the yield strength of the gold alloy increases by a mechanism known as order-hardening.

HEAT TREATMENT PROCEDURE

Stage 1

The alloy is quenched after casting.

Stage 2

- *Homogenization* is done because coring occurs with alloys containing platinum
- The alloy is heated to 700°C for 10 minutes, then quenched
- The alloy is reheated to 400°C and holding it at that temperature for approximately 30 minutes allows the copper atoms to arrange themselves in ordered clusters
- This ordered structure prevents slippage of the atomic layers, which has the effect of raising the yield stress and the hardness of the alloy
- Cooling the alloy from 450°C to 250°C over 30 minutes, followed by quenching
- The copper content must be at least 11% in the gold alloy for order hardening to occur. So it cannot be done in Type I and Type II gold alloys
- Hardening heat treatment causes a reduction in the ductility of the alloy
- The heat-treated alloy is benched, cooled or quenched immediately on casting. This technique is commonly known as self-hardening.

Stage 3

- If any cold working is done to the alloy, a stress relief annealing is carried out
- The effect of this heat treatment on the mechanical properties of these alloys is improved.

Disadvantages of Heat Treatment

- It is not a well-controlled procedure
- Can cause brittleness and fracture if a treated gold clasp is repeatedly bent.

Result of Heat Treatment

- Softening heat treatment decreases in yield strength, tensile strength but increases in ductility
- Hardening heat treatment increases in yield strength, tensile strength, proportional limit and decreases the ductility.

52. Annealing.

DEFINITION

Annealing is a process by which the effects of cold working, such as strain hardening, low ductility and distorted grains, are reversed by heating the metal.

Method of Annealing

- The more severe the cold working, the faster the effects can be reversed by annealing
- The annealing technique depends on the melting range of an alloy and the annealing temperature

- The higher the melting range of the alloy, the higher is the temperature needed for annealing
- Annealing technique uses a temperature that is approximately one half that is necessary to melt the metal on the absolute temperature scale (degrees Kelvin).

Stages in Annealing

- Recovery
- Recrystallization
- Grain growth **(Fig. 40)**.

Recovery Stage

It is the stage at which the cold-work properties begin to disappear without any significant visible changes under the microscope.

Changes

- Slight decrease in tensile strength
- No change in ductility
- There is a recovery of the electrical conductivity
- The residual stress within a cold-worked metal result in warping. When the stresses are released, this tendency for warping disappears in the recovery stage.

Recrystallization Stage

Recrystallization occurs after the recovery stage.

Changes

- At this stage microscopic changes are seen
- The old grains are completely replaced by new set of strain-free grains
- The recrystallization grains nucleate at grain boundaries, or at a deformed lattice area
- The recrystallization strain-free nuclei occupy the distorted matrix faster than the time which the matrix takes to recover
- At the recrystallization stage, the material regains its original soft and ductile condition.

Grain Growth

Normally the recrystallized nuclei has an average grain size.

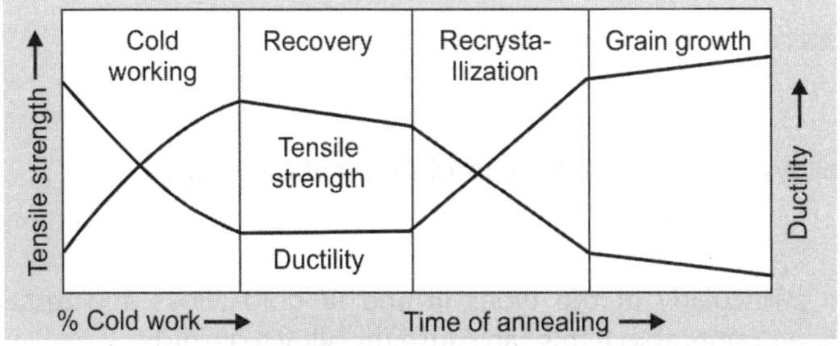

Fig. 40: Stages in annealing

The grain growth depends on the following factors:

- The number of nuclei
- The severity of the cold working
- The amount of nuclei
- Hence recrystallized material can range from fine to coarse
- When a fine grain structure is again annealed, the grains begin to grow minimizing the boundary energy
- When large grains consume the smaller grains, a coarse grain structure is formed and the grain growth process stops.

Factors in grain size

- Excessive annealing causes formation of larger grains as in wrought materials
- A large grain structure is due to excessive casting and mold temperatures
- A large grain structure causes decrease in strength properties as grain boundary dislocations occur
- Small or fine grains increase strength as they prevent grain boundary dislocations
- Small grains cause an increase in strength, hardness and proportional limit during cold work rather than the large grains
- Small grains have low ductility.

53. Type III Gold Alloys.

- These are used for all inlays, onlays, full coverage crowns and short-span bridges, cast posts and cores because of their greater strength
- They are difficult to burnish and have greater chances to fracture compared to types I and II gold alloys.

COMPOSITION OF TYPE III GOLD ALLOYS

Gold

Gold content is less compared to type I and type II

Silver

Strengthens the alloy and counteracts the reddish tint of the copper.

Copper

Imparts strength, particularly of the types III and IV gold alloys and reduces the melting temperature (16%, amounts above this can cause the alloy to tarnish).

Platinum

Increases both the strength and the melting temperature.

Palladium

Same effect as platinum, but is more cheap.

Zinc

Acts as a scavenger during casting, preventing oxidation and improves the castability.

Trace Elements

Indium, ruthenium and rhodium (<0.5%) may be present. These have very high melting temperature and act as nucleating sites during solidification, helping to produce a fine grain size.

HEAT TREATMENT PROCEDURE

Done to strengthen gold alloys.

Stage 1

The alloy is quenched after casting.

Stage 2

- Homogenization is done because coring occurs with alloys containing platinum
- The alloy is heated to 700°C for 10 minutes, then quenched
- The alloy is reheated to 400°C and holding it at that temperature for approximately 30 minutes allows the copper atoms to arrange themselves in ordered clusters
- This ordered structure prevents slippage of the atomic layers, which has the effect of raising the yield stress and the hardness of the alloy
- The copper content must be at least 11% in the gold alloy for order hardening to occur, so that it cannot occur in type I and type II gold alloys
- The addition of copper and hardening heat treatment increase the yield strength by ten-fold
- Hardening heat treatment causes a reduction in the ductility of the alloy
- When the heat treated alloy is quenched, it self-hardens.

Stage 3

- If any cold working is done, a stress relief anneal is carried out
- Homogenized alloys possess a uniform composition throughout the casting.

Disadvantages of Heat Treatment

- It is not as well-controlled as during homogenizing anneal
- Can cause brittleness and fracture if a treated gold clasp is repeatedly bent.

Properties and Applications

- The medium-gold alloys have same applications as types III and IV gold alloys. They have low ductility than type IV gold alloys. Their high-yield stress makes them difficult to burnish

- The low-gold content alloys have lower mechanical properties than the medium-gold alloys and can be used as an alternative to type III gold alloys
- If copper is substituted by indium, alloys with same properties as type III gold alloys are formed. As the gap between the solidus and the liquidus is greater, a less homogeneous structure results, which makes the casting process difficult at high temperature.

54. Galvanic Cell Corrosion.

DEFINITION

Galvanic cell corrosion is a type of electrochemical corrosion which occurs when combination of dissimilar metals are in direct physical contact with each other.

Examples of Galvanic Corrosion

In Dissimilar Metals

- When two dissimilar metals are used for restoration on the opposite arches, a 'galvanic current' or 'galvanic shock' is observed
- For example, amalgam restoration on an upper tooth opposing a gold inlay in a lower tooth. With saliva as media, the contact of these two restorations forms an electrical couple.

Reasons for galvanic shock in dissimilar metals

- An electrical potential (EMF) exists between the two fillings. Saliva forms the electrolyte, with hard and soft tissues forming the external circuit **(Fig. 41)**
- The electric currents measured between a gold crown and an amalgam restoration are approximately 0.5 to 1 mA with EMF of approximately 500 mV
- If a gold restoration comes in contact with an amalgam restoration, the amalgam can form the anode of an electrical cell and starts corroding. The electric couple 'Galvanic Shock' occurs
- The patient senses it as a sharp pain
- This can be minimized by painting a varnish on the surface of the amalgam restoration
- The best procedure is to avoid dissimilar metals to be in contact.

Heterogeneous Composition

- Galvanic currents occur in restorations of dissimilar metals, when there is a difference in surface composition or structure
- Examples: Eutectic and peritectic alloys
- In an eutectic alloy, the metallic grains with the lower electrode potential are attacked and, thus, corrosion results.

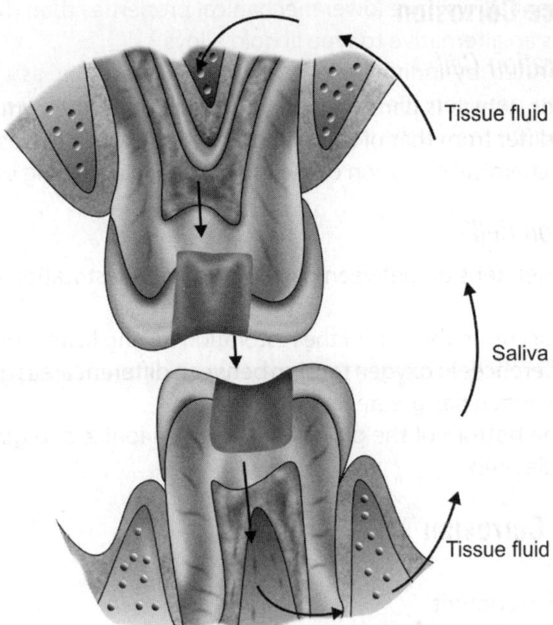

Fig. 41: Path of galvanic current in the mouth

In a Single Isolated Metallic Restoration

- In single restorations, current can form but will be less intense
- This occurs when potential differences are created by saliva and tissue fluids as dentinal fluid or blood which provide a complete external circuit
- Here the internal surfaces of a dental restoration exposed to the dentinal fluid become actively potential
- Coating with varnish decreases these types of galvanic shocks.

55. Concentration Cell Corrosion.

DEFINITION

- An important type of electrochemical corrosion is called concentration cell corrosion, which occurs whenever there are variations in the electrolytes or in the composition of the given electrolyte within the system
- An example of concentration cell corrosion is crevice corrosion.

Examples of Crevice Corrosion

Electrolyte Concentration Cell

In a metallic restoration, which is partly covered by food debris, the composition of electrolyte under the debris will differ from that of saliva and this can result in corrosion of the restoration. This causes an electrochemical corrosion of the metal surface occurring under the food debris.

Oxygen Concentration Cell

- Differences in oxygen tension between parts of the same restoration cause corrosion of the restoration
- Greater corrosion occurs in the part of the restoration having lower concentration of oxygen. When there are differences in oxygen tension between different areas of the same restoration, the area with less oxygen has greater activity (Pits)
- The materials at the bottom of the pit with less oxygen ionize and go into solution (anode) causing the pit to deepen.

Protection Against Corrosion

- Passivation
- Increase noble metal content
- Polishing restorations
- Avoid dissimilar metal restoration.

Other Factors

- Noble metal corrodes less. So, restorations made with noble metals are better than base metals
- Base metals corrode when a surface defect is created
- Two dissimilar metals in direct contact can form an anode to cathode surface area ratio. If protective coatings are used, corrosion decreases
- Certain metals develop a thin, highly protective film by reaction.

56. Inlay Wax.

(ADA SPECIFICATION NO. 4)

Inlay wax is used to make pattern for crown, inlay or bridge that is later casted using lost wax technique.

Availability

(Commercial names—Harvard and Kerr.)

- Inlay waxes are available in deep blue, green, purple rods or sticks about 7.5 cm long and 0.64 cm in diameter
- Inlay wax is available in the form of small pellets, cones or in metal jars.

Composition

Ingredient	%	Function
Paraffin	60%	Aids to establish melting point. Paraffin flakes while trimming; hence, other waxes are added to modify the flakiness.
Carnauba/ Candelilla	25%	Is hard and has high melting point. Along with paraffin, it decreases the flow at mouth temperature and gives glossiness. Candelilla is used to replace carnauba but its melting point is lower and is softer than carnauba.
Ceresin	10%	Partially replaces paraffin and increases toughness. Easy to carve.
Beeswax	5%	Montan has high melting point and finer working qualities; hence, it is used instead of carnauba.
Gum Dummar	1%	Improves smoothness in molding and increases toughness and luster.

Types according to flow

- *Hard*: For direct wax patterns
- *Regular (medium)*: For indirect wax patterns
- Soft.
  The flow can be reduced by adding more carnauba wax or by higher-melting paraffin wax. Resins 1%, also will affect the flow of inlay waxes.

Requirements of Inlay Wax

- Uniform softening should be achieved without granules or hard spots
- Color of inlay wax should contrast with die materials
- Inlay wax should not flake during carving or while molding after softening
- At 500°C (the burn-out temperature), it should burn out completely
- The inlay wax should be rigid and dimensionally stable until it is burned out
- It should be plastic above mouth temperature and become rigid at mouth temperature
- The flow should be more than 70% at 45°C and less than 1% at 37°C.

Technique in Wax Pattern Fabrication

Direct Technique

If the pattern is prepared intraorally.

Indirect Technique

If the wax is heated over a flame/wax bath and adapted to the prepared tooth or die.

Procedure

- A pattern is made first to duplicate the shape and contour of the desired casting
- A sprue is attached to the carved wax pattern and is invested with the sprue leading from the outer surface of the investment mold to the pattern

- After the investment sets, the wax is burned out in a furnace and the mold is conditioned to receive the alloy.

Physical Properties

Residue

Inlay waxes should be able to burn out completely without residue. The limits of the non-volatile residue to a maximum should be within 0.10%.

Flow

- Type I hard wax is for direct patterns in the mouth; hence, the flow for type I wax at 37°C should not be more than 1% to minimize distortion while removing from the cavity preparation
- Type II soft wax is for indirect technic and has greater flow and ease of carving than type I.
- The flow of the type II wax is about 9% at 37°C.

Thermal Expansion

- The maximum linear thermal expansion allowed for both types between 25°C and 30°C is 0.20% and between 25°C and 37°C is 0.60%
- For type I wax, when temperature decreases from 37°C to 24°C, a 0.4% linear contraction is observed
- Thermal conductivity of waxes is low
- Coefficient of thermal expansion: 0.7% with increase in temperature of 20°C.

Carvability

Both types of waxes should not flake during margin formation or carving the pattern.

Warpage of Wax Patterns

- Inlay pattern wax has a tendency to distort when allowed to stand for a long period due to release of residual stress within the pattern
- Inlay wax distorts on cooling due to contraction
- Distortion occurs if occluded gas bubbles are present
- During carving, pooling and removal
- Pattern can distort if stored for a long time at high temperature
- If wax is not melted uniformly, some part thermally contracts than other areas
- If wax is not held under uniform pressure, it can distort
- If wax is added later to the deficient areas of the pattern, the added wax will distort.

Methods to minimize distortion

- Distortion can be minimized by heating wax uniformly at 50°C for at least 15 minutes before use
- By warming the carving instruments before use
- By using a warmed die
- By incremental addition of wax to the die
- The lower the storage temperature, the lesser is the distortion
- The pattern should be invested as early as possible
- If the pattern was stored, the margins should be readapted.

57. Base Plate Wax.

BASE PLATE WAX/MODELLING WAX

ADA Specification No. 24.

Availability

Pink sheets/red sheets of 7.60 × 15 × 0.13 cm. Hard ones are brown in color.

Composition

Paraffin wax/ceresin	75–80%
Beeswax	10–14%
Carnauba wax	1–3%
Natural wax	2–4%
Microcrystalline wax	2.5%

Types

Type I	Soft wax	For building veneers
Type II	Medium	For denture base trials in temperate climate
Type III	Hard	For trial filling in oral cavity in tropical climate

USES

- To form trial denture base to establish vertical dimension, the plane of occlusion and the initial arch form
- To produce the desired contour of the denture after teeth are set in position
- To make patterns for orthodontic appliances and prostheses
- For onlay and crown preparation to check occlusal clearance after occlusal reduction
- To check undercuts in inlay cavity preparation
- As check bites for the various articulating relations in the mouth and to transfer them to articulators.

Physical Properties

- The melting point is 58°C and the transition temperature is 50°C (approx.). Hence, all manipulations should be within the above temperature to minimise stress relief.
- The linear thermal expansion from 26° to 40°C should be less than 0.8%
- They should be easily trimmed with a sharp instrument at 23°C

- They should have a smooth surface after gentle flaming
- They should not leave any residue or color on plastic teeth during processing
- As there is residual stress within the baseplate wax, they should be invested as soon as possible.

58. What are the Causes for the Distortion of Wax Pattern?

INLAY WAX

ADA Specification No 4.

Types of Inlay Wax

Type I and Type II.

Properties of Waxes Required to Prevent Distortion

- The accuracy and fine detail of the wax pattern is required to produce perfect castings
- An ideal wax should burn out completely without any residue remaining in the mold because of incomplete wax burnout (permitted residue 0.10%)
- Type I wax is a hard wax with 1% flow at 37°C; hence, distortion of the pattern is less
- Type II wax is softer and used in indirect technic as it has 9% flow at low temperatures but has greater ease of carving
- Maximum linear thermal expansion allowed between 25°C and 30°C is 0.20%, and between 25°C and 37°C is 0.60%
- Both types should not chip or flake during carving
- *Thermal coefficient of expansion*: A decrease of 12°C to 13°C causes a 0.4% linear contraction of wax.

Distortion of Wax Patterns

- Can be during melting
- Inlay patterns have high coefficient of expansion but also distort after the pattern is made
- The amount of distortion increases as the temperature and time increase due to release of residual stresses developed during pattern formation
- If the pattern was adapted and shaped at high temperature, the distortion is less in the prepared pattern
- During pattern formation
- Overheating the wax can cause the distortion
- Removal of pattern frequently from the die
- Different thicknesses in different areas of the pattern

- Keeping the pattern too long in a humid environment
- Investing the pattern without readapting the margins
- Improper sprue placement
- Sprue should be placed at the thickest portion of wax pattern, at the correct angle and thickness
- The longer the time period of investing the pattern, the more is the distortion
- During investing, lack of using a surface tension reducing agent
- Voids between the investment and pattern
- Thin wax pattern margin.

Methods to Prevent Distortion

- The incorporation of residual stress can be decreased by softening the wax uniformly at 50°C for at least 15 minutes before use
- Warming the carving instruments and the die also decreases chances of distortion
- Addition of wax to the die in small amounts minimizes distortion
- The pattern should be stored at low temperature to prevent distortion
- If inlay wax patterns take more than 30 minutes to invest, they should be kept in a refrigerator but should be brought to room temperature before investing
- Indirect wax pattern should be stored on die or cast to prevent distortion
- The ideal method is to invest it immediately
- During spruing, solid wax sprue or a hollow metal sprue filled with sticky wax is ideal
- The margins should be readapted if the pattern was kept for a period of time
- When wax hardens, it shrinks, during casting the alloy also contracts on setting. This entire shrinkage is compensated by setting, thermal and hygroscopic expansion of investment material.

59. What is the Composition of Investment used for Base Metal Alloys?

Investments used for base metal alloys are phosphate-bonded investments.

COMPOSITION

Investment Powder

Refractory Fillers

- These can be cristobalite, quartz, or a mixture of the two and in a concentration of approximately 80%

- Fillers provide high-temperature thermal shock resistance (refractoriness) and a high thermal expansion
- Filler particle size varies from a submicron level to that of a fine sand.

Binder

- Magnesium oxide (basic) and a phosphate that is acid in nature (mono-ammonium phosphate)
- This can be incorporated into the powdered investment
- Earlier phosphoric acid was used. This reacts with phosphate ions at room temperature.

Ceramic Substrate

For high temperature strength and to harden at room temperature.

Carbon

- Some phosphate-bonded investments contain carbon
- Palladium reacts with carbon at temperatures above 1504°C and cause embrittlement. Hence, a phosphate investment without carbon should be used.

Liquid

Colloidal silica (33% dilution). Freeze stable colloidal silica is also available.

Significance

- They have high strength and can be heated to 950°C or above for 30 minutes without disintegration
- High melting temperature range alloys can be cast with phosphate-bonded investment.

SETTING REACTION

- Magnesia and monoammonium phosphate react to form a colloidal multimolecular $(NH_4MgPO_4 \cdot 6H_2O)n$ around excess MgO and fillers
- $MgO + NH_4H_2PO_4 + H_2O \rightarrow (NH_4MgPO_4 \cdot 6H_2O)n$ MgO and filler particles + H_2O.

During Heating

At 160°C

$(NH_4MgPO_4 \cdot H_2O)n$.

When Heated from 300°C to 650°C

$(Mg_2P_2O_7)$ noncrystalline polymeric phase.

Above 1040°C

$Mg_3(P_2O_4)_2$ (When overheated).

The final products are crystalline $Mg_2P_2O_7$, excess MgO, with unchanged quartz, cristobalite, or both.

Procedure

Phosphate-bonded investment should be heated gradually (at least for half an hour) to 315°C and then rapidly to 750–900°C.

PHOSPHATE INVESTMENTS PREVENT CASTING SHRINKAGE

- Expansion of wax pattern
- Colloidal silica prevents shrinkage and, in turn, increases expansion
- During high temperatures, inversion of cristobalite causes expansion.

Points to Note

Casting pressure

Requires high casting pressure to prevent back pressure porosity due to residual gases present from investment material reaction.

Cleaning

Recovery and cleaning of the casting is difficult with casting from phosphate-bonded investment; hence, need sand blasting

Noncarbon type investment needs to be used or the alloys can become embrittled.

60. Spherical Alloys.

Spherical alloys are made by melting together the desired elements and this liquid metal is atomized into fine spherical droplets.

TECHNIQUE

The liquid metal droplets are made to solidify before hitting the surface to preserve the spherical shape. These atomized powders are called spherical alloy powders.

TYPES OF LOW COPPER ALLOYS

Lathe cut and spherical.

Composition of spherical low copper alloys

Ag	63–70%
Sn	26–28%
Cu	2.5%
Zn	0.2%

Lathe Cut Compared with Atomized Spherical Powder

- Spherical alloys require less mercury than typical lathe-cut alloy
- Spherical alloy powder particles have smaller surface area per volume than do the lathe-cut alloy particles
- Amalgams with a low mercury content have better properties.

Physical Properties

Compressive Strength

The early compressive strength after one hour for the low copper spherical alloy is 141 MPa.

Tensile Strength

The tensile strength is 48–70 MPa.

Particle Size

- Particle sizes of modern powder ranges between 15 µm and 35 µm
- Small average particle sizes produce a more rapid hardening of the amalgam with greater early strength.

61. Hygroscopic Setting Expansion.

DEFINITION

- ADA specification No. 2 for Type II investment
- It is the setting process of gypsum products allowed to set under water
- Generally, plaster or stone is allowed to set in air.

Significance

- Increases the setting expansion more than double in magnitude
- In normal setting, the water of crystallization is given out whereas, in hygroscopic setting expansion, the water from outside maintains the water of crystallization, allowing additional crystal growth
- Hygroscopic expansion is not a chemical reaction.

Stage	Normal setting conditions	Hygroscopic setting conditions
I	Initial mix (showing three round particles of hemihydrate surrounded by water)	
II	The reaction has started and the crystals of the dihydrate are forming and particles are drawn closer due to loss of water.	The water of hydration is replaced and the distance between the particles remains the same. When the crystals of dihydrate grow, setting expansion begins.
III	The crystals grow and the contraction is opposed by the outward thrust of the growing crystals.	The crystals are not inhibited, as the water is available from the outside. Here the crystals grow and the setting expansion occurs.
IV and V	The crystals under normal setting become intermeshed and entangled.	The crystals grow more freely during the early stages until the intermeshing finally prevents further expansion.

Hence, the setting expansion under water has a setting expansion double in magnitude **(Fig. 42)**.

Factors Affecting Hygroscopic Setting

Effect of Composition

- Type and particle size and silica content (α-hemihydrate has more expansion than β-hemihydrate)
- When silica to binder ratio is Increased, hygroscopic expansion increases but strength decreases.

Binder

15% is required to prevent drying shrinkage.

Water : Powder Ratio

The reduction in the W:P ratio increases the hygroscopic setting expansion.

Spatulation

- Increased spatulation results in increased hygroscopic expansion
- The normal setting expansion for dental stone is 0.15%, with a maximum hygroscopic expansion of not more than 0.30%
- For type II investment, the hygroscopic expansion is from 1.2% to 2.2%.

Immersion Time

Before initial set.

Ringless Casting

Casting rings confine the material restricting expansion. Ringless castings give more hygroscopic expansion.

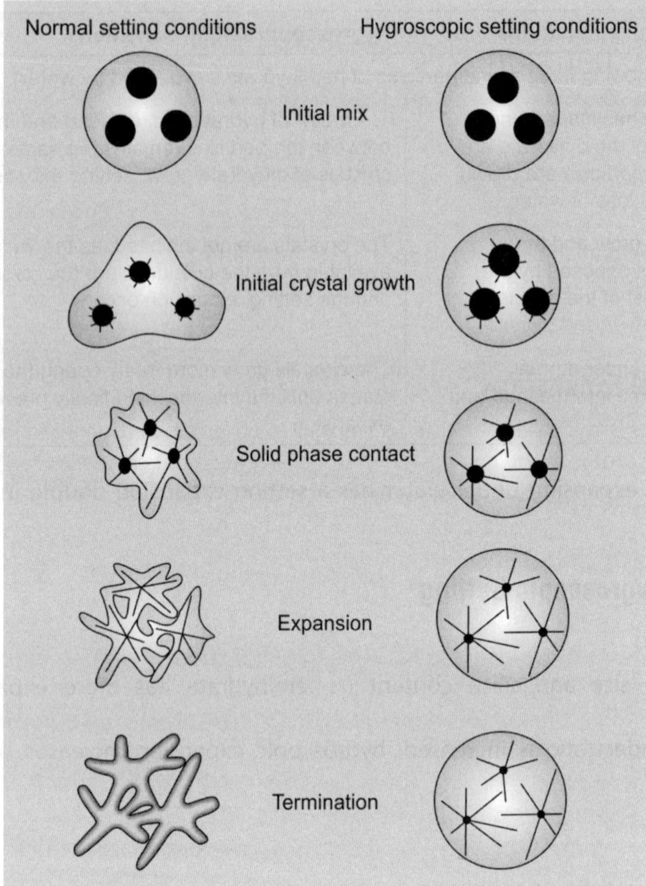

Fig. 42: Theory of hygroscopic expansion

Shelf Life

The longer the investment is kept, the lesser is the hygroscopic expansion.

Temperature of Wax Bath

The higher the temperature of water bath, the more is the wax pattern expansion. Hence, more effective is the hygroscopic expansion.

Strength of Wax and Sprue Position

It critical for hygroscopic expansion.

62. Thermal Expansion.

DEFINITION

Is the normal setting expansion occurring in investments and gypsum products, waxes and resins, due to normal setting reaction and if setting expansion occurs on heating, it is referred to as coefficient of thermal expansion.

Principle of Thermal Expansion

When the temperature is raised either due to normal exothermic setting reaction or due to application of heat, the atoms in the concerned material vibrates, causing an increase in internal energy and interatomic spacing. This causes a thermal expansion of the concerned material.

Dental Materials that Expand

Gypsum-bonded Investment Materials

- Expands when heated from room temperature to 105°C (normal setting expansion) after which it either contracts or remains the same till 200°C
- *From 200°C to 700°C*: Expansion differs depending on the type of silica employed. Cristobalite and tridymite give better expansion due to their inversion from α to β form. These materials also prevent drying shrinkage
- Type I: relies only on thermal expansion and it should be 1 to 1.6%
- Type II: can be by thermal expansion and hygroscopic expansion in which the thermal expansion range is 0 to 0.6% at 500°C.

Phosphate-bonded Investment Material

- Colloidal silica used in manipulation instead of water causes an increase in thermal expansion and also prevents the shrinkage associated with the use of water in gypsum-bonded investment
- Dilution of colloidal silica with water or altering the ratio can cause a decrease in thermal expansion
- Thermal shrinkage of phosphate investments occurs when the binder magnesium ammonium phosphate decomposes and is accompanied by evolution of ammonia
- The amount and type of the refractory filler decreases shrinkage.

Wax Inlay

High coefficient of thermal expansion: 0.7% at 20°C and contraction: 0.35% when cooled from 37°C to 25°C.

63. Ethyl-silicate-bonded Investment.

INTRODUCTION

- This is an investment material used for casting removable partial dentures
- Because of the difficulty in investment procedure and as it is time consuming, they are not commonly used
- In high-fusing base metal alloy removable dentures, they are used for accuracy of fit.

Composition

- Binder is a silica gel. This gel reverts to silica (cristobalite) on heating
- To strengthen the gel, magnesium oxide is added.

Availability

Powder and two types of liquid to mix.

Methods of Producing Silicic Acid Gel Binders

- When an acid or acid salt is added to sodium silicate, the pH is lowered and a silicic acid gel forms
- When ammonium chloride is added to an aqueous suspension of colloidal silica, a silicic gel is formed
- Another method of forming silca gel is from the hydrolysis of ethyl silicate in the presence of hydrochloric acid.

Physical Properties

Thermal Expansion

The investment expands during reheating to the same proportion as initial heating, but second heating can form internal cracks. The investment should have sufficient expansion to compensate for all of the thermal contraction of the alloy.

Strength

- The compressive strength of the investment should not be too high. If high, the investment can resist alloy shrinkage when the alloy is still quite hot and weak. This can cause distortion and even fracture in the casting if the hot strength of the alloy is low
- After burn-out of the mold, the strength of the investment should be sufficient enough to resist the impact of the metal entering the mold
- Increase in compressive strength is due to the amount and the type of the gypsum binder and chemical modifiers

- Strength is affected by the water-powder ratio—if more water is added while mixing, the compressive strength is low
- Investments containing sodium decrease in strength after heating.

Disadvantages

- Expensive
- Releases inflammable components during processing
- Is technique-sensitive and time-consuming.

64. Explain the following Terms:
a. Green Shrinkage
b. Green Strength

GREEN SHRINKAGE

This is a shrinkage occurring in ethyl silicate investments used for investing high-fusing base metal partial alloys.

Method of Formation

- When ethyl silicate is hydrolyzed in the presence of hydrochloric acid, ethyl alcohol and water, a colloidal silicic acid is formed
- This colloidal sol is mixed with quartz or cristobalite to which is added powdered magnesium oxide
- This soft gel is dried at 168°C. During drying, the gel loses alcohol and water causing a volumetric contraction to form hard gel. This contraction reduces the mold size
- This setting shrinkage occurring in ethyl silicate investment during drying process is called green shrinkage.

Method to Compensate for Green Shrinkage

- As the above reaction is time-consuming and not accurate due to shrinkage, another technique is employed
- Here amines are added to the solution of ethyl silicate so that hydrolysis and gelation occur simultaneously
- In this method, the powder is added to hydrolyzed ethyl silicate liquid and vibrated into the mold with an extracollar in which the heavier particles settle down and lighter ones move to the top
- After the set occurs, the excess at top is poured out. This reduces liquid-powder ratio and, hence, the shrinkage is also reduced.

GREEN STRENGTH

Synonyms

Wet strength in gypsum.

Definition

Green strength or wet strength is the strength obtained when the water in excess of that required for hydration of the hemihydrate is left in the test specimen.

Differences between Green Strength and Dry Strength

- Dry strength is the strength obtained after the water within the gypsum has dried off
- Dry strength is many times stronger than the wet strength of a specimen
- The water that was lost from gypsum between 8 hours and 24 hours is approximately 0.6%
- The dry strength is better as fine crystals of gypsum precipitate
- These fine crystals anchor the larger crystals
- There is a weight change from wet strength period to dry strength
- After 24 hours, there was no change in loss of weight
- Wet strength begins from the initial setting period and continues till the final setting of gypsum.

Factors affecting Green Strength

Water-powder Ratio

- If excess water is present, the fine crystals dissolve and strength decreases.

Spatulation Time

- Increase in mixing time can result in crystal break up with less interlocking in the final product, causing decrease in strength.

Addition of Accelerators and Retarders

- Decrease the wet and dry strength because the added salt causes less inter-crystalline cohesion.

Method of Testing Green/Wet Strength

- Strength is related to compressive strength in gypsum, the tensile strength is also tested
- Tests as Gilmore, Vicat, Knoop can be done to indicate setting time and the penetration difference between the wet strength period and dry strength period.

Effect of Drying on Compressive Strength

Drying time	Compressive strength	Loss of weight
At 2 hours	9.6 Mpa	5.1%
At 4 hours	11.7 Mpa	11.9%
At 8 hours	11.7 Mpa	17.4%
At 24 hours	23.3 Mpa	18.0%

Effect of Water-Powder Ratio on Strength

Water-powder ratio	Mixing time	Strength
0.45	0.5 minutes	23.4 MPa
0.45	1.0 minutes	26.2 MPa
0.60	1.0 minutes	17.9 MPa
0.80	1.0 minutes	11.0 MPa

65. Casting Machines and Crucibles Used.

CASTING MACHINES

Casting machines are machines used to cast melted alloys into the mold.

Types of Casting Machines

- Centrifugal casting machine
- Electrical resistance-heated casting machine
- Induction melting and casting machine.

Procedure

- The alloy can be melted in a separate crucible by torch flame or by a resistance or induction furnace
- The melted alloy can be cast into mold by centrifugal force (motor or spring action) or by air pressure vacuum, or both
- Noble metal alloy melted by placing it on the inner sidewall of the crucible so that any gases in the flame is reflected from the surface of the metal than absorbed by the metal
- Fuels that can be used are a mixture of natural, or artificial gas and air, or oxygen and acetylene
- The flame should be nonluminous brush flame, with the different combustion zones clearly seen.

Centrifugal Casting Machine

- Centrifugal casting machine spring is wound two to five turns (depending on the type of machine and speed of casting)
- The metal is melted by torch flame in a ceramic crucible which is attached to the 'broken arm' of the casting machine

- When the metal gives an orange hue, the metal has reached the casting temperature. Meanwhile the heated casting ring is taken from the burnout furnace and positioned in the appropriate area of the centrifugal casting machine
- After the casting ring is correctly positioned, the lever is released and the spring triggers the rotational motion.
- The broken-arm feature accelerates the initial rotational speed of the crucible and casting ring and liquid casting alloy fill the mold
- As the metal fills the mold, a hydrostatic pressure gradient occurs
- The pressure gradient just before solidification begins in about 0.21 to 0.28 MPa (30 to 40 psi) at the tip of the casting
- The greatest heat transfer to the mold is at the tip of the casting, where the pressure is high
- The solidification starts from the thin margin edge to the button surface.

Advantages of Induction Casting Machine

- The metal is melted within a graphite crucible by an induction field surrounded by water-cooled metal tubing than by a torch flame
- Melting within the furnace prevents oxidation of alloys which can increase bond strength in metal-ceramic restorations
- The crucible in the furnace is flush against the casting ring. Hence, the metal button remains molten for a longer time ensuring complete flow of metal before solidification
- A carbon crucible cannot be used to melt alloys with high melting temperatures
- More commonly used for melting base metal alloys.

CASTING CRUCIBLES

Types

- Clay
- Carbon
- Quartz (including zircon-alumina).

Clay Crucibles

These are only used for high noble and noble types.

Carbon Crucibles

These are used only for high noble and higher-fusing, gold-based metal-ceramic alloys.

Quartz Crucibles

These are used for high-fusing alloys as palladium-silver alloys for metal-ceramic copings and nickel or cobalt-based alloys.

66. Porosities/Defects in Noble Metal Castings.

CLASSIFICATION OF DEFECTS

Internal (Fig. 43)

- Solidification defects
- Microporosities
- Pinhole porosities
- Subsurface porosities
- Residual air in the mold.

External

- Surface roughnesses.

Solidification Defects

Solidification Shrinkage

Mainly occurs near sprue-cast junction.

Causes

- Incomplete feeding of molten metal
- Premature solidification of the sprue.

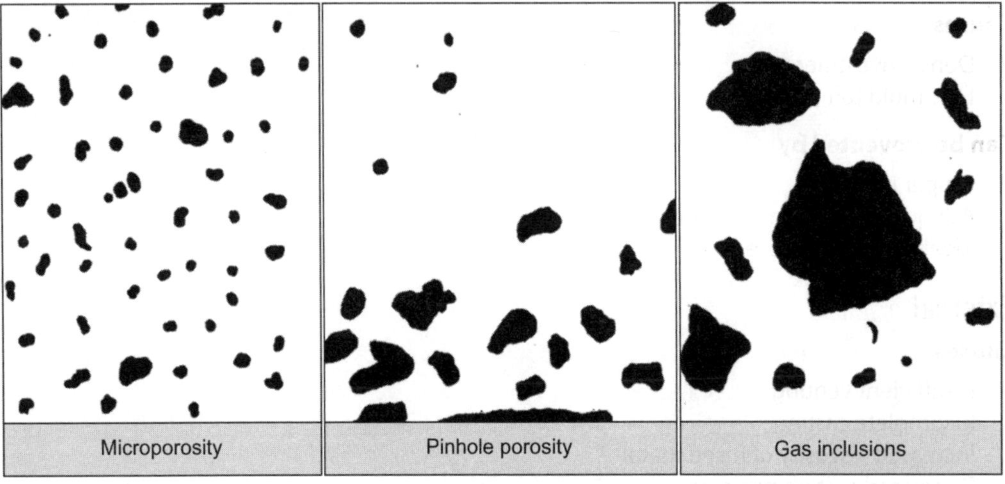

Fig. 43: Types of porosities

Suck Back Porosities

Near area of sprue

- This occurs when a hot metal, impinging from sprue channel on to a point on the mold wall, causes a hot spot. This hot spot causes local region to freeze last resulting in shrinkage of that area leading to a suck back porosity.

Can be prevented by

- Flaring of the area of sprue attachment
- Lowering casting temperature by 30°.

Microporosities

- Occur when solidification occurs too rapidly before the microvoids can reorganize.
- Can prevent by lowering the mold temperature.

Pinhole Porosity

It is spherical in shape whereas gas inclusion porosity is larger. During solidification, absorbed gases are expelled leading to pinhole porosity.

Subsurface Porosities

Cause

- Simultaneous nucleation of solid grains and gas bubbles as the metal freezes at the mold walls
- Can be decreased by controlling the rate of molten metal entry.

Residual Air in the Mold

- It causes back pressure porosity
- It occurs as a large concave depression due to the inability of air in the mold to escape.

Causes

- Dense investments.
- Low mold temperature.

Can be prevented by

- Proper burnout
- Adequate mold temperature
- Ideal casting pressure.

External

Causes

- Insufficient venting
- Incomplete casting
- Increased viscosity of fused metal
- Decreased casting pressure
- Incomplete wax elimination.

RULES TO FOLLOW

Melting can be done by an air/gas torch.

- The alloy should be completely molten or can result in an incomplete casting
- Overheating should be avoided to prevent contamination of castings due to oxidation
- The reducing zone of the flame should be used for melting the alloy
- Flux should be applied to prevent oxidation
- Surplus alloys of different types should not be mixed
- The alloy should not be reused more than two times, otherwise zinc (a scavenger for oxygen) may be lost by volatilization
- A mixture of new and used alloys is commonly used.

67. Sprue Former.

DEFINITION

- Sprue is a metal or plastic that connects a casting to the residual sprue button
- A sprue former is a wax, plastic or metal pattern used to form the channel allowing the molten metal to flow into the mold to make a casting
- Spruing is the procedure of attaching a sprue to the wax pattern.

Types of Spruing

- Single spruing
- Multiple spruing for long span bridges.

Materials Used as Sprues

- *Wax*—Commonly used
- *Plastic*—Only the hollow plastic sprues to be used
- *Metal*—If used, should be removed before casting with care.

Rules for Spruing

- A short thick sprue helps the metal to be molten for a longer duration and keeps feeding the mold with metal without solidification at the sprue area. A thin long sprue can cause shrink spot porosity
- Sprue should be attached to the bulkiest portion of the pattern (10 gauge sprues for molar crowns)
- Sprue diameter should be larger than the bulkiest portion

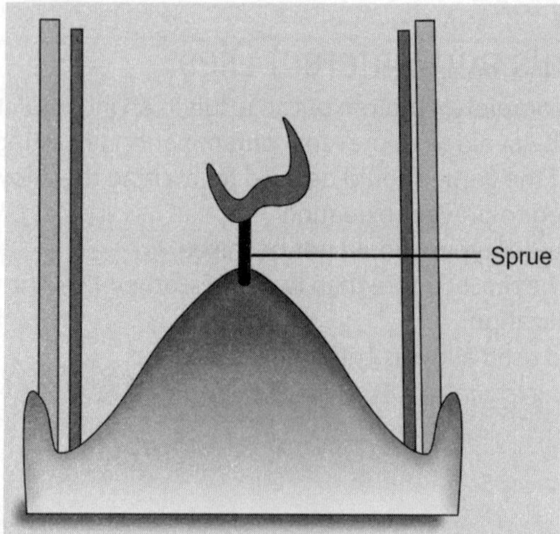

Fig. 44: Wax pattern with sprue placed inside the casting ring

- Sprue should not be attached perpendicular to the wax pattern
- Sprue should be firmly attached to the wax pattern
- A reservoir should be placed in the sprue for complete casting
- Sprue must allow molten wax to escape completely.

Sprue Placement

- It should be attached at 45° angulation to the thickest portion of the pattern. This prevents porosities and air entrapments
- The area of sprue attachment is flared for smooth flow of metal.

Sprue Attachment

- One end of the sprue is attached to the wax pattern with a reservoir
- The other end is attached to the crucible former's cone-shaped structure
- The wax pattern should have 6 mm space between the tip of pattern and casting ring. The space allows for the air to escape out of the pores in investment
- The wax pattern should have uniform space within the casting ring (it should be placed in the center of the casting ring) **(Fig. 44)**.

68. Die Materials and Different Dies.

MATERIALS USED

- Gypsum
- Epoxy resin
- Electroplated dies.

Gypsum

Advantages

Inexpensive, easy to use and able to produce consistent results.

Disadvantage

Decreased accuracy and resistance to abrasion.

Variation of Technique

It is to impregnate the surface of the die with a low viscosity resin, (cyano-acrylate), to improve abrasion resistance.

Epoxy Resin

Advantages

- Good strength
- Good abrasion resistance
- Can be cured at room temperature
- No complicated equipment required
- Dimensionally stable
- Retainers adapt better when made on epoxy dies
- Silicone and polyether are compatible with epoxy.

Disadvantages

1. More expensive than gypsum.
2. Polymerization shrinkage.
3. Polysulfide and hydrocolloid are not compatible.

Variation

Epoxy resin, which is heat-treated after setting, is also available.

Electroplated Die

Advantages

Good abrasion resistance.

Disadvantage

- Silicone and polyether impressions are difficult to electroplate.
- Polysulfide can be silver plated, but cannot be copper plated.
- Silver plating uses cyanide solution, which is extremely toxic.

Technique

- Finely powdered silver or graphite is brushed on to the impressions to make them conduct electricity.
- The impression is then placed in the electroplating bath.
- A layer of pure metal is deposited on the impression which is supported with type IV stone or resin.

69. Dispersion Alloys.

DEFINITION

- These are alloys containing spherical silver copper particles to 'dispersion harden' amalgams. They are made from admixed powder and are called dispersion or dispersant amalgam alloys.
- They are also called admixed alloys as the final powder is a mixture of two or more kinds of particles.

Importance

- Amalgam made from admixed powders is stronger than amalgam made from lathe-cut low-copper powder
- The strength is due to the silver copper particles in 'dispersion hardened' amalgam.

Mechanism of Dispersion Hardening

It is a strengthening seen in metals when a large volume fraction of ultrafine particles (typically less than 1 mm) is dispersed throughout the metal.

- The silver copper particles in admixed amalgams are small or closely spaced to produce dispersion hardening
- Silver-copper particles act as strong fillers strengthening the amalgam matrix similar to composites with fillers

- Restoration with admixed amalgam show better resistance to marginal breakdown than low copper amalgam restoration
- Admixed alloy powder usually contains 30–55 wt% spherical high copper powder with total copper content ranging from 9 to 20 wt%.

70. Porosities in Casting.

GROUPED UNDER

A. Distortion.
B. Surface roughness and irregularities.
C. Porosity.
D. Incomplete casting.

A. Distortion

Factors Causing Distortion

1. Due to distortion of the wax pattern.
2. Uneven setting and hygroscopic expansions of the investment.
3. Configuration of the pattern, type of wax and thickness.
4. Distortion during the carving, pooling and removal of wax.

B. Surface Roughness and Irregularities

- *Surface roughness* is defined as finely spaced surface irregularities, whose height, width and direction establish predominant surface pattern
- *Surface irregularities* are isolated, generally caused by improper mixing technique.

Causes

Air bubbles

- Air bubbles on margin of casting prevents proper seating
- This can be prevented by proper vacuum mixing, application of wetting agent and applying an initial layer of investment on pattern.

Water films

- These appear as ridge or veins
- This occurs due to high water-powder ratio of investment material
- Application of wetting agent to wax pattern before investment can reduce water films.

Rapid heating

- Seen as fins or spines
- When the invested material develops tensile stresses inside and compressive stresses outside, the investment cracks and forms fins.

Underheating

It is due to incomplete wax elimination.

Water-Powder ratio

Increased water-powder ratio causes rough casting and decreased ratio causes voids.

Prolonged heating

This causes sulfur compounds that contaminate the surface of the casting.

High temperature

Above 700°C causes breakdown of the investment and results in rough casting.

High casting pressure

Ideal casting pressure is 0.10 to 0.14 MPa (3–4 turns in the centrifugal casting machine).

Composition of investment

If coarse silica is present, it can cause rough casting.

Foreign bodies

Incorporated from rough crucible, sprue former, investment pieces, bits of carbon from flux.

Impact of molten alloy

Due to improper spruing.

Wrong pattern placement in the casting ring

Too many patterns placed together and patterns placed too close in the same ring should be avoided.

C. Porosities

Internal

- Solidification defects
- Microporosities
- Pinhole porosities
- Subsurface porosities
- Residual air in the mould **(Fig. 45)**.

External

- Surface roughnesses.

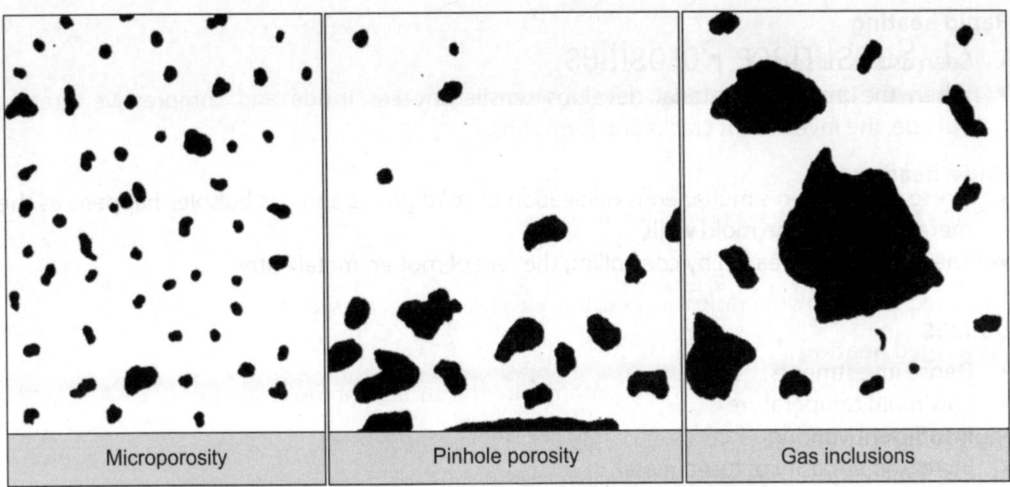

Fig. 45: Types of porosities

Solidification Defects

Solidification shrinkage

Mainly occurs near sprue-cast junction.

Causes

- Incomplete feeding of molten metal
- Premature solidification of the sprue.

Suck Back Porosities

- Near the area of sprue
- This occurs when a hot metal, impinging from sprue channel onto a point on the mold wall, causes a hot spot. This hot spot causes local region to freeze last resulting in shrinkage of that area leading to a suck back porosity.

Can be prevented by

- Flaring of the area of sprue attachment
- Lowering casting temperature by 30°.

Microporosities

- These occur when solidification occurs too rapidly before the microvoids can reorganize
- These can prevent by lowering the mold temperature.

Pinhole Porosity

It is spherical in shape whereas gas inclusion porosity is larger. During solidification, absorbed gases are expelled leading to pinhole porosity.

71. Subsurface Porosities.

- These occur when simultaneous nucleation of solid grains and gas bubbles happens as the metal freezes at the mold walls
- These can be decreased by controlling the rate of molten metal entry.

Causes

- Dense investments
- Low mold temperature
- Insufficient venting
- Increased viscosity of fused metal
- Decreased casting pressure
- Incomplete wax elimination.

Can be prevented by

- Proper burnout
- Adequate mold temperature
- Ideal casting pressure.

72. Metal Ceramics/Types of Bond/Technique.

TYPES OF BOND

- Mechanical retention
- Compression
- Chemical bonding.

Mechanical Retention

- Mechanical retention occurs when ceramic flows into the microscopic spaces in the surface of the metal
- The roughness of the metal surface can be increased by air abrasion or by grinding, hence increasing mechanical bond and also aids in better wetting of the ceramic onto the metal.

Factors affecting mechanical bond

- *Impurities on the surface*—Before application of the ceramic, the coping is degassed, which removes impurities and trapped gasses at the interface
- If the thermal mismatch is too large, then the bond strength decreases.

Compression

- Residual compressive stresses are incorporated to prevent stress concentrations and crack propagation
- If tensile stresses are formed within a treated ceramic (residual compressive stress incorporated) material, the amount of residual compressive stress present in the material decreases, neutralizing the tensile stress
- A treated ceramic is much stronger than untreated ceramic
- A treated ceramic requires high tensile forces to fracture and exhaust the entire residual compressive forces.

Different methods to induce residual compressive forces are:

- Ion exchange
- Thermal tempering
- Thermal compatibility.

Ion exchange (Chemical tempering)

- Ion exchange involves the exchange of larger potassium ions for the smaller sodium ions by placing the sodium containing glass in a bath of molten potassium nitrate
- The larger potassium ions (35% larger than sodium) squeezes into the areas previously occupied by smaller sodium ions creating large residual compressive stresses (roughly 700 MPa [100,000 psi]).

Points to note:

- The above treated material cannot be ground
- It should not be allowed to come into contact with acidulated phosphate fluoride for more than 3 hours
- Alumina core ceramics, dicor glass ceramics are resistant to ion exchange when in contact with acidulated phosphate fluoride.

Thermal tempering

- Thermal tempering is done by heating a material to create residual surface compressive stresses and then cooled rapidly (quenched) while it is hot and in molten state
- Quenching forms a rigid outer surface and an inner molten core. When the molten core solidifies, it shrinks, but the outer skin remains rigid
- The pull of the solidifying molten core creates residual tensile stresses in the inner core and residual compressive stresses in the outer surface
- Thermal tempering strengthens glass materials. Quenching is done in silicone oil or other special liquids for uniform cooling.

Thermal compatibility

- The thermal expansion of the metal and porcelain are adjusted so that the porcelain is under slight compression and the alloy selected contracts slightly more than the porcelain on cooling to room temperature and forms a residual compressive stress within

- To create a compressive force, a three-layer technique with different thermal coefficient contraction is used
- In three-layer technique, the outer two layers have the same composition and thermal contraction coefficient, whereas the middle layer has different composition and a higher thermal contraction coefficient.
- Hence, on cooling to room temperature, the inner layer produces compressive stresses in the outer layers.

Chemical Bonding

- Chemical bond is created between the ceramic and the oxide coating on the metal
- During firing, the ceramic flows and fuses with the oxides on the metal surface by migration of the oxides into the ceramic
- In gold alloy copings, small amounts of oxide forming elements (tin and indium) are added to the alloy that aids in oxide forming
- Oxide bond increases the bond strength.

Procedure for Bonding

Steps in preparation of metal

- Surface grinding
- Heating under partial vacuum
- Acid pickling
- Heating in air.

Surface grinding

- Surface grinding is done to remove residual investment bonded to the surface of the casting, unwanted oxides, small porosities and projections
- Grinding process also increases the surface roughness, improving micro-mechanical interlocking
- Grinding should not result in formation of deep fissures, porosities or undercuts
- Grinding is done using fissure burs or carbide burs
- Surface contaminants are removed by placing into carbon tetrachloride in ultrasonic bath.

Heating under partial vacuum

- Short heating cycle forms thin or partial oxide coating, decreasing bond strength
- Long heating cycles cause depletion of the oxidising elements and no bond will be formed
- In base metal alloys, the metals oxidise readily and too much oxide is formed
- Heating under partial vacuum allows the proper wetting of ceramic.

Acid pickling

- The heat treatment of gold alloys produces other oxides apart from tin oxide
- To remove these unnecessary oxides, acid pickling is done
- Acid pickling removes the dark surface of the alloy and the alloy is lightened from grey to white due to increased concentration of tin oxide on the alloy surface
- Commonly used acids are 50% hydrofluoric acid or 30% hydrochloric acid (more preferred)
- Not done for base metal alloys.

Heating in air

- Heat treatment in air is done to form an oxide coating of the correct thickness and quality
- The oxide film should have a mat, greyish white appearance, consisting of tin oxide
- If the treated surface has a glossy appearance, re-treatment is required or else the bond strength will be poor.

73. Choice of Alloys in Ceramics, Benefits, Requirements and Drawbacks of Bonded Ceramics.

TYPES OF ALLOYS AND THEIR BENEFITS

High-gold Alloys

- In high-gold alloys, platinum and palladium are added to raise the melting temperature
- Copper is not included in ceramic alloys as it can lower the melting temperature and cause a green discoloration, hampering the esthetics of the restoration
- High-gold alloys have good bond strength with ceramic.

Disadvantages

- High-gold alloys have low melting temperatures and are susceptible to creep at high temperatures
- They have low elastic moduli and require a minimum of 0.5 mm coping thickness.

Gold-palladium Alloys

- These alloys were introduced as high gold alloys were expensive
- They possess better castability
- They provide better fit and are corrosion-resistant
- Some of these alloys are not compatible with porcelain due to large thermal mismatches.

High-palladium Alloys

- The main component is palladium, to which are added copper, gallium and tin
- Copper (up to 15%), when present in palladium alloys, does not form greenish discoloration on porcelain
- Possess poor sag resistance and hence are contraindicated for long-span bridges.

Palladium-silver Alloys

- They have good sag resistance, good elastic modulus and low flexibility of castings
- Compared to gold alloys, their castability and fit are poor but an accurate technique can produce good results

- Silver in these alloys can cause discoloration
- Repeated firings should be avoided in order not to overheat the alloy.

Nickel-chromium Alloys

- Ni-Cr alloys have high elastic modulus nearly 2.5 times higher than that of high-gold alloys
- Because of their high modulus, their coping thickness can be reduced to 0.3 mm.
- Can be used for long-span bridges as they have good strength, high melting temperature and good sag resistance
- Difficulty in castability, poor fit compared to other alloys and high casting shrinkage.
- Ceramic to metal bond is poor.

Advantages

Metal-bonded ceramic crowns are three times stronger and the microcracks can be eliminated.

The crown consists of a cast metal coping on which the ceramic veneer is fired. The metal prevents the propagation of cracks due to its high fracture toughness.

REQUIREMENTS OF ALLOYS/CERAMICS TO BE USED AS METAL CERAMICS

- The alloy should have a high melting temperature, so that the ceramic can be fired on to the alloy
- The metal/alloy should possess high elastic modulus and high yield stress
- The high stiffness of the metal prevents excessive occlusal loading on ceramic
- Good bond strength with ceramic
- A slightly greater thermal coefficient than ceramic
- If repeated firings are employed, the number and size of the leucite crystals will increase, which, in turn, will increase the coefficient of expansion of the ceramic
- This can decrease the bond strength between the metal and ceramic
- Slow cooling also produces the same effects
- If firing technique is not precise, ceramic can devitrify, which can esthetically alter the color of ceramic
- Both soda (Na_2O) and potash (K_2O) are added to increase the coefficient of expansion to 12 ppm/°C
- Increase in Soda and Potash forms a crystalline phase known as leucite, which has high coefficient of thermal expansion
- The amount of precipitated leucite is controlled to 30 to 40% of volume to provide the ceramic with the correct coefficient of expansion
- After the ceramic frit is prepared, it is held at an elevated temperature for a specific time to allow the formation of leucite crystals.

DRAWBACKS OF METAL CERAMICS

1. Excessive tensile stresses within the material can cause microcracks leading to failure of the restoration.

   Eliminating microcracks can be done by
   - Glazing the internal fitting surface.
   - Bonding ceramic to a metal substrate.

2. They are brittle in nature.
3. Metal bonded ceramics can fail if ceramic separates from the metal due to interfacial breakdown.
4. If the thermal mismatch between the metal and ceramic is great, then stresses will build up during the cooling, resulting in crazing or cracking of the ceramic.

74. Acid Pickling.

DEFINITION

Pickling is a process that removes a surface film from the casting, which has dark surface oxides and tarnish.

Cause of Oxide Formation on Casting

When the cast gold alloys are quenched to retain their superior physical properties, the water that contacts the hot investment, causes reaction that makes the investment soft and granular. This causes a darkening of the casting.

Advantages of Pickling

1. Removes any clinging investment.
2. Removes the oxide coating and tarnish.

Disadvantage of using Hydrochloric Acid

Fumes from the acid corrode office and laboratory metals.

Other agents that can be used are:
- Solution of sulfuric acid with traces of potassium dichromate
- Ultrasonic cleaners.

PICKLING PROCEDURE

- The discolored casting is heated in an acid such as 50% hydrochloric acid for gypsum-bonded investments
- The casting is placed in a test tube or dish and heated acid is poured over the casting
- The acid is poured off and the casting is removed
- Pickling solution should be renewed frequently.

Rules to Follow

1. Casting, if gripped with steel tongs, will get contaminated because the pickling solution contains small amounts of copper dissolved from previous castings, which when contacted by the tongs, deposits copper on the casting.
2. The casting, if heated, can melt the delicate margin or when plunged into the acid, the casting can get distorted by sudden temperature variation.
3. After pickling, the casting should be washed thoroughly to remove traces of the acid.

75. Condensation and Firing of Porcelain Jacket Crown.

CONDENSATION

Fine porcelain powder is mixed with water and condensed into the desired form.

Dense Condensation Provides

1. Lower firing shrinkage.
2. Less porosity in the fired porcelain.

Methods of Condensation

Vibration

Mild vibration to densely pack the wet powder upon the underlying framework.
The excess water is blotted with a clean tissue.

Spatulation

A small spatula is used to apply and smooth the wet porcelain.

Brush Technique

- Dry porcelainpowder is added to the surface with brush to absorb the water
- Porcelain must never be allowed to dry out until condensation is complete.

FIRING

- The thermochemical reaction is complete during fritting
- Firing is done to fuse the particles of powder together, a process called sintering.

Method

- The condensed porcelain mass is placed in a preheated furnace, approximately 650°C (1200°F) for 5 minutes
- This removes the remaining water.

Stages in Firing

In Low-bisque (Low-biscuit) Firing

The glass grains have softened and have started to flow.

In Medium-bisque (medium-biscuit) Firing

The glass grains have flowed to the extent that the powder particles exhibit complete cohesion.

In High-bisque (high-biscuit) Firing

- The shrinkage is complete and the mass exhibits a smoother surface
- The lesser the firing cycles, the higher will be the strength and esthetics.

GLAZING

Air-fired porcelain cannot be polished.

Application of Over-glaze/Self-glaze

- Self-glazing, which was previously fired to a high bisque, is heated rapidly (10–15 minutes) to its fusion temperature
- It is maintained at that temperature for approximately 5 minutes before it is cooled
- Glass grains flow over the surface to form a vitreous layer
- Glazed porcelain is much stronger and reduces crack propagation than the unglazed variety.

Cooling

- Because of the low thermal conductivity of the porcelain, the differential between the thermal dimensional change of the outside and inside can introduce stresses, which embrittle the porcelain
- The ideal cooling method for a porcelain restoration from its firing temperature to room temperature is controversial.

76. Methods of Strengthening Ceramics.

REASONS FOR STRENGTHENING CERAMICS

- Any *stress concentration* at the tips of minute scratches or flaws causes the localized stress to increase leading to crack formation. This crack propagates through the material, weakening the entire material
- Ceramics are basically brittle with low tensile strengths and so they cannot yield to stress without fracture as metals do
- Ceramics possess good esthetic qualities, hardness, compressive strength, chemical durability and excellent biocompatibility
- Ceramics are brittle, have low fracture toughness and low tensile strength.

METHODS TO OVERCOME ABOVE DEFECTS

- By strengthening brittle materials
- By designing components to minimize stress concentrations and tensile stresses.

Methods to Strengthen Brittle Materials

- Development of residual compressive stresses within the surface of the material
- Interruption of crack propagation
- Dispersion of crystalline phase
- Transformation toughening.

Development of Residual Compressive Stresses

- To introduce residual compressive stresses, the residual stresses must be first negated by developing tensile stresses
- If residual compressive stresses are formed within a treated ceramic material the amount of residual compressive stress present in the material decreases the tensile stress and neutralises it
- A treated ceramic is much stronger than untreated ceramic
- A treated ceramic requires high tensile forces to fracture and exhaust the entire residual compressive forces.

Methods to induce residual compressive forces are:

- Ion exchange
- Thermal tempering
- Thermal compatibility.

Ion Exchange (Chemical Tempering)

- Ion exchange involves the exchange of larger potassium ions for the smaller sodium ions by placing the sodium containing glass in a bath of molten potassium nitrate

- The larger potassium ions (35% larger than sodium) squeeze into the areas previously occupied by smaller sodium ions creating large residual compressive stresses (roughly 700 MPa [100,000 psi]).

Points to note

- The above treated material cannot be ground
- It should not be allowed to come into contact with acidulated phosphate fluoride for more than 3 hours
- Alumina core ceramics, dicor glass-ceramics are resistant to ion exchange when in contact with acidulated phosphate fluoride.

Thermal Tempering

- Thermal tempering is done by heating a material to create residual surface compressive stresses and then cooled rapidly (quenched) while it is hot and in molten state
- Quenching forms a rigid outer surface and an inner molten core
- When the molten core solidifies, it shrinks, but the outer skin remains rigid
- The pull of the solidifying molten core creates a residual tensile stress in the inner core and residual compressive stresses in the outer surface.

Significance

Thermal tempering strengthens glass materials. Quenching needs to be done in silicone oil or other special liquids for uniform cooling.

Thermal Compatibility

- *Metals expand* linearly as the temperature increases, whereas expansion of porcelain is unpredictable
- Hence, the thermal expansion of the metal and porcelain are adjusted so that the porcelain is under slight compression for which the alloy selected contracts slightly more than the porcelain on cooling to room temperature
- To create a compressive force within the technique commonly employed is a three-layer technique with different thermal coefficient contraction
- Here the outer two layers have the same composition and thermal contraction coefficient and the middle layer has different composition and a higher thermal contraction coefficient. Hence, on cooling to room temperature, the inner layer produces compressive stresses in the outer layers.

Disruption of Crack Propagation

A stronger reinforcing material is dispersed within the glasses and ceramics so that a crack is stopped from propagating through the material.

Two types

1. The first type utilizes the toughness of the particle to absorb energy and preventing the crack from propagating
2. The second type utilizes materials that can undergo crystal structural change to absorb energy under stress from the crack.

Dispersion of a Crystalline Phase

- When a tough, crystalline material alumina (Al_2O_3) in particulate form is added to a glass, the glass is toughened and strengthened
- Here the crack cannot penetrate the alumina particles as easily as it can penetrate the glass.

Example:
- Aluminous porcelains/dicor glass-ceramic
- In dicor, during casting, the temperature causes micron-sized mica crystals to grow in the glass which disrupt crack propagation, thereby strengthening the crown.

Transformation Toughening

Incorporation of a crystalline material that changes in crystal structure when placed under stress.

Example:
- Partially stabilized zirconia (PSZ)
- The energy for the transformation of PSZ is taken from the energy of crack to propagate.

Disadvantage

The index of refraction is higher than the surrounding glass matrix. Hence, PSZ scatters light through the bulk of the porcelain and causes an opacifying effect.

Design of Dental Restorations for Ceramics

- Design should accommodate for bulk of material to increase strength
- The preparation should not have sharp margins/angles to prevent stress concentration.

77. Aluminous Porcelain/Dicor.

AVAILABLE AS

- Solid ceramic ingots, which are cast using lost-wax and centrifugal-casting technique
- Only one shade is available
- Staining is done to obtain proper shading of the final restoration.

Picon

This is a polycrystalline glass-ceramic material, in which glass is heat-treated under controlled crystallization.

Procedure

- When solid ceramic ingots are cast at 1350°C, a transparent glass crown is obtained
- This crown is then heat-treated at 1075°C for 10 hours
- 'Ceramming' causes partial crystallization (55 percent) of tetra-silicic-mica-like crystals.
- For final restoration, colorant stains are baked on the surface of the glass-ceramic material.

Advantages

- Easier as it is a lost wax technique
- The transparent crown after heat treatment at 1075°C for 10 hours forms an opaque crown, which increases fracture resistance and strength
- Less abrasive to opposing tooth structure.

Dicor Plus

This is a shaded feldspathic porcelain veneer applied to the Dicor substrate.

Disadvantages

- Abrasive to opposing teeth
- Requires a special high-temperature, electric-heated casting unit
- Fracture of the restorations is common.

78. Explain the following:

a. Greening in Porcelain.
b. Green State.

GREENING IN PORCELAIN

- It is the discoloration occurring in porcelain due to silver
- The colloidal dispersion silver atoms entering the body and incisal porcelain or the glazed surface from vapor transport or surface diffusion causes a green, yellow-green-yellow-orange, orange or brown hues. This discoloration is referred to as greening.

Common Factors

- Porcelains with high sodium content is more prone to silver diffusion
- Porcelains with low opacifier content and high sodium have more greening effect
- Greening is seen more in cervical region as surface diffusion from metal margins is more in this region

- Greening increases when silver oxide gas vaporizes from alloy and deposits in cooler areas of furnace
- During heating and cooling, silver vaporizes and condenses on restoration and especially on porcelain metal margins
- Greening can also occur in silver free alloys if the furnace is contaminated from previous firings of silver containing alloys
- Multiple firing procedures, body porcelain contacting alloy, vacuum firing cycles and high silver content porcelains, all cause greening.

Greening Effect can be Prevented by

- Discoloration is mostly due to neutral silver atoms than silver ions. Hence, porcelains with high affinity to oxygen are used that can convert neutral silver atoms to silver ions
- Will-Ceram and Pen craft porcelain are resistant to discoloration with 38% of silver content
- Greening can be prevented by using graphite blocks to maintain reducing atmosphere near the alloy, to prevent silver oxide formation
- Metal coatings as pure gold film on metal substrate reduce discoloration
- Ceramic conditioner can be applied on metal substrate to form a barrier between alloy and porcelain
- An ultra low fusing porcelain or a nongreening porcelain can be used.

Alloys

- Gold-silver palladium alloys containing 5 to 12% silver are more prone to greening
- High noble metal and noble metal alloys cause less greening
- Gold-platinum-palladium alloys with 5 to 8% silver have less greening effect.

GREEN STATE CERAMICS

- This term refers to as pressed condition before sintering
- Cercon is a presintered zirconia ceramic milled to an enlarged size in green state by scanning of a wax pattern.

79. Ring Liners/Ringless Castings.

TYPES OF RING LINERS

- Asbestos
- Nonasbestos

Asbestos

Asbestos was commonly used as a ring liner until evidences of it being a carcinogenic potential was established (making it a biohazard).

Nonasbestos

a. Aluminum silicate ceramic liner.
b. Cellulose (paper) liner.

Significance of Ring Liners

- To provide space for investment expansion. If the setting expansion is not permitted, the casting can be smaller than the actual size, as metal contracts **(Fig. 46)**
- Increasing expansion is achieved by using a split ring or flexible rubber ring
- Ring liners achieve perfect fit of the casting by providing uniform expansion of investment material
- Ring liners also permit easy removal of the casting.

Method of Using Ring Liner

- The liner is wrapped on the outside of the casting ring to form an idea about the length of the liner required to line the inside of the ring
- The measured amount of liner is cut using a sharp pair of scissors and is fit on the inside diameter of the casting ring with no overlap
- Liner can be used as dry or wet. In the dry technique, the liner is tacked in position with sticky wax
- If wet technique is used, the liner is dipped in water and the excess water is shaken away.
- In wet technique, the liner should not be squeezed as this can lead to uneven expansion.

Differences in Liners

Cellulose liner absorbs water whereas a ceramic liner does not absorb water, but the ceramic fiber network can retain water on the surface.

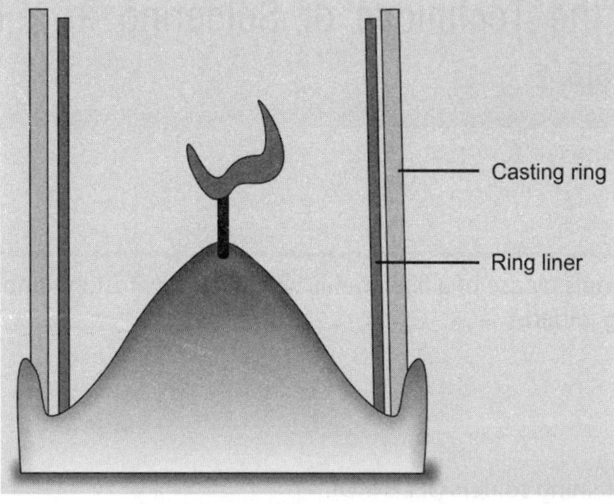

Fig. 46: Casting ring with ring liner

Advantages of Wet Liners/Number of liners

- Wet liners provide for greater normal setting expansion in the investment. The larger the amount of water present in the liner, the greater is the semihygroscopic expansion
- The use of one liner increases the normal setting expansion. If two liners are placed, a greater semihygroscopic expansion occurs.

RINGLESS CASTING SYSTEM

Powercast Ringless System (Whip Mix Corporation, Louisville, KY, USA)

Consists of

- Three sizes of tapered plastic rings and formers
- Preformed wax sprues and shapes
- Special investment powder and a special investment liquid.

Advantages

- It provides maximum expansion of investment
- This system can be used for casting alloys that require greater mold expansion
- The tapered plastic rings can be easily removed after the investment material has set. Hence, there is no confining pressure (negative pressure) on the invested mold and so maximum setting expansion can be achieved.

80. Define Solders. Give Examples, Composition and Uses. Explain the Technique of Soldering in a Bridge Work Prosthesis.

DEFINITION

It is the joining of metals by use of a filler metal, which has low fusion temperature than that of the metal parts being joined.

Types

Group I

Traditional gold-containing solders (JELENKO).

Group II

Presoldering

Used for joining the components before porcelain application.

Postsoldering

Used for joining the components after porcelain application.

Preceramic solders

These are high-fusing alloys, with temperature slightly beneath the softening point of the parent alloy to be joined and should flow well above the fusion range of applied porcelain

Solder flow is increased by the addition of silver and decreased by the presence of copper.

Postceramic solders

These should flow well below the pyroplastic range of the porcelain.

Composition of Solders

Gold, silver, copper, zinc and tin.

Requirements of Solder

1. Should resist tarnish and corrosion.
2. The fusion temperature of solder should be lower than metal.
3. Should be free flowing with proper adhesion to metal.
4. Solder should not cause pitting of soldered joint.
5. Strength of solder should be equivalent to the parts to be soldered.
6. Color of solder should match the parts to be soldered.
7. It should be corrosion-resistant.
8. It should have adequate mechanical properties to withstand the forces.
9. It must have a low surface tension when molten.

Soldering Techniques

A. Torch soldering
B. Oven soldering
C. Electrosoldering
D. Microwelder/laser welding
E. Infrared soldering.

Torch Soldering

- After preheating the assembly, a gas-air torch is used as the heat source to melt the solder. The flame is kept moving to prevent uneven heat distribution
- Oxidization of the joint surfaces is prevented by using the reducing zone of the flame and by applying an appropriate flux.

Advantages

- Solder flow is controlled and solder flows to the hottest point only

- Ideal for badly designed connector in wax, which can be connected well by varying the temperature of solder manually.

Advantages of Oven Soldering/Electrosoldering over Torch Soldering

a. The temperature is uniform throughout the procedure.
b. The temperature is known throughout the procedure.
c. Application of vacuum can control oxidation.
d. Close monitoring is possible.

Electrosoldering Technique

- Easier to use than torch soldering
- Permits the use of very high-fusing alloy solders.

Laser Welding

Used for joining cast titanium components in implant superstructures.

Infrared Soldering

- These can be used for low-fusing connectors as well as for preceramic soldering.
- A pointer is used to direct heat source to the connector after the application of flux.
- While activating the infrared heat source, a protective shield to prevent eye injury is used.

FLUXES

Fluxes containing fluoride must be used.

Soldering Investment

- Gypsum and phosphate-bonded investments containing fused quartz with low thermal expansion are used as casting investments
- Invested units should expand at the same rate as the castings.

Soldering in Fixed Partial Denture

Preceramic Soldering

Advantages

- The connected prosthesis can be tried in the mouth in the unglazed state
- Adjustments can be made before final glazing.

Disadvantages

- Needs support to prevent high-temperature deformation or sag on long span
- Difficult to contour the proximal embrasures.

Postceramic Soldering

- Indicated when regular gold and metal-ceramic units are being combined
- Final staining and glazing must be completed before the soldering.

Advantages

- Proximal areas are more esthetic as they are shaped before soldering
- Sag does not occur and, hence, support is not required.

Disadvantage

Adjustment cannot be made after soldering. If made, they need to be reglazed and resoldered.

Soldering Steps in Fixed Partial Denture

A. Preparation of connector.
B. Occlusal soldering index.
C. Investing.
D. Wax removal and preheating.

Preparation of Connector

- After removing surface oxides from the connector surfaces with a stone, evaluate the seating of restoration in the mouth or cast
- The soldering gap should be 0.25 mm.

Occlusal Index

- This can be made using plaster, resin or zinc oxide eugenol in a small tray or on a sheet of base plate wax.
- The index should not cover the margins and the margins should be exposed prior to investing.

Investing

- The cervical aspect of the restorations is placed into a warmed wax sheet and sealed along the axial wall to protect the porcelain from contact with the soldering investment
- After sealing the porcelain, the entire assembly is boxed and filled with soldering Investment, forming into a patty on a slab
- The restorations are seated angled forward so that the solder can be placed above the joint.

Wax Removal and Preheating

Wax removal

- After the investment has completely set, remove the index by placing it in boiling water (if plaster or ZOE index was used)
- Flow a little flux into the joint space while the soldering block is still warm
- The joint space must be free of investment
- Acrylic resin indexes are removed by heating slowly to 300°C till the resin is burned out and then heat the block to 650°C and then transfer it to the soldering oven for soldering.

Preheating

Preheat the investment in a burnout furnace to 650°C for low-heat soldering and 850°C for preceramic soldering.

81. Flux/Antiflux.

FLUX

Definition

Flux is a substance applied to surfaces to be soldered by joining to increase fluidity and reduce oxidation of a molten metal.

Significance of Flux

1. It removes oxides and prevents oxidation.
2. It allows the solder to wet the metal surface.
3. It helps the solder to adhere to metal surface uniformly.

Availability

- Powder form
- Liquid form
- Paste form is commonly used (Flux powder mixed with petrolatum).

Composition

1. Borax glass ($Na_2B_4O_7$)/Sodium pyroborate—55 parts.
2. Boric acid—35 parts.
3. Silica—10 parts.
   Borax glass + boric acid + silica are fused and ground to form flux powder.

Rules to Follow

Fluxes should not contact porcelain surfaces (Discoloration and pitting results).

ANTIFLUX

Definition

Antiflux is a material that confines solder attachment or flow.

Significance

1. Limits flow of solder (Prevents spreading of solder).
2. Applied before application of flux.
3. Helps to confine the solder to the required area.
4. Maintains the connector shape and thickness.

Types of Antiflux

1. Graphite.
2. Iron oxide in chloroform (Painted with small brush).

82. Beilby Layer.

This phenomenon was observed by a scientist called Beilby.

DEFINITION

- The polishing agents remove material from the surface molecule by molecule
- In the process, fine scratches and irregularities are filled by powdered particulates being removed from the surface
- This microcrystalline layer is referred to as polish layer or beilby layer.

Method of Polishing

- First a coarse abrasive is used to remove gross surface irregularities
- Then a finer abrasive is used to remove the deep scratches to form fine scratches
- Finally a polishing agent is used to eliminate the fine scratches giving it a smooth finish
- During final polishing, the fine irregularities are filled by powdered particulate forming a microcrystalline layer called Beilby layer.

Surfaces in which Beilby layer can be observed

- Metal surfaces
- Enamel surfaces.

Beilby layer on enamel surfaces

- High polish dentifrices increase enamel lustre, decreasing plaque and calculus formation
- Highly polished tooth is also more resistant to cariogenic action.

83. Hard Solders.

- Hard solders have higher melting temperature, greater strength and hardness
- They can be melted only by a blow torch or electric oven.

Uses

- For soldering wires in orthodontics
- For joining components in fixed partial denture
- To repair perforations in crown and bridge
- To develop contact points in crowns
- For soldering clasps in removable partial denture.

Types

- Gold solders.
- Silver solders.

Composition of Gold Solders

- Gold—45 to 81%.
- Silver—8 to 20%.
- Copper 10–15%.
- Tin—2 to 4%.
- Zinc—2 to 4%.

Composition of Silver Solders

- Silver—10 to 80%.
- Copper—15 to 50%.
- Zinc—4 to 35%.

  Trace elements as cadmium or phosphorus may be present.

Properties

Fusion Temperature

- The fusion temperature should be at least 50°C lower than parent metal
- Gold solders—690 to 870°C
- Silver solders—620 to 700°C.

Flow

- Solders with short melting range have better flow
- Gold and silver-based alloys have better flow than nickel-based alloys
- Any impurities as oxide layer on the parent metal reduce the flow.

Color Match

Solders should match in color with the parent metal.

Tarnish/Strength

- Gold solders have good tarnish and corrosion resistance than silver solders
- Well formed joint should have a boundary at microscopic level
- If due to prolonged heating, the solders are diffused with parent metal, then the joint becomes weak.

84. All-Ceramic Restoration.

- The first all-ceramic crowns were introduced by Land in 1903
- In 1965, McLean and Hughes formulated aluminous porcelain, in which 50% aluminum oxide increases the strength and baking temperature.

DEFINITION

- Ceramics are defined as man-made solid objects formed by baking raw materials at high temperatures
- Derived from Greek word 'Keramos', meaning 'burnt stuff'.

COMPOSITION OF ALL CERAMICS

Feldspathic dental porcelain with high amounts of alminum oxide.

CLASSIFICATION OF ALL-CERAMIC SYSTEMS

- Conventional powder-slurry ceramics—Optec HSP, Duceram LFC
- Castable ceramics—Picon, Dicor Plus
- Machinable ceramics—Cerec vitablocs Mark I, Mark II, Dicor MGC, Celay
- Pressable ceramics—IPS Empress, Optec Pressable Ceramic
- Infiltrated ceramics—In-Ceram.

Conventional Powder-slurry Ceramic

Available as

- Powders to which water is added to produce a slurry
- Available in various shades and translucencies, with characterizing stains and glazes.

Manufacturing

- Leucite crystals are dispersed in a glassy matrix by controlling their nucleation and crystal growth
- The leucite and glassy matrix fuse together during the baking process
- The build-up and contouring of the crown can be done by using the powder-slurry technique on semipermeable die material.

Advantages

- Greater strength than conventional feldspathic porcelain due to its leucite content
- Does not require a core as with aluminous porcelain jacket crowns
- The body and incisal porcelains can be pigmented to provide desired shade and translucency
- Does not require special processing equipment
- These restorations fit accurately.

Disadvantage

Their high leucite contents can cause increased wear to the opposing teeth.

Duceram LFC

- Hydrothermal low-fusing ceramic
- Composed of an amorphous glass containing hydroxyl ions.

Advantages

- Greater density, higher flexural strength, greater fracture resistance and lower hardness than feldspathic porcelain
- No special laboratory techniques or equipment required.

Uses

For fabrication of ceramic inlays, veneers and full-contour crowns.

Procedure

Base layer

Duceram Metal Ceramic—(a leucite-containing porcelain)—is placed on a refractory die using powder-slurry techniques and baked at 930°C.

Over-base layer

Duceram LFC is applied using the powder-slurry technique and baked at a relatively low temperature (660°C).

Castable Ceramic Systems

Available as

- Solid ceramic ingots, which are cast using lost-wax and centrifugal-casting technique
- Only one shade is available
- Staining is done to obtain proper shading of the final restoration.

Picon

This is a polycrystalline glass-ceramic material, in which glass is heat-treated under controlled crystallization.

Procedure

- When solid ceramic ingots are cast at 1350°C, a transparent glass crown is obtained
- This crown is then heat-treated at 1075°C for 10 hours
- 'Ceramming' causes partial crystallization (55%) of tetra-silicic-mica-like crystals
- For final restoration, colorant stains are baked on the surface of the glass-ceramic material.

Advantages

- Easier as it is a lost wax technique
- The transparent crown after heat treatment at 1075°C for 10 hours forms an opaque crown, which increases fracture resistance and strength
- Less abrasive to opposing tooth structure.

Dicor Plus

This is a shaded feldspathic porcelain veneer applied to the Dicor substrate.

Disadvantages

- Abrasive to opposing teeth
- Requires a special high-temperature, electric-heated casting unit
- Fracture of the restorations is common.

Machinable Ceramics

Available as

- Ceramic ingots in various shades
- Used in computer-aided design and computer-aided manufacturing (CAD-CAM) procedures
- The machined restorations are stained and glazed to the desired characterization.

Cerec Vitablocs Mark I

- This is a feldspathic porcelain, used with the Cerec system
- Composition and properties are the same as feldspathic porcelain used for porcelain-fused-to-metal restorations.

Cerec Vitablocs Mark II

This is a feldspathic porcelain of increased strength with less abrasive wear of the opposing tooth structure.

Dicor MGC

- It contains fluorosilicic mica crystals in a glass matrix
- It has greater flexural strength than the castable Dicor and Cerec
- Less abrasive wear of the opposing tooth structure than Cerec Mark I.

Celay

- It can be used for CAD-CAM and copy-milling technique
- Identical in physical properties to Cerec Vitablocs Mark II.

Disadvantage

Marginal fit is not good.

Pressable Ceramics

Available as

- Ceramic ingots, which are melted at high temperatures and pressed into a mold created by lost-wax technique
- These can be made to full contour, or can be built up using feldspathic porcelain.

IPS Empress

- This is a feldspathic porcelain supplied in ingot form
- The ingots are heated and molded under pressure to produce the restorations.

Procedure

- The ceramic ingot is placed under the plunger and heated to 1150°C
- The plunger presses the molten ceramic into the mold
- The final shade of the crown is done by staining or veneering (Cut back technique of wax pattern).

Optec Pressable Ceramic

This is a type of feldspathic porcelain with increased leucite content, processed by molding under pressure and heat.

Advantages of IPS and OPC

- Produce strong, translucent, dense and etchable ceramic restorations
- Useful in fabricating ceramic veneers.

Disadvantage

Require special equipment to fabricate the restorations.

Infiltrated Ceramics

Available as

- Powder (aluminum oxide or spinel), which is fabricated into a porous substrate and a glass, which is infiltrated at high temperature into the porous substrate
- The infiltrated ceramic is then veneered using conventional feldspathic porcelain technique.

In-Ceram

- The spinel cores are more translucent than the aluminum oxide cores

- The core is made from fine-grained particles that are mixed with water to form a suspension referred to as a 'slip'.

Procedure

- The slip is placed on a gypsum die and baked at 1120°C for 10 hours to produce the opaque, porous core
- An appropriate shade of glass powder is applied to the core, which is baked again at 1100°C for four hours
- During this process, the molten glass infiltrates the porous alumina core by capillary action.

Advantages

- Extremely high flexure strength
- The aluminum oxide or spinel crystals limit crack propagation and the glass infiltration reduces porosity
- Provides an accurate fit.

Disadvantages

- Cannot etch internal surface; hence a resin cement such as Panavia 21TC is recommended
- Not as esthetic as other systems
- Requires specialized equipment to fabricate a restoration.

85. Weld Decay.

DEFINITION

The joining of two or more pieces by applying heat, pressure or both, or without a filler metal to produce a localized union across the interface through fusion or diffusion of ions.

WELD DECAY

- Joining of stainless steel can be done either by soldering or by welding
- Silver solders containing silver and copper and other elements to lower the fusion temperature are used for soldering
- High temperature during soldering can result in overheating of the alloy, causing recrystallization of grain structure with a lack of springiness
- Overheating of 18/8 austenitic stainless steel causes the chromium to react with carbon forming chromium carbides above 500°C, which precipitate at the grain boundaries. This reaction causes a brittleness in stainless steel
- Chromium loses its passivating property after forming chromium carbides at grain boundaries

- The chromium present has migrated to the boundaries to form carbides causing a decrease in corrosion resistance of stainless steel alloys. This process is known as 'weld decay'.
- Weld decay results in a loss of corrosion resistance around the soldered joint causing them to be brittle
- The solder itself can corrode as it is of eutectic-type composition.

Technique of Welding

- Welding is done by pressing two pieces of wire together while two electrodes pass an electric current which is sufficient to melt wires at the point of contact joining them together
- High temperatures, sufficient for welding, require high values of electrical resistance at the junction. Hence, it is not suitable for joining gold wires.

Prevention of Weld Decay

- The electrical current and the time for which the current flows must be controlled
- Overheating leads to weld decay and a degree of recrystallization, causing a loss of fibrous grain structure. Hence, overheating should be prevented
- Addition of titanium to prevent chromium carbide formation gives what is known as 'stabilized austenitic stainless steel'
- In stabilized austenitic stainless steel, addition of titanium causes the carbon to react preferentially with dispersed titanium such that chromium remains where it is at its most effective sites.

86. Classify Steels. Add a Note on 18/8 Stainless Steel.

STAINLESS STEELS

- These are Chromium-containing steels with 11% to 30% chromium
- Other elements present are iron and carbon
- This composition gives a wide variation in composition and properties of the stainless steels.

Classification of Stainless Steels/Composition

(Space Lattice)	Chromium %	Nickel %	Carbon %
Ferritic (BCC)	11.5–27	Almost nickel-free	0.20 max.
Austenitic (FCC)	16–26	7–22	0.25 max.
Martensitic (BCT)	11.5–17	0–2.5	0.15–1.20

Silicon, phosphorus, sulfur, manganese, tantalum and niobium can be present as trace elements and the rest is iron.

Properties

- Their yield strengths may range from 211 MPa to more than 1760 MPa
- They resist tarnish and corrosion by forming a chromium oxide layer that is thin, transparent, tough and impervious
- If this protective oxide layer is ruptured, another oxide layer forms again in an oxidizing environment.

Ferritic Stainless Steels

American Iron and Steel Institute (AISI) designated these as Series 400 stainless steels along with the martensitic alloys.

Properties

- The ferritic alloys have good corrosion resistance
- They are economical and have less strength
- This alloy cannot be subjected to heat treatment
- Ferritic stainless steel is not work hardenable and not used much for dental purposes.

Martensitic Stainless Steels

- They can be heat-treated
- They possess high strength and hardness
- They are used for surgical and cutting instruments
- The yield strength of a high-carbon martensitic stainless steel ranges from 492 MPa and in the annealed condition, it is 1898 MPa
- The hardness ranges from 230 to 600 BHN
- Corrosion resistance of the martensitic stainless steel is less than other types
- As the strength and hardness increase, ductility decreases to as low as 2% elongation for high-carbon martensitic stainless steel.

Austenitic Stainless Steels

Austenitic stainless steels are the most corrosion-resistant alloys and used as stainless instruments and crowns in pediatric dentistry. The austenitic structure for the AISI series is 300.

Composition

- 16% to 26% chromium
- 7% to 22% nickel
- 0.25% carbon (maximum).

Both 302 and 304 stainless steels are designated as 18/8 stainless steels used to form bands and wires.

Type 316L (0.03% maximum carbon) is used for implants.

Properties of Austenitic Stainless Steel

- Greater ductility and ability to undergo cold work without fracturing
- Ease of welding

- Strength increases during cold working
- Ease in forming
- Less critical grain growth
- Ability to overcome sensitization.

Sensitization

- Corrosion resistance is reduced when chromium reacts with carbon forming chromium carbide at the grain boundaries
- The formation of chromium carbide is at 650°C. This is sensitization
- Two methods can be used to minimize sensitization when austenitic stainless steel is heated to elevated temperature range.

First method

- Is to reduce the carbon content of the steel so that carbide precipitation does not occur
- If the stainless steel is cold worked, the carbides are uniformly distributed from grain boundaries and chromium are less localized so that the resistance to corrosion is greater
- Used in the processing of orthodontic stainless steel wires.

Second method

Stabilization

- It is a method to prevent the sensitization of austenitic stainless steel at elevated temperature by introducing another element with passivating property along with chromium, as niobium, titanium or tantalum
- Stainless steels that are treated in this manner are said to be stabilized
- If titanium is introduced six times the carbon content, the precipitation of chromium carbide is inhibited for a short period at soldering the temperatures.

Mechanical Properties

- The elastic modulus is 180 gigapascals (GPa)
- Yield strength is 1600 MPa
- Ultimate tensile strength is 2100 MPa
- Strength and hardness may increase with a decrease in cross-section dimensions.

Recovery Heat Treatment

An increase in the elastic properties of a stainless steel wire can be obtained by heating to temperature between approximately 400°C and 500°C after it has been cold-worked.

87. Wrought Stainless Steel Alloys.

TYPES

- Wrought cobalt-chromium-nickel alloy (Elgiloy)
- Wrought nickel-titanium alloy (Nitinol)
- Wrought beta-titanium alloy.

WROUGHT COBALT-CHROMIUM-NICKEL ALLOY (ELGILOY)

Availability

Wire and band forms which are cold-worked and heat-treated (7 minutes at 482°C) available as soft, ductile, semi-spring temper and spring temper.

Composition

Cobalt	40%
Chromium	20%
Nickel	15%
Molybdenum	7%
Manganese	2%
Iron	15.8%
Carbon	0.15%
Beryllium	0.04%

Points to Note

- Elgiloy can be soldered using silver solder in the presence of fluoride flux or spot wielded
- The angle at which during bending the permanent deformation takes place increases from soft to spring temper types
- The permanent set after 90° bend decreases from soft to spring-temper types
- Heat treatment at 482°C for 7 minutes causes increase in angle at permanent deformation but decreases the permanent set.

Properties of Elgiloy Spring-tempered Wire

Proportional limit	1610 MN/m^2
Yield strength	1930 MN/m^2
Tensile strength	2540 MN/m^2

WROUGHT NICKEL-TITANIUM ALLOY (NITINOL) (IN 1972)

- It is a wire with high resiliency and limited formability
- When heated from below transition temperature to above transition temperature, a crystallographic transformation occurs and the alloy returns to its original shape.

Composition

Nickel	55%
Titanium	45%
Cobalt	1.6% (To lower transition temperature to 37°C)

Points to Note

- Nitinol cannot be bent but can be used with pretorqued, preangulated brackets
- This alloy cannot be soldered or welded, but wires are joined mechanically
- Nickel-titanium has the lowest elastic modulus and yield strength, but the highest spring back
- Nitinol has the highest resiliency. Hence, constant forces can be applied with increased working range.

WROUGHT BETA-TITANIUM ALLOY (1979)

Beta-titanium exists as body-centered cubic crystal lattice which can be stabilized at room temperature when alloyed with molybdenum.

Composition

Titanium	78%
Molybdenum	11.5%
Zirconium	6%
Tin	4.5%

Points to Note

- They have low elastic modulus, maximum elastic spring back, low yield strength, good ductility, weldability and corrosion resistance
- They can be shaped easily
- They can be welded by electrical resistance welding
- It has larger working range than stainless steel and Elgiloy wires.

88. Wrought/Dental Casting Alloys.

- Compared to wrought alloys, cast alloys can be easily melted, cast and finished, possess good corrosion, tarnish resistance and are biocompatible
- Wrought alloys are work-hardened and used when superior mechanical properties are required as in the form of wires.

WROUGHT ALLOYS

- Gold alloy wires used for clasps and root canal posts
- Cobalt-chromium-nickel wires used for clasps and root canal posts
- Stainless steel wires used for orthodontic applications
- Nickel-titanium wires for orthodontic applications.

Uses

- Work-hardened gold (Direct-filling gold) can be used for filling teeth in the form of gold foil
- Alloys can also be work-hardened by swaging, i.e. by adapting an alloy sheet to the shape of the palate on a suitable die, as wrought denture base.

TYPES OF CASTING ALLOYS

Precious Metal Alloys

- Gold alloys of high content and medium content
- SIlver-palladium for bridges, crowns and porcelain fused to metal
- High-content palladium for porcelain fused to metal.

Base Metal Alloys

- Cobalt-chromium for framework of partial dentures
  Cobalt-chromium alloys (Co-Cr)
- Nickel-chromium for bridges, crowns and porcelain fused to metal
  Nickel-chromium-beryllium (Ni-Cr-Be).

PRECIOUS METAL ALLOYS

Gold Alloys

High and Medium Gold Alloys

Used since 1907.

Composition

- Main composition is gold
- It has platinum content of 8%

- Palladium 4.6%
- Silver 1.3%
- Tin, indium and iron to promote oxide bonding, harden the alloy and refine the grain structure.

Advantages

- Excellent bonding to porcelain
- Good castability
- Resistance to tarnish and corrosion
- Freedom from toxicity
- No discoloration.

Disadvantages

- Expensive
- Low elastic modulus and poor sag resistance.

Gold-Palladium-Silver Alloy

Composition

Gold 42–50%
Palladium 25–32%
Silver 6–16%
Indium and tin contribute 8%.

Advantages

- Substituting palladium for gold raises the melting range and lowers the coefficient of expansion
- Less susceptibility to dimensional changes with good corrosion resistance and clinical working.

Disadvantage

Greening effect due to the silver content.

Gold-Palladium Alloy

Composition

- Gold 42–55%
- Palladium 36–40%
- Minor quantities of tin, indium and gallium.

Advantages

- Greening effect not present
- Lower coefficient of thermal expansion of gold and, hence, more compatible with porcelain
- Strength is improved
- Corrosion resistance is good with better sag resistance.

Disadvantage

Thermal expansion incompatible with higher expansion porcelain.

Palladium-based Alloys

Used since 1970s.

Palladium-silver Alloys

Composition

- Palladium 50–60%
- Silver 30–40%
- Traces of tin and indium
- Palladium increases strength, reduces the cost and produces white color.

Advantages

- Good tarnish and corrosion resistance
- Good bond strength
- Lower sag tendency.

Disadvantage

Porcelain discoloration.

Palladium-copper Alloys

Used since 1982.

Composition

- Palladium 70–80%
- Copper 15%.

Disadvantage

Copper discolors porcelain.

Palladium-Cobalt Alloys

Available as silver-free, nickel-free, gold and beryllium-free commercial alloys.

Composition

- Palladium 78–88%
- Cobalt 4–10%.

Disadvantage

Difficult to melt and has high thermal expansion.

Palladium-Tin Alloys

- The silver is substituted with tin and gallium
- Recent clinical use, hence clinical data is not available.

Nonprecious Alloys

Base Metal Alloys

Due to the high cost of gold and palladium, base metal alloys were developed.

Nickel-chromium Alloys

Composition

- Nickel 70–80%
- Chromium 13–20%
- With or without small quantities of beryllium (0.5–2%).

Advantages

- Good strength, hence can be used in thin sections permitting excellent crown contour
- Physical properties as hardness, yield strength and modulus of elasticity is superior to all noble metals with regard to sag resistance.

Disadvantages

- High casting shrinkage of 2.4%
- Questionable biocompatibility
- Requires modified casting techniques.

Cobalt-Chromium Alloys

These base metals may contain 55–68% cobalt and up to 25–27% chromium but no beryllium.

Cobalt-Chromium-Nickel Alloy

Advantages

- Base metal alloys are cheaper than noble alloys
- They have good strength
- They can be used along with metal ceramics.

Disadvantages

- Fusion temperature is high
- Marginal fit is poor compared to gold alloys
- Cannot be burnished
- Nickel containing alloy can cause allergy to some.

89. Silver-palladium Casting Alloys (White Gold).

WHITE GOLD

Properties

- Silver and palladium have complete solid solubility
- Palladium (*Pd*) is a platinum group metal possessing strong affinity for hydrogen gas
- Melting point of palladium is 1552°C and Silver (*Ag*) has a melting point of 62°C, but tarnishes in the presence of hydrogen sulfide
- The tarnishing of Silver is prevented by the addition of palladium
- They consist of ternary *Ag-Pd-Cu* systems and can be single-phase or multiphase
- The alloys can be heat treated to increase surface hardness (precipitation hardening)
- *Ag-Pd* alloys for precision castings require careful melting of the alloy in an inert gas atmosphere
- Values for the 0.1% proof stress and surface hardness are relatively high
- White alloys have relatively high melting range of the materials and low density
- Cannot be used as metal backup for porcelain as they impart a greenish tint to the ceramic
- The alloys become age-hardened during the porcelain-firing cycle.

Composition

- *Ag*: 45% (wt) Main metal
- *Pd*: 25% (wt) Solid solution hardening; tarnish protection
- *Cu*: 15% (wt) Precipitation hardening
- *Au*: 14% (wt) Solld solution hardening
- *Zn*: 1% (wt) Protection of Cu on melting
- Palladium in alloys increases strength, reduces the cost and produces white color.

Advantages

- Good tarnish and corrosion resistance
- Good bond strength
- Lower sag tendency.

Disadvantage

Porcelain discoloration.

Casting Ag-Pa alloys

- The materials should be melted using an induction technique and in an inert gas atmosphere
- Melting these alloys in a carbon/graphite crucible is contraindicated, as carbon uptake alters the physical property of these metals
- These alloys should be in clay or aluminum oxide crucibles.

Bonding Alloys to Tooth Material

Silicoating

A thin *Si-oxide* layer is coated onto the surface of the alloy. This coating aids in forming a bond to resin *via* a silane-bonding agent.

Coating method

- The fitting surface is grit-blasted and coated by placing the surface in the oxidizing portion of a tetraethoxysilane-propane-oxygen flame (flame spraying)
- After coating is applied, silane bonding agent is applied.

90. Nickel-Titanium Alloys (Shape Memory and Super-elasticity).

ALLOYS WITH SHAPE MEMORY

- Nitinol—a nickel-titanium alloy and titanal, titanol.
- β-titanium wire.

Nickel-titanium Alloys

Mechanical Properties

- The modulus of elasticity is 41.4 GPa
- Yield strength is 427 MPa
- Ultimate tensile strength is 1489 MPa
- The orthodontic forces applied are low when compared with stainless steel appliances
- The low stiffness with moderately high strength gives large working range.

Composition

- 54% nickel
- 44% titanium
- 2% or less cobalt.

Other Properties

- At high temperatures, *austenitic phase (BCC lattice* is stable), but on cooling or application of stress, a transformation to a hexagonal martensitic phase is induced
- When a transition from austenitic to martensitic phase occurs, it is accompanied by a volumetric change, shape memory and superelasticity

- A change from austenite martensitic causes a reduction in Young's modulus
- In titanol wire, Young's modulus decreases with strain (*superelastic effect*)
- NiTi wires have a low Young's modulus and cannot be soldered or welded.

Shape memory

- Memory effect is obtained by first shaping at temperatures near 482°C
- If the same orthodontic arch wire is then cooled and formed into a second shape and again heated at a low transition temperature, the wire will return to its original shape
- The low transition temperature is controlled by addition of cobalt.

Superelasticity

Inducing the austenite to martensitic transition by stress produces superelasticity.

Significance

- Orthodontic nickel-titanium wires result in low forces and a large working range or springback. *Removal of the stress* results in the reverse transition and recovery
- Endodontic files fit snugly into sharp curvy root canals and on retrieving the file from the canal regains its shape without deformation and minimizes the risk for perforation of the root by the file.

β-Titanium Alloys

Composition of β-Titanium alloys

- Titanium 6%
- Aluminum 4%
- Molybdenum.

Properties

- Pure titanium has different crystallographic forms at high and low temperatures
- At low temperature based on the HCP lattice, the yield strength is as high as 965 MPa. Addition of molybdenum stabilizes the alloy down to room temperature
- At lower temperatures than 885°C, the hexagonal close-packed (HCP) form is stable, whereas at higher temperatures, the metal rearranges into a BCC, or β-crystal, lattice
- The HCP lattice has modulus value of 110 GPa and yield strength values of 379 MPa
- β-Titanium can be cold-worked and, hence, can be easily bent
- The mechanical properties of titanium alloys can be altered by heat treatments.

Wrought Wire Titanium Form

Composition

- Titanium 11%
- Molybdenum 6%
- Zirconium 4%
- Tin.

Properties

Wrought titanium orthodontic wire has an elastic modulus of 71.7 GPa and yield strength between 860 and 1170 MPa.

91. Swaging.

DEFINITION

Swaging is to shape a sheet of metal by adapting it to a die under hydraulic pressure, or by pressing it between a die and counter die.

Importance

- Swaging is accompanied after work hardening
- Used for the production of a denture base in stainless steel
- A denture base in stainless steel when compared with PMMA has high rigidity in thin section, high impact resistance, no monomer toxicity and good thermal conductivity.

Procedure

- A sand mold is formed and poured in plaster
- This mold is poured in zinc, to form the die
- A counter-die is formed by again pouring zinc onto the fitting surface of the die
- The sheet 18/8 stainless steel is sandwiched between die and counter-die in a hydraulic press and pressure applied
- Stainless steel ribbon is then spot-welded onto the denture base to retain the PMMA gumwork which is processed normally
- A difficulty with the process is that 18/8 austenitic stainless steel work-hardens quickly and an intermediate annealing process at 1050°C for 2 minutes, followed by rapid cooling for adequate fit to the die takes place.

92. Types of Implants.

CLASSIFICATION OF IMPLANTS

Depending on Tissue Placement

- Subperiosteal (periosteal)
- Endosteal—Root form and plate form
- Transosteal—Passes the entire alveolar bone height.

Depending on Materials Used

- Bioinert—Titanium and its alloys, cobalt-chromium and alloys
- Bioactive—Ceramics, hydroxyapatite and carbon.

Depending on Edentulous Spaces

- Misch and Judy classified spaces with different bone volumes (similar to Kennedy's classification)
- Classified as FP-1, FP-2, FP-3, RP-4 and RP-5
- The first three classifications were for fixed prostheses and the other two were for removable prostheses
- In fixed prosthodontics, the endosteal root form implants are commonly used.

Subperiosteal Implants

Implants placed on top of resorbed alveolar ridges are called subperiosteal implants.

Types

Total or full subperiosteal implants. They can be noncoated or coated with hydroxyapatite.

Materials

Surgical vitallium, titanium or titanium alloy, Wironium, bionium and nickel-free cobalt-chromium alloy.

Endosteal Implants

An endosteal implant is an alloplastic material surgically inserted into residual ridge, primarily to serve as prosthodontic foundation.

Commonly available as

- Pin, needle, screw, cylinder.
- Plate or blade or blade vent implant.

Types based on design

- Cylindrical-microscopic retention, bonding to bone
- Screw root forms
- Combination root forms (both cylinder and screw design).

Other types

- Immediate function or of later function as loaded after a healing time
- Totally submerged or partially submerged
- Functions with a direct bone interface or functions with a periimplant connective tissue ligament.

Types based on design

Blade or Plate-form Implants: (by Linkow, 1970)

- Latticework design and closed bottoms, both these types can be coated with materials such as hydroxyapatite or plasma-sprayed titanium
- Their ease of insertion led to extensive use.

Screw, Root and Pin-form Implants

- Smooth
- Threaded (These types can either be coated or uncoated)
- Hollow submergible or nonsubmergible
- Solid
- Perforated.

Root-form implants

- Cylinder type, which is tapped in **(Fig. 47)**
- Screw type, which is threaded or nonthreaded, coated or non-coated **(Fig. 48)**.

Mechanism of Integration

- **Osseointegration—(Ingvar Brånemark)**
- **Fibro-osseous attachment—(Weiss)**
  In which a fibro-osseous ligament is formed between bone and implant interface
- **Biointegration**
  Occurs when the material is coated with hydroxyapatite, which forms a physiochemical bond with bone.
- **Periosteal integration**
  The ideal attachment is osseo-integration, which is an apparent direct attachment of osseous tissue to an inert alloplastic material without intervening connective tissue.

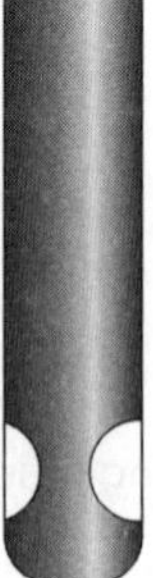

Fig. 47: Cylinder-type implant

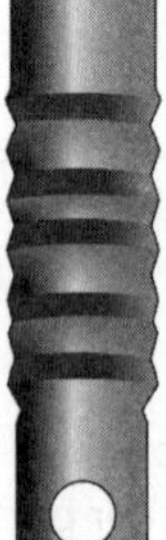

Fig. 48: Screw-type implant

93. Implant Materials.

MATERIALS USED

- Metals
- Stainless steel
- Cobalt-chromium-molybdenum alloy
- Titanium and titanium-aluminum-vanadium alloy
- Metal with surface coatings
- Ceramics
- Polymers and composites
- Zirconium and tungsten
- Wironium, bionium and nickel-free cobalt-chromium alloy.

Metals

Surgical grade stainless steel and cobalt-chromium alloy were used. Now they are replaced by pure titanium or titanium alloys as they have better physical properties, good corrosion resistance and biocompatibility.

Stainless Steel

Composition

- Iron
- Carbon (0.05%)
- Chromium 18% (imparts corrosion resistance)
- Nickel 8% (stabilizes the austenitic structure). (Contraindicated in patients with nickel allergy).

Properties

- Used in wrought and heat-treated conditions
- Possesses high strength and ductility
- Surface passivation increases corrosion-resistance
- If a noble metal or base metal alloy comes in contact with stainless steel alloys, it can cause galvanic corrosion.

Cobalt-Chromium-Molybdenum Alloy

- These alloys are used in as-cast or cast and annealed condition
- Used as framework for subperiosteal frames.

Composition

- 63% cobalt
- 30% chromium
- 5% molybdenum (serves to stabilize the structure)
- Trace of carbon (acts as a hardener), manganese and nickel.

Properties

- Good resistance to corrosion
- Have a high modulus
- Least ductile of all the alloy systems
- Proper quality control ensures excellent biocompatibility
- Low cost and long-term clinical success.

Titanium: Commercially Pure Titanium (cpTi)

- Titanium is a highly reactive metal—and it oxidizes (passivates) on contact with air or normal tissue fluids. Hence, it is highly corrosion-resistant
- Any cut or nick on the surface of pure titanium forms an oxide layer 10μA thick within a millisecond (*self-healing*)
- The oxide coating can be thickened and made durable by placing titanium in a bath of nitric acid
- Pure titanium contains 0.5% oxygen and minor amounts of nitrogen, carbon and hydrogen.

Alloys of Titanium: Titanium-Aluminum-Vanadium Alloy

Composition

- 90 wt% titanium
- 6 wt% aluminum
- Vanadium.

Properties

- Titanium has a density of approximately 4.5 g/cm^3 (40% lighter than steel)
- Possesses a high strength : weight ratio
- Titanium has a modulus of elasticity one-half of stainless steel or cobalt-chromium alloys but 5–10 times higher than bone
- The mechanical properties of the alloy are superior to pure titanium
- Though titanium is highly biocompatible, the titanium oxide surface releases titanium ions at a low rate into blood and saliva
- Any contamination of the surface will affect the success of the implant.

Metal with Surface Coatings

Titanium and other implant materials can be plasma-sprayed or coated with a thin layer of a calcium phosphate ceramic.

Significance of coating

- Bioactive materials are inorganic materials that form an adherent, bonded interface with bone
- A coating of the implant, with tricalcium phosphate or hydroxyapatite, enriches the implant material in calcium and phosphorus, to produce a bioactive surface which promotes bone growth and aids in a direct bond between the implant and the bone tissue
- Materials as ceramics have good elastic modulus but low ductility and tensile strength and, hence, are brittle in nature but coating increases its physical properties
- Coatings enhance the bond strength of the implant to bone and increase the rate at which attachment occurs

- Coating provides a roughened, biologically acceptable surface for bone in-growth, increasing the anchorage in the jaw.

Ceramics

They are brittle and tend to fracture but are highly biocompatible.

Types

Bioactive: Hydroxyapatite and bioglass (rich in calcium and phosphate).

Nonreactive: Include alumina and sapphire (They do not participate in the process of bone deposition).

Hydroxyapatite

Hydroxyapatite is a mineral with the formula $Ca_{10}(PO_4)_6(OH)_2$, that is similar to that of bone and teeth. Used as an implant material for augmenting alveolar ridges or filling bony defects.

Availability

- Block or granular form
- Dense or porous form
- Block or granular form is packed into the bony site, to provide a scaffold for new bone growth
- As it is difficult to keep the granular form localized at the site of implantation, presently collagen is added as a matrix to hold the particles together in the defect
- Porous material contains porosity of 100–300 μm in size, which is adequate for bone in-growth
- Ceramic materials can be used in very-low-stress applications only
- Hydroxyapatite as a coating for titanium overcomes the mechanical deficiencies of the titanium and makes it bioactive by the coating.

Bioglass

- Bioglass is a dense ceramic material made from CaO, Na_2O, P_2O_5 and SiO_2
- Local pH changes on the surface of bioglass surface cause sodium, calcium and phosphate ions to be dissolved from it. Meanwhile, hydrogen ions from the local tissue fluids replace the lost sodium in the bioglass
- The replacement on the surface of bioglass forms a silica-rich gel
- The silicon depletion is accompanied by the migration of calcium and phosphate ions to the silica gel surface, to form a calcium-phosphorus layer
- As phosphorus concentration increases on the surface, osteoblasts begin to proliferate, producing collagen fibrils that form into the calcium-phosphorus gel and are anchored by the calcium-phosphorus crystals
- This bonding layer is 100–200 μm thick and exceeds 100 times the thickness of layers formed on hydroxyapatite.

Nonreactive Ceramic from Aluminum Oxide (Al_2O_3)

Available as

- Polycrystalline form
- Single crystal (sapphire).

Properties

- It possesses high strength, stiffness and hardness
- These implants are designed with a screw or blade shape and used as abutments for partially edentulous mouths.

Polymers and Composites

Available as

- Porous
- Solid forms.

Uses

- For tissue attachment
- Replacement augmentation
- As coatings for force transfer to soft and hard tissues as internal force distribution connectors.

Other Implant Materials

- Gold, palladium, tantalum, platinum and alloys of these metals
- Recently, zirconium and tungsten and carbon compounds.

94. Dentifrices.

TYPES

- Toothpastes
- Gels
- Powders.

Significance of Dentifrices

- They possess abrasive and detergent actions that efficiently remove debris, plaque and stained pellicle
- They polish teeth to provide increased light reflectance and good esthetics
- The high polish prevents further accumulation of microorganisms and stains
- Dentifrices act as vehicles for the delivery of therapeutic agents such as fluorides, tartar control agents and desensitizing agents
- Fluorides improve caries resistance and enhance the remineralization of incipient enamel lesions

- Tartar control agents such as potassium and sodium pyrophosphates reduce the rate of new calculus deposits supragingivally
- Desensitizing agents such as strontium chloride and potassium nitrate decrease tooth sensitivity in patients.

Composition

- The abrasive concentrations in paste and gel dentifrices are 50%–75% lower than those of powder dentifrices
- Hence, powders should be used sparingly to avoid excessive dentinal abrasion and pulpal sensitivity.

Component	Pastes and Gels	Powders	Materials	Purpose
Abrasive	20–55	90–98	Calcium carbonate Dibasic calcium phosphate dihydrate Hydrated alumina Hydrated silica Sodium bicarbonate Mixtures of listed abrasives	Removal of plaque/ stain Polish tooth surface
Detergent	1–2	1–6	Sodium lauryl sulfate	Aids debris removal
Colorants	1–2	1–2	Food colorants	Appearance
Flavoring	1–2	1–2	Oils of spearmint, peppermint, wintergreen or cinnamon	Flavor
Humectant	20–35	0	Sorbitol Glycerine	Maintains moisture content
Water	15–25	0	Deionized water	Suspension agent
Binder	3	0	Carrageenan	Thickener Prevents liquid-solid separation
Fluoride	0–1	0	Sodium monofluorophosphate, sodium fluoride, stannous fluoride	Dental caries prevention
Tartar control agents	0–1	0	Disodium pyrophosphate. Tetrasodium pyrophosphate Tetrapotassium pyrophosphate	Inhibits formation of calculus above the gingival margin
Desensitization agents	0–5	0	Potassium nitrate Strontium chloride	Promotes occlusion of dentinal tubules

Factors in Abrasivity

- An ideal dentifrice should provide good cleaning action with low abrasion rates
- Dentifrices should have low abrasion rates, otherwise, in tooth that are exposed, cementum and dentin are abraded at rates of 35 and 25 times more than that of enamel

- An abrasivity ratio is calculated by comparing the amounts of radioactive phosphorus (^{32}P) released by each dentifrice and this value is multiplied by 1000
- A dentifrice must obtain an abrasivity score of 200–250 or less to meet ADA and ISO specifications.

Points to Note

- Lab test cannot account for all variables
- A test dentifrice must abrade dentin at 20%–25% of the rate of the reference standard to be considered safe
- Dentifrices containing sodium bicarbonate cannot be tested because the particles completely dissolve in 1 minute into the 8-minute test.

95. Tooth-cutting Instruments.

DEFINITION

- Tooth-cutting instruments such as dental burs are rotary cutting instruments used for finishing metal restoration, for tooth preparation and surgical removal of bone
- Burs are designed to take advantage of the properties of the material used.

SHAPE

Refers to head contour.

Commonest shapes are (Fig. 49)

- Round
- Inverted cone
- Pear
- Straight fissured
- Tapering fissured.

Size

Refers to the head diameter and specific shape.

Example

A No. 37 bur is an inverted cone bur with a head diameter of 0.056 inch.

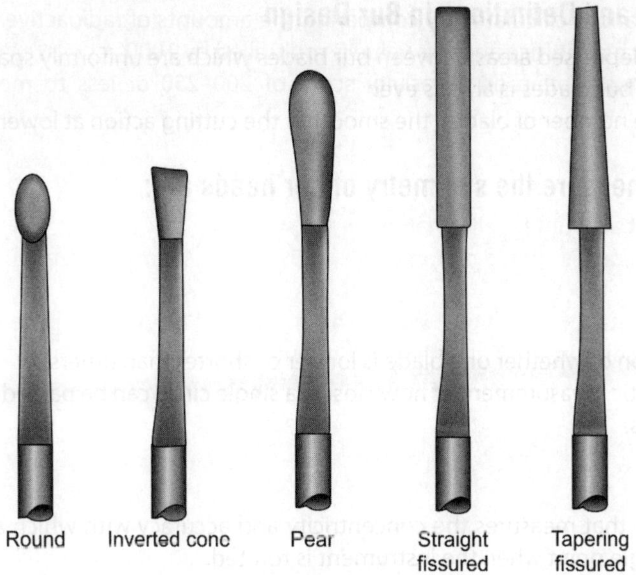

Fig. 49: Types of burs

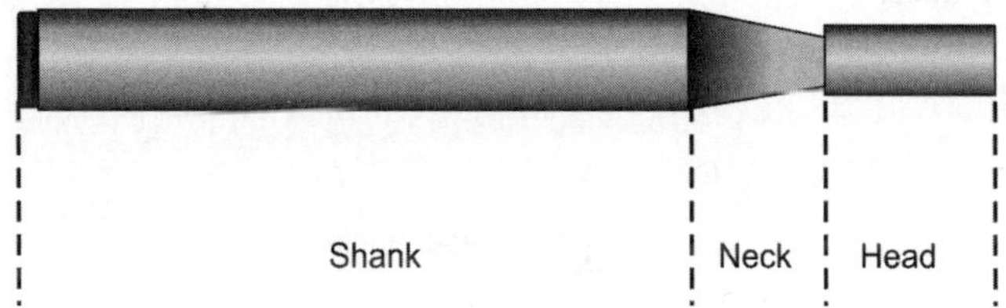

Designation of the three parts of rotary cutting instruments
Fig. 50: Design of a dental bur

New Designs

- Reduced use of crosscuts
- Extended heads on fissure burs
- Rounding of sharp tip angles.

Factors Determining the Clinical Effectiveness of a Bur Design (Fig. 50)

- Head size
- Head shape
- Head length
- Head diameter
- Neck diameter
- Taper angle
- Spiral angle
- Cross cut size and spacing.

Common Terms and Definitions in Bur Design

- Flutes are the depressed areas between bur blades which are uniformly spaced
- The number of bur blades is always even
- The greater the number of blades, the smoother the cutting action at lower speeds.

Terms used to measure the symmetry of bur heads are:

- Concentricity
- Run out.

Concentricity

- It is an indication of whether one blade is longer or shorter than others
- It is a direct, static measurement of how closely a single circle can be passed through the tips of all the blades.

Run out

It is a dynamic test that measures the concentricity and accuracy with which all the blade tips pass through a single point when the instrument is rotated.

Blade Design (Fig. 51)

Each blade has two faces:

1. Rake face
2. Clearance face.

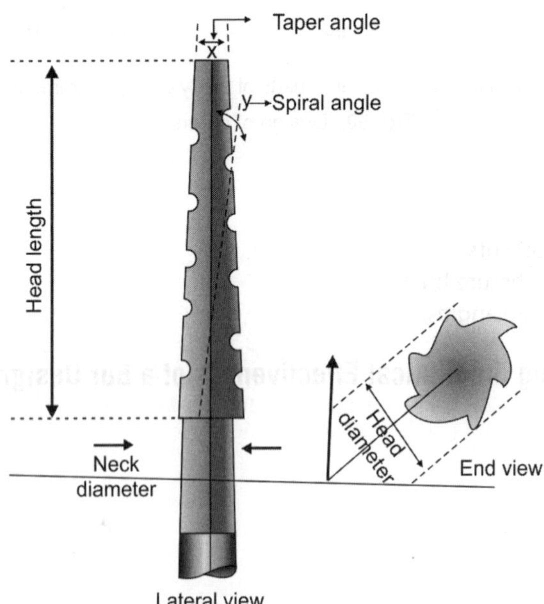

Fig. 51: Design features of a bur head

Rake Face

It is the face which is in the direction of rotation and makes contact with the tooth structure being removed.

Clearance Face

It is the other face of the blade which follows behind the edge as the bur rotates.

Cutting Edge

Cutting edge of the blade is at the interaction of rake and clearance face.

Rake Angle

It is the angle between the rake face and the line connecting the edge to the axis of the bur. The rake angle is the most important design aspect of a bur blade.

Edge Angle

It is the internal angle at the edge formed by the rake and clearance faces of the bur blade. The edge angle of a bur blade is closely related to resistance of the blade to fracture.

Clearance Angle

It is the angle between the clearance face immediately behind the edge and a tangent to the path of rotation.

The clearance angle serves three functions

i. It eliminates rubbing friction of the clearance face of the blade against the new tooth surface exposed behind the cutting edge.
ii. Clearance angle provides a stop to prevent the bur edge from digging into the tooth structure excessively.
iii. It reduces the radius of the blade back of the cutting edge so as to provide adequate flute space or clearance space for the chips formed ahead of the following blade.

DESIGN OF DENTAL INSTRUMENTS

- Carbide burs normally have blades with slight negative rake angles and edge angles of about 90%
- Their clearance faces either are curved or have two surfaces to provide a low clearance angle near the edge and a greater clearance space ahead of the following blade.

96. Polishing Agents/Types of Abrasives.

DEFINITIONS

Abrasion

Consists of physical scratching and removal of the surface layer of a substance, usually by use of hard, rough particles called an abrasive.

Polishing

It is the process of smoothing a surface, by causing plastic flow of micro roughnesses, usually achieved by swift rubbing with a soft agent in particulate form mounted in a brush or cloth.

TYPES OF ABRASIVES

- Natural abrasives
- Remnants of living organisms
- Manufactured abrasives.

Natural Abrasives

- Arkansas stone
- Chalk
- Corundum
- Diamond
- Emery
- Garnet
- Pumice
- Quartz
- Sand
- Tripoli
- Zirconium silicate.

Remnants of Living Organisms

- Cuttle
- Kieselguhr.

Manufactured Abrasives

- Silicon carbide
- Aluminum oxide
- Synthetic diamond
- Rouge
- Tin oxide.

Arkansas Stone

- It is a siliceous light gray semi-translucent, sedimentary rock mined in Arkansas
- It is hard and uniformly textured containing microcrystalline quartz
- Small pieces of this mineral are attached to metal shanks and trued to different shapes.

Uses

For fine grinding of tooth enamel and metal alloys.

Chalk

It is a mineral form of calcite and is white in color. It is composed of calcium carbonate.

Uses

It is used as a mild abrasive paste to polish tooth enamel, gold foil, amalgam and acrylic resins.

Corundum

This consists of aluminum oxide and is white in color. This natural abrasive has been replaced by synthetically manufactured aluminum oxide, which has better physical properties.

Uses

Used for grinding metal alloys and is available as a bonded abrasive in several shapes.

Diamond

It is transparent, colorless and composed of carbon. It is the hardest substance known and is called a superabrasive as it can abrade any other known substance.

Uses

- Diamond abrasives are available as bonded abrasive rotary instruments, flexible metal-backed abrasive strips and polishing pastes
- They are used to polish ceramic and resin-based composite materials.

Emery

It is a greyish-black corundum. Emery is fine grained and coated on disks which is available in variety of grit sizes.

Uses

For finishing metal alloys and plastic materials.

Garnet

- Garnet consists of different minerals with similar physical properties and crystalline forms such as silicates of aluminum, cobalt, iron, magnesium and manganese
- The garnet abrasive is dark red in color
- Garnet is extremely hard and, during grinding, it fractures forming sharp, chisel-shaped plates, increasing the effectiveness of the abrasive
- Garnet is available on coated disks and arbor bands.

Uses

Used in grinding metal alloys and resins.

Pumice

- It is a light-gray, highly siliceous material formed from volcanic activity
- It is available in grit form, rubber-bonded abrasives and as powder (flour).

Uses

To polish resins. Flour of pumice is fine-grained volcanic rock derivative from Italy and is used in polishing tooth enamel, gold foil, dental amalgam and acrylic resins.

Quartz

- It is very hard, colorless and transparent
- Quartz crystalline particles are pulverized to form sharp, angular particles and are coated on abrasive disks.

Uses

Used to finish metal alloys and sometimes to grind dental enamel.

Sand

- Is a mixture of small mineral silica particles in different colors
- Sand particles are either rounded or angular in shape.

Uses

- Applied under air pressure to remove refractory investment materials from base metal alloy castings
- Also available as paper disks for grinding of metal alloys and plastic materials.

Tripoli

- Derived from a lightweight, friable siliceous sedimentary rock, which can be white, gray, pink, red or yellow in color
- The gray and red types are commonly used in dentistry.

Uses

The rock is ground into very fine particles and is formed with soft binders into bars of polishing cake and is used for polishing metal alloys and resins.

Zirconium Silicate

It is as an off-white mineral which is ground to various particle sizes and is coated on abrasive disks and strips.

Uses

As a component of dental prophylaxis pastes.

Cuttlefish, Cuttlebone or Cuttle

It is a white calcareous powder made from the pulverized internal shell of a Mediterranean mollusc of the genus *Sepia.*

Uses

It is available as a coated abrasive for polishing metal margins and dental amalgam restorations.

Kieselguhr

- It is composed of the siliceous remains of aquatic plants known as diatoms
- The coarser form is called diatomaceous earth, which is used as a filler in many dental materials.

Uses

- Used as a mild abrasive
- Respiratory silicosis is reported by chronic exposure to airborne particles of this material. Hence, mouth masks are worn during its handling.

Silicon Carbide

- It is a hard and brittle synthetic abrasive which was the first of the synthetic abrasives to be made
- Green and blue-black types are commonly available
- The green form is preferred as substrates are more visible against the green color
- Particles are sharp and break to form new sharp particles increasing the grinding efficiency.

Uses

- Used to polish alloys, ceramics and plastic materials
- Silicon carbide is available as an abrasive in coated disks and vitreous-bonded and rubber-bonded instruments.

Aluminum Oxide

- This was the second synthetic abrasive to be developed after silicon carbide
- Synthetic aluminum oxide is a white powder which is harder than corundum
- Different grain sizes are available and can be used to make bonded abrasives, coated abrasives and air-propelled grit abrasives.

Uses

- White stones made of sintered aluminum oxide are used for adjusting dental enamel and for finishing both metal alloys and ceramic materials
- Pink and ruby colors are aluminum oxide abrasives which are made by adding chromium compounds to the original melt as vitreous-bonded form on mounted stones are used for the preparation of metal-ceramic alloys to receive porcelain
- As per Yamamoto (1985) review, carbide burs are best to finish metal ceramic alloys as they do not contaminate the metal surface with entrapped abrasive particles.

Synthetic Diamond Abrasives

Manufactured as diamond saws, wheels, burs, blocks with embedded diamond particles for truing other types of bonded abrasives, diamond polishing pastes (particles smaller than 5 μm in diameter) are used in polishing ceramic materials.

Uses

Used to abrade tooth structure, ceramic materials and resin-based composite materials.

Rouge

Iron oxide is the fine, red abrasive component of rouge and is blended with soft binders into a cake form.

Uses

Used to polish high noble metal alloys.

Tin Oxide

- It is a fine abrasive used as a polishing agent for polishing teeth and metallic restorations in the mouth
- It is mixed with water, alcohol or glycerin to form a mildly abrasive paste.

97. Platinum Group.

PLATINUM GROUP METALS

These constitute:

- Platinum
- Palladium
- Iridium
- Rhodium
- Ruthenium
- Osmium.

Physical Constants

Element	Symbol	Atomic Weight	Melting Point (°C)	Boiling Point (°C)	Density (g/cm^3)	Linear Coefficient of Thermal Expansion $\times 10^{-6}/°C$
Iridium	Ir	192.2	2454.0	5300	22.5	0.068
Palladium	Pd	106.4	1552.0	3980	12.02	0.118
Platinum	Pt	195.09	1769.0	4530	21.45	0.089
Rhodium	Rh	102.91	1966.0	4500	12.44	0.083

ALLOYS CONTAINING PLATINUM

- Gold alloys contain platinum as a component in them to improve the physical properties. Gold alloys contain 75% (wt) gold and metals of the platinum group
- Type IV contains gold and alloying elements such as silver (Ag), copper (Cu), platinum (Pt) and palladium (Pd)
- Iridium (Ir) may be present as a grain refining agent 0.005% (approx.)
- This alloy is used as the framework for partial denture.

EFFECTS OF PLATINUM GROUP IN IMPROVING PHYSICAL PROPERTIES OF ALLOYS

- *Silver*: Reduces the melting range of the alloy
- *Palladium*: May replace platinum
- *Copper* and *platinum*: Order hardening effects (for Cu content of > 8% (wt) approx.)

HEAT TREATMENT PROCEDURE

Hardening

- Heat to 450°C.
- Hold for 10 minutes.
- Air-cool.

Softening

- Heat to 700°C for 10 minutes.
- Water quench.

Order hardening

- Copper less than 8% along with platinum forms AuCu at a suitable composition
- At a temperature above 450°C, the Cu and Au atoms migrate to preferred sites in the solid
- The effect is that the random substitutional solid solution breaks down and is replaced part by the lattice (AuCu*)*
- When these dislocations are introduced into the casting, they prevent plastic deformation, in turn, increasing the strength of the material.

Quenching

- Quenching retains the casting in the 'soft' condition preventing the atoms to migrate in the solid to form AuCu (order hardening)
- Just before quenching, the fit of the casting can be checked and burnishing of the edges can be done
- Before cementation in the mouth, the casting is re-heated to 450°C for 10 minutes, to allow the ordering effect to occur and is allowed to air cool
- If required, the casting may be softened again by re-heating to 700°C
- Copper content of the alloy needs to be > 8% (wt) for order hardening to take place. (Types III and IV).

98. Duplicating Impression Materials.

- Duplicating materials are used to duplicate the plaster or stone cast of the patient's mouth
- Duplication is common in the preparation of partial dentures.

SIGNIFICANCE OF DUPLICATION

- Duplication is done as to reproduce the cast on which the wax pattern of the metal framework is formed
- The duplicated cast is poured with a refractory investment material which can withstand the casting temperatures of gold or base metal alloys
- For gold alloys, gypsum-bonded refractory material is used
- For base metal alloys, a phosphate-bonded investment material is used
- The original cast poured in dental stone is required to check the accuracy of the metal framework and to acrylize the plastic portion of the partial denture.

DUPLICATING MATERIALS

- Agar
- Alginate.

Composition of Duplicating Materials

- The composition of duplicating hydrocolloid materials are the same as hydrocolloid impression materials
- Duplicating hydrocolloid materials are mixed with more water in manipulating when compared with hydrocolloids impression materials
- An impression material is diluted with as much as one to three times its weight of water and used as a duplicating compound.

Procedure

Agar Manipulation

- An impression of the original cast is made in an elastic duplicating material
- This duplicated impression is poured with a refractory investment and is called a refractory cast
- 200–400 mL of material is required for each duplication
- The agar duplicating materials are stored in the sol state at 54°–66°C and used when needed
- After a duplication procedure, the gel is chopped up and reheated to be added to the material being stored at 54°–66°C
- The material can be reused about 20 times before it is discarded.

Duplication Procedure

- The blocked out master cast is placed on the base of a duplicating flask

- The duplicating flask has a metal base on which the master cast is fixed. The metal base aids in cooling of the agar
- Agar at the proper temperature is poured into the flask and is cooled in a regulated cooling tank for an hour
- The flask is then disassembled and the master cast is removed.

Refractory Cast

- Gypsum-bonded investments are poured into the mold for type IV gold partial denture
- Phosphate-bonded investments are used for chrome-cobalt alloy denture base
- After the refractory material sets, the cast is removed and placed in a drying oven at 93°C
- When dry, the cast is trimmed to within 6 mm of the proposed design.

Disadvantages of Agar

- The set material is a gel and can undergo dimensional changes if stored in air or water. The material should be stored in 100% relative humidity
- The duplicated mold should be immediately poured with refractory material
- The agar is an polysaccharide which will hydrolyze at storage temperatures leading to loss of elasticity and stiffness.

Advantages of Agar

- They are reversible and can be reused a number of times
- They have adequate strength and elastic properties so that the duplication of undercut areas is possible
- The accuracy of the agar duplication compounds is good
- Alginate has similar advantages and disadvantages as the alginate impression materials.

99. Pulp Response of Restorative Dental Cements.

RESTORATIVE MATERIAL MAY IRRITATE THE PULP DUE TO

- Exothermic heat, evolved during setting.
- Chemical toxicity.
- Acidity.
- Poor marginal adaptation.

RESPONSE TO

- Cements
- Amalgam

- Restorative resins
- Gold restoration.

Cements

Zinc Phosphate Cement

- Pulp response is moderate
- Due to phosphoric acid content, there is high acidity at the time of insertion
- Three minutes after mixing, pH is 3.5
- pH reaches neutrality in 24–48 hours
- Damage to pulp can occur during first few hours after insertion
- Dentin thickness of even 1.5 mm can be penetrated by the acid in the cement
- In deep cavities, pulpal reaction is minimized by lining with either zinc oxide, calcium hydroxide or cavity varnish.

Zinc Oxide Eugenol

- Pulp response is mild
- pH is 6.6–8.0, hence most biocompatible cement
- It has bacteriostatic and obtundent properties
- They inhibit growth of bacteria and have an anodyne or soothing effect in pulp in deep cavities, reducing pain, if present
- Eugenol is a toxic phenol derivative
- If applied directly to pulp, it produces thrombosis of blood vessels
- Provides good marginal seal.
- Excellent thermal insulating properties. It is in the range of cork and asbestos. It is about 3.95 $\times 10^{-6}/°C$
- Solubility is the highest among other dental cements. They disintegrate in oral fluids.

Glass Ionomer Cement

- Pulpal response is mild
- Type II GIC is biocompatible
- Pulpal reaction is greater than zinc oxide eugenol but lesser than zinc phosphate
- Water settable cements show higher acidity when compared to powder/polyacrylic acid
- Type I (luting) is more acidic due to low powder/liquid ratio.

Zinc Polycarboxylate Cement

- Pulpal response is mild
- pH is 1.0–1.7 and pH of freshly mixed cement is 3.0–4.0
- After 24 hours, pH is 5.0–6.0
- It is less irritant than zinc phosphate cement
- Penetration of polyacrylic acid into dentinal tubule is less
- More reparative dentin is observed than zinc oxide eugenol.

Calcium Hydroxide Cement

- Cement is alkaline in nature
- Higher pH of 9.2–11.7

- Formation of secondary dentine due to alkalinity
- It has antibacterial and protein-lysing effect.

Silicate

- Disintegrate in oral fluids due to high solubility
- Severe irritant to pulp. Act as standard for comparing pulpal response to other materials
- So, pulp protection is done with ZnO/E/Ca $(OH)_2$ or varnish
- Reduced incidence of secondary caries
- Reduced incidence of contact caries due to fluoride release.

Amalgam

- In deep filling, pulpal inflammation occurs, if unlined
- Thermal sensitivity can occur due to expansion or contraction of fluid between cavity wall and amalgam
- Fluid movement causes nerve fiber stimulation giving rise to pain
- Use of base cavity varnish, seals dentinal tubules preventing pain.

Restorative Resins

- Marginal leakage around resin restoration is reduced by acid etching and use of bonding agent or primer
- Cavity liner should be used or it can irritate pulp due to bacterial contamination beneath the restoration.

Gold Restoration

- Can cause hypersensitivity, pulpal inflammation, necrosis, depending on force and direction of flow from mallet during condensation
- It can cause trauma to vascular supply at apical foramen.

100. Sensitization.

- Austenitic stainless steel loses its resistance to corrosion if heated between 400°C and 900°C depending on its carbon content
- The decrease in corrosion resistance is caused by the precipitation of Chromium-Iron carbide at the grain boundaries.

MECHANISM

- The small carbon atoms rapidly diffuse to the grain boundary regions to combine with the chromium and iron atoms in solid solution and form $(CrFe)_4C$, resulting in the loss of corrosion resistance
- Formation of $(CrFe)_4C$ is most rapid at 650°C. Below this temperature, the diffusion rate for carbon is slower, whereas decomposition of $(CrFe)_4C$ occurs at higher temperatures
- Corrosion resistance is reduced in regions adjacent to the grain boundaries in which the chromium level is below 12%.

METHODS TO MINIMIZE SENSITIZATION

First Method

Reduce the carbon content of steel to an extent such that carbide precipitation cannot occur. (Not employed).

Second Method

- If the stainless steel is severely cold-worked and heated within the sensitization temperature, iron carbides form instead of chromium carbides
- Iron carbides form uniformly rather than forming a network of grain boundary precipitates.

Third Method

Stabilization

The common method to prevent sensitization of austenitic stainless steels is to introduce one or more elements that form carbide at high temperatures in preference to chromium, such as:
- Niobium (or) Titanium + Tantalum
- Stainless steels treated in this manner are said to be stabilized
- This method is not used for stainless steel orthodontic wires due to the cost factor.

101. Eames Technique.

SYNONYMS

- Minimal mercury technique
- Squeeze cloth technique as the squeezing out of mercury is needed here.

Eames Technique

It is the method for reducing the mercury content of the restoration by reducing the original mercury:alloy ratio.

Advantages

- Less mercury content improves the physical and mechanical properties of amalgam
- Sufficient mercury is required in the original mix to provide a coherent and plastic mass after trituration.
- Excess mercury need not be removed during condensation
- The mercury content of the finished restoration is comparable to that of the original mercury: alloy ratio.

Manipulation by Eames Technique

- The recommended mercury: alloy ratio for most modern lathe cut alloys is 40:60%
- In Eames technique, the manipulation is done with powder and mercury in the ratio of 1 : 1 parts by weight.

Methods of Dispensing

- Volumetric dispensers
- Preweighed pellets or tablets
- Preproportioned capsules

The most accurate method is to weigh the mercury and alloy components using a balance which is not presently done.

Volumetric dispensers

- Dispensing by volume is unreliable, hence only fine-grained types can be volumetrically dispensed
- The dispenser should be held vertically. Tilting the bottle to a 45°-angle results in unreliable mercury to alloy ratio
- The dispenser should be at least half full, if not, the weight of mercury dispensed may be wrong
- Entrapment of contaminants (air/voids) in the dispensers can alter ratio of mercury dispension.

Preweighed pellets/tablets

Alloy powder is compressed in tablets of uniform weight which is used with the measured amount of mercury.

Pre-proportioned capsules

- The alloy is available as pellet forms or as preweighed powder form, with the correct amount of mercury in a separate compartment separated by a membrane
- Just before mixing, the membrane is broken by compression of the capsule or is automatically activated when placed in an amalgamator.

The capsules may be:

- Reusable.
  - Disposable.
- Containing pestle.
  - Not containing pestle.

102. Ethoxy Benzoic Acid Cement.

INTRODUCTION

- Ethoxy benzoic acid (EBA) is ortho-ethoxy benzoic acid
- Was formulated to improve mechanical properties of zinc-oxide eugenol cement A higher powder/liquid ratio can be used.

Composition

Powder	Liquid
Zno—60%	Ethoxy benzoic acid—50–60%
Aluminum/quartz—20–30%	Eugenol—40%
Rosin—5–10%	
Zinc acetate—0.4%	

- The ratio of ortho-ethoxy-benzoic acid to Eugenol is 2:1
- These two form chelate compounds with zinc ions.

Powder

- Zinc oxide—60% (primary reactive ingredient)
- Quartz/aluminum—35% (reinforcing agent)
- Hydrogenated rosin—5% (reinforcing agent)
- Zinc acetate—0.4%.

Liquid

- Ortho-ethoxybenzoic acid—62.5%
- Eugenol—37.5% (reactive ingredient).

Properties

- Compressive strength is 55 MPa
- Tensile strength is 4.1 MPa
- Modulus of elasticity is 2.5 GPa
- Film thickness is 25 μm
- Solubility and disintegration in water—0.05% weight
- Compressive strength is increased by reinforcement.
  - Resin-bonded — 40–60 MPa.
  - EBA — 85–90 MPa.

Other Properties

- Strength is more
- Solubility is less
- Low film thickness is used for permanent cementation.

Setting time

Resin-bonded — 5–9 minutes.
EBA — 7 minutes.

P/L ratio

Resin-bonded — 4:1.
EBA — 7:1.

Manipulation

The dispensed powder is incorporated into the liquid in bulk on a glass slab for 30 seconds and stropped with the spatula for an additional 60 seconds with broad strokes.

Setting time

5–9 minutes.

Applications

- Primarily used as luting cements
- As cavity liners for amalgam condensation—as they have adequate strength and resistance to flow.

103. Resin-modified Glass Ionomer Cement/Hybrid Ionomer.

MODIFIED GLASS IONOMER

- These are hybrid material with a significant acid-base reaction as part of their overall curing process
- It has a double action molecule capable of reacting with a polyalkenoic acid as well as with the vinyl group of certain resin.

Composition

Powder

- Ion leachable fluoroalumino silicate glass particles
- Initiator for light curing and for chemical curing.

Liquid

- 15–25% resin component hydroxyethyl methacrylate (HEMA)
- Less than 1% polymerizable group
- Photo-initiator.

Reaction

The original acid-base reaction continues and the resin component provides an umbrella effect, protecting the cement from early loss of water and further uptake of water through the dissolution of certain polyacrylate.

104. Percolation.

DEFINITION

If a tooth containing a nonadhesive plastic restoration is cooled by drinking of cold liquid, the restoration contracts more than the tooth and a small space results at the junction between two materials. Oral fluids can penetrate this space. This phenomenon is called percolation.

Factors in Percolation

- Temperature changes in mouth result in dimensional changes of restorative dental materials, which cause a differential expansion of restorative material that does not match with that of tooth structure resulting in the leakage of oral fluids between the restoration and tooth
- Linear coefficient of thermal expansion can be calculated by finding out the difference in length of specimen at two different temperatures $\{(lt_2 - lt_1/lt_1)/(t_2 - t_1)\}$
- The values for amalgams and composites are 2–5 times that of human teeth. The values for unfilled plastics are 5–7 times those of teeth
- Dental amalgam is unusual in that percolation decreases with time after insertion, as a result of the space being filled with corrosion products from the amalgam restoration
- Percolation can cause possible irritation to dental pulp and recurrent decay.

Coefficients of thermal expansion of various materials used in dentistry are as follows:

Materials	Coefficient × 10^{-6}/°C
Inlay wax	350–450
Silicone impression material	210
Polysulfide impression material	140
Pit and fissure sealants	71–94
Acrylic resin	76
Mercury	60.6
Resin compounds	14–50
Zinc oxide eugenic cements	35
Amalgam	25
Silver	19.2
Copper	16.8
Gold	14.4
Porcelain	12
Tooth (crown)	11.4

105. Single-composition Alloys/Admixed Alloys.

SYNONYMS

Unicompositional alloys.

DEFINITION

- Admixed amalgams are a variety of high-copper alloys
- Admixed alloy powders have same particle and same chemical composition; hence also called single-composition alloys.

Composition

- Silver—60%
- Tin—27%
- Copper—13%
- Traces of indium and palladium.

Reactions in Admixed Alloy

- The phases in single-composition alloy are the β-phase (Ag-Sn), α-phase (Ag_3Sn)
- Some alloys may contain Σ-phase (Cu_3Sn) and some γ-phase (Cu_6Sn_5)
- Atomized particles have dendritic structures, consisting of fine lamellae
- When triturated with mercury, silver and tin, form the Ag-Sn phases
- The amount of copper dissolving in mercury is less
- The α_1 crystals grow forming a matrix with partially dissolved alloy particles
- The α_1 crystals are found as meshes of rod-like crystals at surface of alloy particles
- Undesirable γ_2 phase can form if atomized powder has not been heat-treated or if treated for too long at a high temperature.

Reaction

Ag-Sn-Cu alloy particles + Hg $\rightarrow \gamma_1 + \eta$ + Unconsumed alloy particles.

Properties

- Amalgam made from these powders is stronger than the amalgam made from lathe-cut low copper powder because of the increase in residual alloy particle and decrease in matrix rather than dispersion strengthening mechanism
- Silver and tin act as strong fillers in amalgam
- Admixed amalgam is more resistant to marginal breakdown than low copper amalgam restoration
- Admixed alloy particles usually contain 30 wt% to 55 wt% spherical high—Cu powder. Total copper content in admixed alloys ranges approximately from 9 wt% to 20 wt%.

106. Trituration.

Trituration is a term used to wet all the surfaces of the alloy particles with mercury.

FACTORS AFFECTING TRITURATION

- If alloy particle surface is not clean, improper wetting of the alloy surface occurs
- The oxide film on the surface of the alloy powder prevents the mercury from coming into direct contact with alloy powder
- Surface tension of mercury is high (465 dynes/cm) which prevents the wetting of the alloy particle
- Trituration with the application of sufficient pressure removes the oxide coating and reduces the surface tension of mercury, thus increasing the wetting of the powder by mercury.

Methods of Mixing

- Hand mixing.
- Mechanical mixing.

Hand Mixing

- For hand trituration, a glass mortal and pestle with roughened surface are used
- A low alloy:mercury ratio (around 5:8) is required to produce a workable mix
- Trituration time—45–60 seconds
- Trituration pressure—800–1000 gm/cm^2
- Excessive pressure should be avoided to prevent splintering of alloy particles which can alter the character of the mix
- A fist grasp (palm and thumb) is used to hold the pestle
- Following trituration, excess mercury is squeezed out using a gauze cloth.

Mechanical Mixing

Amalgamators are the devices used for mechanical mixing.

Three levels in amalgam manipulation

- After proportioning, the mercury and alloy are placed in a capsule held by a holder in the amalgamator and vibrated
- Mechanical mixing in a semiautomatic machine, which proportions the mercury and alloy, is also possible
- The use of encapsulated, preproportioned materials in the amalgamators are used but are more expensive.

Factors affecting mixing

- Trituration time, speed and force applied during trituration
- Types of alloys being used and the dispensing and mixing systems
- The spherical alloys tend to mix more readily and are easier to wet and have a shorter trituration time than the lathe-cut particles
- The trituration time for a system running at a speed of 4,000 rpm and a throw of 50 mm is 5 seconds
- For a slower system of 2,600 rpm, time will be 20 seconds.

Undertriturated Mix	Normal Mix	Overtriturated Mix
Dull, grainy, crumbly in appearance	Shiny and homogeneous in appearance	Soupy in appearance
Give rough surface after carving	Give smooth surface after carving	Loss of strength
Tarnish and corrosion are accelerated	Increased resistance to tarnish and corrosion	Creep is increased
Loss in strength	Greatest strength	Excessive contraction
High setting expansion	Mix separates in a single max and may be warm when removed from the capsule	Mix tends to stick to the inside of the capsules and is hence, difficult to remove and handle

Advantages of Mechanical Trituration

- A uniform and reproducible mix
- A shorter trituration time
- A greater alloy-mercury ratio can be used, which negates the need to express excess mercury after trituration
- Encapsulate materials reduce the risk of atmospheric mercury contamination.

107. Mulling.

Is continuation of trituration.

It is done to

- Improve homogeneity of the mix
- Get a consistent mix.

Methods in Mulling

Using Palm and Thumb

The amalgam mix is placed in a rubber dam sheet, covered and kept on the palm and rubbed with the thumb for 2–5 seconds.

Mechanical

After trituration, the pestle is removed from the capsule and the capsule is vibrated for 2–3 seconds at lower speeds to produce a uniform texture throughout the mass.

108. Condensation.

CONDENSATION OF AMALGAM

- It is the insertion of the amalgam mass into the prepared cavity
- It should be done within 3 minutes of trituration.

Need for Condensation

- For adaptation of the amalgam mass to the cavity walls
- Brings excess mercury to the surface layer, which on removal reduces the final mercury content in the restoration. This influences the properties of dimensional change, creep and compressive strength
- Reduces voids and improves the strength.

Methods of Condensation

- Hand condensation
- Mechanical condensation.

Hand Condensation

- Hand condensation utilizes suitably sized condensers in relation to cavity size
- Use of optimum force (approximately 3–4 pounds)
- Placement of small increments with minimum voids
- Removal of excess of mercury
- Small and large condenser tips of different shapes are available.
  For example, round, triangular, oval, square, trapezoidal and crescent.

Method of hand condensation

- The mixed material is carried to the prepared cavity using an amalgam carrier and each increment is condensed with sufficient pressure using overlapping technique
- Condensation is started at the centre and the condenser is stepped slowly toward the cavity wall by overlapping method
- Condensation brings out excess mercury to the surface layer, the removal of which reduces the final mercury content
- The size of the condenser tip and the direction and magnitude of force applied depend on the alloy used.

Lathe-cut alloy → Small-tip condenser (1–2 mm tip) greater force, vertical condensation pressure.

Spherical → Larger condenser, less force, lateral direction.

If small tips are used with spherical alloys, the particles tend to roll over each other, the tip penetrates the amalgam and the mass does not adapt well to the cavity.

Mechanical Condensation

These devices are more useful for condensing lathe-cut alloys where high condensation forces are required

- Most of these devices are based on the principle of vibration
- Others have tapping or malleting action
- Ultrasonic condensers are not recommended as they increase the mercury vapor level to values above the safety standard.

109. Carving/Polishing.

OBJECTIVES OF CARVING AN AMALGAM RESTORATION

- To remove the mercury-rich layer on the amalgam surface
- To rebuild the anatomy of the tooth
- To re-establish contact with the opposing dentition.

Factors Affecting Carving in Amalgam restoration

- Amalgam prepared from a coarser grain alloy is difficult to carve
- After restoring, it should be sufficiently hardened to start carving
- Improper condensation delays hardening, which, in turn, affects carving
- If carving is done too soon, there will be danger of 'dragging out' significant amounts of material from the surface
- If carving is delayed too long, the material can chip at the margins during carving
- Amalgam needs to be cut back to the cavity margins to prevent fracture under occlusal loading
- Occlusal contact pattern should be checked while carving a restoration
- When the amalgam is still soft, rubbing the surface with cotton wool produces a mat finish
- High contacts are located by asking the patient to tap their teeth together or move them from side to side, which show up as bright burnished spots
- These bright burnished spots need to be reduced.

POLISHING

Polishing is carried out to achieve a lustrous surface having a more acceptable appearance and better corrosion resistance.

Points to Note

- The filling should not be polished until the material has achieved good mechanical strength, or it can fracture at the margins
- The strength of most material is good after 24 hours after placement
- Advantage of 8-minute polishing is that a second appointment is not required
- A well polished restoration is smooth and has less plaque accumulation
- Rough surfaces cause galvanic action on the surface of the restoration to develop tarnish and corrosion
- Final polish at a second appointment is developed through a series of final polishing and finishing steps
- Polishing can be done by flours of pumice with water as carrier
- Final polish is accomplished through the application of a sequence of operations that includes the use of fine stones and abrasive disks or chips

- During the final polishing, the restoration should be kept moist to avoid overheating from dry polishing surfaces
- Since the amalgam is weak in tension and shear resistance, it should not be drawn over the margin by burnishing or drawing operations
- For spherical high copper alloys, which have high early strength, finishing and polishing may be done at the same appointment.

Steps Involved in Polishing

- Contour (Green stones, abrasive disks, burs)
- Finish margins (Green stones, abrasive disks, burs)
- Smooth alloy surface (Rubber abrasive points, pumice, sluice).

110. Amalgam Bond.

Amalgam bond is an adhesive used to increase the bond between Amalgam and Tooth structure.

DISADVANTAGES OF AMALGAM

Dental amalgam does not bond to dentin or enamel and restoration is retained by undercuts and roughness in the cavity design

As a result, amalgam restorations leak around the margins, especially after they have been recently placed

As amalgam does not bond to tooth structure, the strength of clinical crown is not restored to the level of the sound tooth

Hence, an adhesive increases bond to tooth structure.

Composition of Amalgam Bond

- Amalgam bonds are fluid resins containing a compound with 4 META or 4 methacryl oxyethyl trimethitaic anhydride
- *Example*: Amalgam bond plus, meta-bond and all-bond, all produce shear bond strengths. They possess a bond strength of approximately 10 MPa.

Advantages of Amalgam Bond

- They reduce marginal leakage and strengthen the tooth structure
- Aids in amalgam retention
- The bond strength has been shown to be 10 MPa, which is about half the bond strength of composite to tooth structure

- Fracture resistance of teeth containing amalgam-bonded MOD restoration is more than twice more retentive than unbonded amalgam MODs
- Retention of amalgam-bonded MODs with proximal boxes was as great as pin-retained restorations
- Amalgam-bonded restorations were found to decrease marginal leakage in Class V restorations.

111. Amalgam Capsule.

For ease of dispensing the alloy, the alloy powder is compressed into tablets of controlled weight which is used with measured amount of mercury. This is called an amalgam capsule **(Fig. 52)**.

Method of Use

- This is the most accurate method of dispensing
- Preproportioned capsules containing alloy particle and mercury in compartment separated by a membrane are available
- Before use, the membrane is ruptured by compression of the capsule and the capsule is placed in a mechanical amalgamator.

Advantages

- The right ratio of mercury to alloy is maintained (as this is prefixed by the manufacturer)
- Less danger of mercury spillage during the handling stages

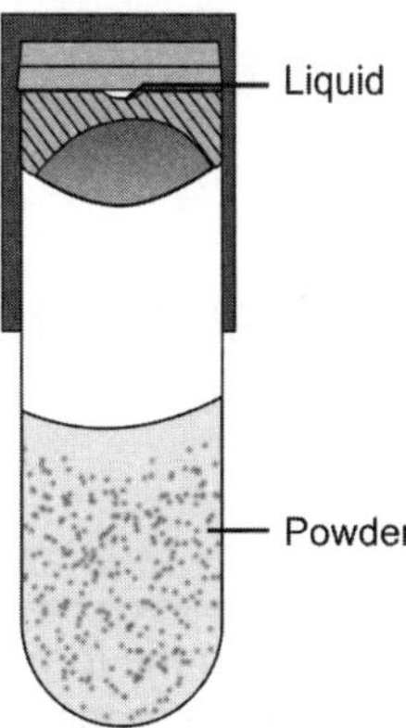

Fig. 52: Cross-sectional view of amalgam capsule

- Saving of proportioning here
- Accuracy in manipulation; hence improved physical properties.

Disadvantages

- It is expensive
- Mercury alloy prepackaged in disposable capsules may leak during trituration
- The dentist is forced to use one alloy-mercury ratio for all situations when using disposable capsules
- Disposable capsules can never be reused, since fracture or leakage of capsule may occur
- Capsules, which does not require the use of a press, are called self-activating capsules.

Manipulation of Amalgam (Considerations)

- Alloy and mercury are dispensed in a capsule, which is placed in a holder
- A housing is placed in a holder over the capsule to confine any loss of mercury from the capsule during mixing
- The holder is attached to a motor, which rotates the holder and capsule or a pestle may be included in the capsule for mixing
- When tablets of alloy are used, a pestle is required to break up the tablet so that mercury can contact the particles of alloy and develop a smooth mix
- Low copper alloys, spherical or lathe cut, maybe amalgamated in a slow-speed, low-energy amalgamator, but high-copper alloys require a high-speed amalgamator for trituration
- Care should be taken in the choice of capsule-pestle combination and in the setting of the timer and speed controller for amalgam being mixed
- Reusable capsules should be thoroughly cleaned after each mix to present amalgam particles from hardening inside the capsule
- After constant use, the interior surfaces of the capsules become scarred and the capsules should be replaced
- For ensuring efficiency of mixing, it is important to periodically calibrate dental amalgamators
- Electrical amalgamators have digital controls to permit programming of settings.

112. Mercury Hazard and Mercury Hygiene.

MERCURY HAZARD

The danger from mercury exposure depends on the form in which mercury is present as liquid, vapor, intermetallic compound, organometallic compound and the quantity and frequency of exposure.

Mercury Exposure in Dentistry

- Accidental spills
- Direct skin contact with mercury
- Mixed but unhardened amalgam during trituration and insertion
- While removing old restoration
- During manipulation.

Mercury hyper-sensitivity can cause sensitivity reaction, which is mild and not life-threatening and disappears in a few days.

Concentration of Mercury

- Maximum amount of mercury in the workplace—0.05 mg/m^3 (threshold limit value)
- Lowest dose of mercury that elicits atoxic reaction—307 mg
- Hearing loss and death—4000 mg/kg body wt
- These values are much greater in magnitude than the exposure to mercury from amalgam
- Mercury levels in blood of patients with amalgam restoration 0.7 mg/mL compared with a value of 0.3 mg/mL for subjects with no amalgam restoration.

Symptoms of Mercury Toxicity

Systemic	Local
Excitability	Allergic contact dermatitis
Inability to concentrate	Stomatitis
Depression	Gingivitis
Headache	Loosening of teeth
Fatigue	Excessive salivation
Weakness	
Loss of memory	
Drowsiness	
Tremors of hands, lips, trunks and jaws	

MERCURY HYGIENE

- It is the process of handling mercury health hazards
- Daily exposure of mercury in small amounts can build up to toxic levels in the body over time
- In dentistry, the main route of exposure is by inhalation of mercury vapor, which is absorbed through the alveoli in the lungs.

Properties of Mercury

• Melting point	–39°C
• Boiling point	357°C
• Density	13.6 g/cc (very high)
• Surface energy	460 ergs/cm^2
• Vapour pressure	–20 mg/m^3 at 25°C

Exposure to mercury can occur from many different sources including diet, water, air and occupational exposure.

DENTAL MERCURY HYGIENE RECOMMENDATIONS

- Train all the personnel in handling of dental amalgam
- Make the personnel aware of the potential sources of mercury vapor in the dental operator, e.g. spills, open storage of amalgam scrap
- Work in well ventilated spaces with fresh air exchanges and outside exhaust
- Periodically check the dental operatory atmosphere for mercury vapor with the aid of dosimeters
- Use proper work area design to facilitate spill consummation and clear up. Floor coverings should be nonabsorbent, seamless for easy clean-up.
- Use only precapsulated alloys; discontinue the use of bulk mercury and bulk alloy
- Use an amalgamator with a completely closed arm
- Avoid skin contact with mercury or freshly mixed amalgam
- Use high-volume evacuation while finishing or removing amalgam
- Salvage and store all scrap amalgam in a tightly closed container, either dry or under radiographic fixer solution
- When feasible, recycle amalgam scrap and waste amalgam
- Dispose of mercury-contaminated item in sealed bags according to the applicable regulations
- Cleanup spilled mercury properly using trap buttes, or gas to pick up droplets and commercial clean-up kits
- Remove professional clothing before leaving the workspace.

113. Cohesive Gold Foil and Manipulation of Gold Foil.

They are supplied as gold, free of surface contaminant and, thus, are cohesive and are called cohesive gold foil.

MANIPULATION

Degassing

- Before insertion of gold foil into a cavity, it is heated to remove absorbed gases as oxygen from the metal surface and to improve the weldability
- Gold foil can be heated on a container, above a gas or alcohol flame, or in an electric furnace at 250–350°C
- This procedure is termed degassing

- The time of heating depends on the individual material and the degree of surface contamination.

Compaction/Condensing

The clean and decontaminated gold is packed into the cavity in increments by any of the following methods:

- A plugger and hand mallet
- A pneumatic vibratory condenser
- An electrically driven condenser.

Significant Points in Condensing

- The first of these methods usually requires the greatest time and may be the most traumatic
- The area of the condenser point needs to be of correct size
- If too large, there is less pressure and adaptation may not be achieved
- If too small, the condenser will punch a hole in the metal rather than adapt it
- The area of the condenser point should be between 0.3 mm and 1.0 mm
- Force of compaction should be applied perpendicular to the surface of the foil
- Failure to do this will result in shear stresses, which may cause a piece of foil to become dislodged.

114. Advantages and Disadvantages of Composite Resin Restoration.

ADVANTAGES

Adhesion to Tooth Structure

Adhesion to tooth structure seals the margins of restoration and reinforces the remaining tooth structure against fracture.

Low Thermal Conductivity

It has an insulating effect that helps to decrease postoperative temperature sensitivity.

Elimination of Galvanic Currents

Composites do not contain metal and so will not initiate or conduct galvanic currents.

Radiopacity

Most of the modern composites have radio-opacity greater than that of enamel and, thus, can evaluate the contours and marginal adaptation of the restoration, caries and tooth structure.

Mercury-free Alternative to Amalgam

Composites are a safe alternative to amalgam.

Esthetic

They are one of the most esthetic restorative materials available.

Need to Remove Less Tooth Structure

Its property of adhesion to tooth structure offsets the need to remove more tooth structure.

DISADVANTAGES

Polymerization Shrinkage

- Modern composites undergo a volumetric polymerization shrinkage of approx. 2.6–7.1%
- This causes the material to pull away from the least retentive cavity margin and, thus, forming a gap.

Secondary Caries

Marginal gap can lead to ingress of bacteria and secondary caries.

Postoperative Sensitivity

This may occur due to polymerization shrinkage.

Decreased Wear Resistance

Composites cause a general abrasive wear by the food particles during mastication and attrition due to direct contact with the opposing tooth.

Water Sorption

Water is absorbed preferentially into the resin component, weakening the filler resin bond, causing a hydrolytic breakdown.

115. Macrofilled Composites.

DEFINITION

Macrofilled composites are also referred to as conventional or traditional composites (because of the large size of the filler particles).

Composition

- These consist of finely-ground amorphous silica and quartz as filler
- *Filler particle size:* Average size is 8–12 µm but particles as large as 50–100 µm may also be present
- Filler loading generally is 70–80 wt% or 60–70 vol%.

Properties of Macrofilled Composites

The macrofilled composites have improved properties, when compared to unfilled restorative resins.

Compressive Strength

It is four to five times greater than that of unfilled resins.

- 250–300 MPa.
- 36,250–43,500 Psi.

Tensile Strength

It is double that of unfilled acrylic in resins.

- 50–65 MPa.
- 7,250–9,425 Psi.

Elastic Modulus

It is four to six times greater.

- 8–15 GPa.
- 1.16–2.18 × 10^6 Psi.

Hardness

It is considerably greater than that of unfilled resins.

- 55 KHN.

Water Sorption

It is less than that of unfilled resins.

- 0.5–0.7 mg/cm^2.

Coefficient of Thermal Expansion

The high filler-to-resin ratio reduces the expansion co-efficient significantly.

- $25–35 \times 10^{-6}$/C.

Esthetics

Polishing of the macrofilled composite resulted in a rough surface due to the selective wear of the softer resin matrix leaving the hard filler particles elevated. This results in stain over a period of time.

Radio-opacity

Composites that contain quartz or amorphous silica as fillers are radiolucent.

DISADVANTAGES OF CONVENTIONAL COMPOSITES

- Polishing is difficult
- Poor resistance to occlusal areas
- Tendency to discolor, the rough surface tends to retain stains
- Not hard enough; hence undergoes occlusal surface wear
- Not indicated as posterior restorative material.

116. Acid Etch Composite Resins/Technique.

COMPOSITION

- A continuous phase (Resin-matrix phase)
- A disposed phase of filler particles
- Coupling agents
- Initiator-activator
- Inhibitors
- Optical modifiers
- Matrix phase.

Resin Matrix

- It is either an aromatic or urethane diacrylate oligomer
- Oligomers are viscous liquids
- Common oligomers used are dimethacrylate (BIS-GMA-Bis phenol-A-glycidyl methacrylate) and urethane dimethacrylate (UDMA).

Disadvantage of BIS-GMA and UDMA

- Highly viscous liquid
- O_2 or air inhibits polymerization
- High water sorption
- Difficulty in synthesizing the material.

To overcome these problems, alternative monomers are used, such as:

- Monofunctional methyl methacrylate (MMA)
- Di-functional ethylene glycol dimethacrylate (EDMA) or TEGDMA.

Diluents

- As the monomers as Bis-GMA are extremely viscous at room temperature, diluents as triethylene glycol dimethacrylate (TEGDMA) are added to reduce the viscosity
- Addition of TEGDMA increases the polymerization shrinkage.

Fillers

Filler particles in resin matrix increase the strength, hardness, rigidity, modulus of elasticity and decrease the coefficient of thermal expansions and polymerization shrinkage.

The Routinely used Fillers

Quartz

Used in early composites. They are extremely hard, making it difficult to grind into fine particles which were difficult to polish and even abraded opposing tooth structure.

Silica

Pyrogenic and precipitated form of colloidal silica have been used. Aluminosilicate and borosilicate glasses are also used.

Coupling Agents

- Coupling agents are used to bind filler particles to resin matrix
- They also allow the more flexible polymer matrix to transfer stresses to the stiffer filler particles
- They provide hydrolytic stability by preventing water from penetrating along the filler-resin interface.
  For example, organic silane such as r-methacryloxy trimethoxysilane.

Initiator-Activator

For chemically activated resins

- Initiator – Benzoyl peroxide
- Activator – Tertiary amine (N, N-dimethyl-p-toluidine).

ACID-ETCH TECHNIQUE

- Developed by Buonocore in 1955
- Phosphoric acid (37%) is used for etching

- It is supplied in the form of a colored gel, which can be applied by a brush or, when supplied in a syringe, it can be dispensed on enamel
- The acid-etch technique improves the bond and marginal seal between resin and enamel.

Mode of Action

- It creates micro-porosities by selective dissolution of enamel rod centers
- Etching increases surface area
- Etched enamel has high surface energy, allowing the resin to wet tooth surface better and penetrate into microporosities
- When polymerized, it forms resin tags.

Procedure

- Classically the tooth is cleaned and polished with pumice and acid is applied on enamel for 60 seconds, but now 15 seconds provide as a strong bond
- Acid is rinsed thoroughly with a stream of water for 15 seconds and enamel is dried
- After drying, enamel has a white frosted appearance.

Bond Strength

Bond strength of etched enamel ranges from 16 MPa to 22 MPa.

Three enamel etching patterns have been described as follows:

Type I

- Predominant dissolution of prism cores
- Honey-comb pattern.

Type II

- Predominant dissolution of prism peripheries
- Cobblestone pattern.

Type III

- No prism structures are evident
- The most commonly used etchant is 37% H_3PO_4
- Concentrations higher than 50% result in the formation of monocalcium phosphate monohydrate that inhibits further dissolution.

Alternative Enamel Etchants

Total-Etch systems, in which enamel and dentin are etched simultaneously, weaker acids are applied to the enamel, such as:

- 10–40% H_3PO_4
- 2.5% HNO_3
- 10% citric acid.

117. Light-cured Composites.

TYPES

Visible Light-activated Resins

Components

• Activator	Blue light with a peak wavelength of 470 nm
• Photoinitiator	Camphoroquinone
• Accelerator	Organic amine (Diethyl amino ethyl methacrylate)

Available as a single paste system.

Significance

- Reinforcing the composites helps in high scattering and transmission
- Filler materials are made radiopaque by addition of glasses and ceramics containing heavy metals such as barium, strontium and zirconium
- Recently, fillers containing fluoride as ytterbium fluoride are also tried
- The translucency of the filler must be similar to tooth structure
- Mostly glasses have a refractive index of 1.5 c as compared to dentin (1.52) and enamel (1.62).

Reaction

- Visible light activation is initiated by energy transfer to the di-ketone (camphoroquinone) which forms an excited triplet state
- The excited triplet attract the accelerator (DMAEMA) molecules and form excited complexes that convert both the camphoroquinone and the DMAEMA molecules to free radicals that initiate addition polymerization.

UV Light-curing System

Components

• Initiator	Benzoyl peroxide
• Activator	Benzoin methyl ether
• Inhibitors	Butylated hydroxytoluene—0.01 wt%
• Hydroquinone	Inhibits chain propagation by terminating the ability of free radicals to initiate polymerization
• Optical modifiers	Metal oxides—TiO_2 (0.001—0.008 wt%)/Al_2O_3.

The UV light-activated resins have been replaced by the visible light-curing systems.

Chemistry of Setting

- Self-cured/chemically cured —(Type from Activator-initiator).
- Visible light cured —(Type from Activator-initiator).

Dual-cured

- This combines cold-curing and visible light-curing components in the same material
- They consist of two light curable pastes, one of which contains benzoyl peroxide and a tertiary amine added to the other
- When the two parts are mixed and exposed to light, both light-curing and cold-curing achieved with the same material.

USES

- Anterior esthetic restorative material
- Posterior restorative material in less stress-bearing areas
- For more retention (Dual-cured resins)
- To veneer metal crowns and bridges
- Pit and fissure sealant
- Core build-up of teeth.

118. Microfilled Resins and Small-sized Resins.

- Microfilled composites were developed to overcome the problem of surface roughness associated with conventional composites
- Microfilled composites consist of colloidal silica particles as the inorganic filler
- Filler particle size is 0.02–0.04 μm, which was 200–300 times smaller than the average quartz particle in conventional composites.

Disadvantages

- Cannot be adequately wetted by the resin matrix and, hence, results in undue thickening of the resin matrix
- Hence, it was not possible to attain the same filler loading as conventional composites.

Types

- Sintered prepolymerized microfilled complexes
- Spherical polymer-based microfilled complexes
- Agglomerated microfilled complexes.

Sintered Prepolymerized Microfilled Complexes

- Made by incorporating 60–70 wt% silica into a resin matrix
- This is then heat-cured and milled into particles of 1–200 μm.

Spherical Polymer-based Microfilled Composites

Manufactured by incorporating pyrogene silica into partially-cured polymer spheres 20–30 μm. This small-size filler permits a dense packing.

Agglomerated Microfilled Composites

They consist of artificially agglomerated microfillers in the range of 1–25 μm. These particles are purely inorganic.

Clinical Performance

- Microfilled composites can be polished to the highest luster and has the smoothest surface compared to all composites
- Primary indication is for esthetic and nonstress-bearing areas
- Their low modulus of elasticity allows them to flex during tooth flexure
- Good for restoring Class V cervical lesions.

SMALL-SIZED RESINS

Composition

- Fillers used are glasses containing heavy metals. Average filler size ranges from 1–5 μm and they have a broad size distribution, which facilitates higher filler loading
- Filler content—65–77 volume%, 80–90 wt% (more than conventional composites).

Properties

Compressive strength	350–400 MPa—Highest among the composition
Tensile strength	75–90 MPa—Double that of microfilled and 50% greater than conventional
Modulus of elasticity	15–20 GPa—Highest
Hardness	50–60 KHN; similar to conventional; but has improved wear resistance
Coefficient of thermal expansion	19–26 × 10^{-6}/°C; lowest; twice that of tooth structure
Water sorption	0.5–0.6 g/cm^2 similar to conventional
Esthetics	Better surface smoothness than conventional
Polymerization shrinkage	Comparable to or less than conventional
Radio-opacity	Radiopaque as glasses containing heavy metals are used as fillers.

Clinical Performance

- Due to their improved strength and abrasion resistance, they are used in stress-bearing areas such as class-IV restorations
- They are not as good as the microfilled as regards smoothness.

Methods to Increase Filler Loading

To sinter the colloidal silica particles

The larger agglomerate has a reduced surface area, allowing more filler particles to be incorporated.

Addition of prepolymerized fillers

- Prepolymerized fillers known as organic fillers are prepared by adding 60–70% of silane-coated colloidal silica to the monomer, which is held at a slightly higher temperature to reduce its viscosity
- It is then heat-cured and ground to the same size as the quartz fillers used in microfilled composites
- Filler content is 80 wt% or 70 vol%, but the actual inorganic filler content is only 50 wt%.

119. Hybrid Composites.

INTRODUCTION

Was developed to obtain smoother surfaces than that provided by small particle composites and to maintain the properties of the latter.

Composition

The organic matrix is reinforced with microfillers to decrease the differences in properties between inorganic macrofillers and unfilled organic matrix.

Kinds of filler particles employed are

- Colloidal silver—10–20 wt% of the total filler content
- Ground particles of glass containing heavy metals.

Colloidal silica and ground particles of glass constitute a filler content of 75–80% by weight. There is a blend of submicron (0.04 μm) and small particle (1–4 μm) fillers with an average size range of 0.6–1 μm.

Properties

Physical and mechanical properties range between conventional and small-particle composites and are superior to microfilled composites.

Compressive strength	300–350 MPa; slightly less than small particle
Tensile strength	70–90 MPa, comparable to that of small particle
Modulus of elasticity	7–12 GPa, between conventional and microfilled
Hardness	50–60 KHN, similar to small particle
Coefficient of thermal expansion	30–40 × 10^{-6}/°C; less than microfilled
Water sorption	0.5–0.7 mg/cm^2, similar to conventional
Esthetics	Surface smoothness and esthetics comparable with microfilled composites
Radio-opacity	The presence of glasses containing heavy metals makes them radiopaque

Clinical Performance

- They are widely used for anterior restorations due to their good esthetics
- Due to their improved physical and mechanical properties, they are used in stress-bearing areas as class-IV and class-II.

120. Describe the Improvements in the Development of Newer Composite Resins.

Though composites are highly esthetic restorative material, they have few disadvantages, which needed to be improved.

DISADVANTAGES OF COMPOSITES

- High polymerization shrinkage
- Lack of ability to condense
- Lack of wear resistance.

ADVANCES IN COMPOSITES

Recently introduced composite materials are:

- High viscosity composites (condensable/packable)
- Flowable composites
- Smart composites
- Polymeric rigid inorganic matrix material (PRIMM)
- Nanocomposites.

High Viscosity Composites (Condensable/Packable)

- These composites contain a wide range of filler particles (0.04 μ–20 μ) and has a 60–70% filler by volume.
- These materials can be compacted.
- For example, solitaire, surefil.

Flowable Composites

- Are 'painted on' in small increments, thereby building the restoration
- They have low filler loading and the particle sizes are small (less than 50% by volume)
- They have very low modulus of elasticity, which allows then to flex and flow
- They can also absorb polymerization stresses
- For example, revolution.

Uses

- Class-V cavities
- Pit and fissure sealant
- Base for classes I, II and III.

Smart Composites

For example, Ariston PHC (PH Control)

They release fluoride ions, hydroxyl ions and calcium when the pH in the restoration, in this material, falls to less than 5.5. This neutralizes the acid and counteracts decalcification.

Polymeric Rigid Inorganic Matrix Material (PRIMM)

- This has a resin and a ceramic component
- It consists of a continuous network of ceramic fibers (Al_2O_3 + SiO_2) of diameter 2 μ which are fused together at various sites to produce a continuous network of small chambers into which BISGMA/UDMA flow.

Advantages

- Low polymerization shrinkage
- Are packable
- Depth of polymerization—6 mm (light conducting through ceramic fibers).

Nanocomposites

- They have size below the wavelength of visible light
- These do not scatter/absorb light
- These small particles fill spaces between larger filler particles and allow increased filler loading (95% by weight). This reduces polymerization shrinkage
- They also provide a means for incorporating radio-opacity without interfering in the esthetics.

121. Nanocomposites.

DEFINITION

New ultra small fillers are being investigated that are from 0.005–0.01 micron in diameter and are called nanofillers.

Significance

- New composites are being incorporated with nanofillers that range in size from 0.005–0.01 microns, which is below the wavelength range for visible light
- Nanofillers do not interact with visible light and they do not produce scattering or significant absorption
- Nonsilicate-based compositions can be used for nanofillers because they are effectively invisible
- Nonsilicate fillers do not tend to agglomerate or cluster, like typical silica-based fillers
- Nanofillers are so small that they fit between several polymer chains
- These characteristics aid them to achieve very high filler loading levels in composites while still maintaining workable consistencies.

122. Gutta-percha.

Introduced by Bowman in 1867, gutta-percha is used most often as a solid core filling.

Chemically Pure Gutta-percha Exists in Two Forms

1. Crystalline forms: alpha and beta
2. Processed form (beta form) is used in root fillings.

Properties

- It has the property of plasticity
- It does not shrink after insertion unless it is plasticized with a solvent or heat
- It is radiopaque

- It is easily sterilized and does not encourage bacterial growth
- It is impervious to moisture
- It is nonstaining
- It is least toxic and least irritating to periapical tissue compared to all root canal-filling materials
- It can be removed easily from the root canal.

Disadvantages

- It is difficult to introduce gutta-percha into a narrow root canal
- It does not seal a canal apically or laterally unless it is combined with a root canal cement or sealer
- It has limited shelf life
- It becomes brittle with age
- The more the gutta-percha is plasticized, the greater will be the shrinkage of the filling material.

Use

Root Canal Obturation

- For root canal obturation, gutta-percha is available in standardized and nonstandardized cone sizes
- Standardized cone sizes co-ordinate with ISO sizes of root canal file sizes 15 through 140 and are used primarily as main core material for obturation with similar color coding
- Nonstandardized sizes are designated as extra-fine, fine, medium fine, fine, fine-medium, medium, medium-large, large and extra-large
- Gutta-percha is normally applied using some form of condensation pressure
- The most practical method of sterilizing gutta percha is immersing it in 5% sodium hypochlorite for 1 minute.

Two types of gutta-percha cones are available

1. Core points—used as master cones
2. Auxiliary points—used for lateral condensation.

123. Dentin-bonding Agent.

DEFINITION

An agent or series of substances which mediate a bond to the dental hard tissue without relying on the interlocking effect or retention of the prepared cavity.

CLASSIFICATION

On the basis of chronology from generations I to VI.

I Generation

- Based on NPG-GMA (N-phenylglycine-glycidyl methacrylate)
- This could mediate water-resistant chemical
- Bonds resin to dentinal calcium
- Bond strength—low (2 MPa).

II Generation

- Phosphate bonding systems
- There is ionic interaction between chlorophosphate group and calcium but this was not strong enough to resist the hydrolysis resulting from saliva exposure or moisture from dentin itself
- Bond strength—4–6 MPa.

III Generation

- Based on oxalate bonding system
- Here, dentin conditioning was done to modify removal of the smear layer
- Dentin primers were used, for example, hydrophilic resin monomers (HEMA) (Multistep Adhesive System)
- Bond strength—10 MPa.

IV Generation

- Hallmark of this generation was the introduction of Total Etch Concept by Fusayama (1979—etching both enamel and dentin)
- Based on 4-META
- Concept of wet/moist dentinal bonding was introduced
- Intertubular and dentinal tubules were used for bonding
- Bond strength—18 MPa.

V Generation

- Two different types of adhesive material:
  1. One bottle systems (containing primer and adhesive).
  2. Self-etching primer (conditioner and primer).
- Monofillers are present
- The self-etching primers eliminate the need to wash out the acidic gel.

VI Generation

- One-step bonding system
- Device consists of 2 chambers, the first and uppermost contains methacrylated phosphoric esters, initiator and stabilizers
- The second chamber contains a fluoride complex water and stabilizer
- The system is activated by squeezing the upper chamber first and then the second chamber, forcing the material into the pocket which contains the application device. This bonding agent is rubbed onto the tooth surface
- *Advantages*: No acid etching; no washing/air dispersing and no light-curing of bonding agent.

Dentin Bonding System consists of 3 Components

1. Dentin conditioner
2. Dentin primer
3. Dentin adhesive.

Dentin Conditioning

- After surface alteration of dentin, the creation of dentin cutting debris, termed smear layer, is present
- This needs to be removed by conditioning
- Conditioning can be done by using:
  - Acids, e.g. H_3PO_4(37%), HNO_3 (2.5%)
  - Chelators
  - Lasers
  - Microabrasion.

Dentin Primer

This is an adhesion promoter in a solvent, such as water, ethanol or acetone.

Dentin Adhesive/Bonding Agent

Usually contains both hydrophilic and hydrophobic groups and thus is able to interact with the moist dentinal surface as well as to the restorative resin.

MECHANISM OF BONDING

- Acid etching/conditioning leaves a layer of dentin-anchored collagen fibers on the surface of demineralized dentin
- Into this the hydrophilic resins (dentin primer) infiltrates forming a hybrid layer consisting of resin-infiltrated dentin
- The adhesive then bonds to the primer leaving the hydrophobic groups exposed to create a favorable surface for the restorative resins
- Most of the presently used bonding systems belong either to the IV, V or the latest VI, generation.
- Improvements in the bonding systems make them to be used in fewer steps in less time.

124. Ozokerite Waxes.

DEFINITION

- Ozokerite waxes are synthetic waxes that are predominantly complex hydrocarbons formulated into specialty waxes.
- Ozokerites are blends of true waxes which produce a dry wax with high solvent absorption and gel values.

Companies Developing Ozokerite

Ozokerite wax is a bituminous product occurring near petroleum deposits in Poland, Austria, Russia, Ukraine, Utah and Texas.

- Strahl & Pitsch Inc.

PROPERTIES

- Ozokerite waxes melt at the higher range of 140–200°F. They are nontoxic and nonhazardous
- Unlike the paraffin and microcrystalline waxes, ozokerite waxes have long fibers.
- As ozokerite is a hydrocarbon product, it is less recommended in cosmetics
- Ozokerite comes in white and yellow and its melting point varies according to grade (most flakes melt at 1520 to 650°F)
- True ozokerite is no longer available. It has been replaced with blends of petroleum-derived paraffin and microcrystalline waxes
- These blends are designed to meet the specific physical properties required by the application involved

- Ozokerite waxes are compatible with all vegetable waxes, variety of natural, animal, synthetic waxes, glycerides and fatty acids.

USES

- As adhesives
- In cosmetics
- In polishes.

125. Coupling Agent.

DEFINITION

Coupling agents are bonding agents applied to the filler particle to ensure chemical bonding to the resin matrix.

COMPOSITION OF COUPLING AGENTS

Although titanates and zirconates can be used as coupling agents, organosilanes, such as r-methacryloxypropyl trimethoxy silane are used.

CHEMISTRY

- In the presence of water, the methoxy groups (-OCH_3) are hydrolyzed by silanol (-Si-OH) groups that can bond with other silanols on the filler surfaces by formation of a siloxane bond (-Si-O-Si-)
- The organosilane methacrylate groups form covalent bonds with the resin when it is polymerized. This completes the coupling process
- Proper coupling by means of organosilanes is important to the clinical performance of resin-based composite restorative materials.

SIGNIFICANCE OF A COUPLING AGENT

- Allows more flexible polymer matrix to transfer stresses to higher modulus (more rigid and stiffer) filler particles
- The bond between the two phases of the composite is provided by a coupling agent
- Improves the physical and mechanical properties of the resin
- Provides stability by preventing water from penetrating the filler-resin interface.

126. Cement for Temporary Restoration.

- Temporary restorations are often required before the placement of a permanent restoration
- Cements used for temporary restorations last for a few days or a few weeks
- They may serve as treatment while the pulp heals or while the permanent restoration is fabricated and inserted
- Temporary restorations provide good initial sealing ability and pulpal response.

Materials used for Temporary Restorations

Zinc Oxide Eugenol

Useful when a sedative treatment is required until the pulp has healed to the point where permanent restorations can be placed.

Unmodified Zinc Oxide Cements

Several cotton fibers may be added to the mix and setting is accelerated.

Modified Zinc Oxide Eugenol

For long-term fillings
Hybrid ionomer
Zinc polycarboxylate.

Gutta-percha

It was the material previously used. It is not used presently.

Ideal Properties

- The strength of temporary cement must be low so that it permits easy removal
- The specification for compressive strength of temporary cements ranges from no requirement for nonsetting material to a maximum of 31 MPa for materials that attain a hard set.

Zinc Oxide Eugenol Cements

- Used as temporary restorations, soft tissue packs in oral surgery and periodontics and as root canal sealers
- The unmodified zinc oxide eugenol and noneugenol zinc oxide cement are two paste systems
- Powder is often incorporated into the dispensed amount of liquid until a consistency is achieved
- The EMA alumina modified cements can be used as temporary restorations as they did not chip during trimming and showed no pulpal symptoms
- The EBA alumina modified cement, despite its low solubility in water, disintegrated and wore excessively in the mouth

- A thick mix of polymer modified zinc oxide eugenol was more serviceable than the EBA modified type
- All temporary restorations of zinc oxide eugenol were serviceable for 2–10 months of observation.

127. Explain the Role of Various Cements and their Indications.

Cement	Indication	Precaution
Zinc phosphate	Under amalgam restoration in normal cavities	If it is used in deep cavities, use a cavity liner on the pulpal floor before its use. In routine use, apply cavity varnish before and after placement of base
Zinc oxide eugenol	Reinforced ZOE may be used as a base under amalgam restoration	Not indicated under composition as eugenol interferes with the polymerization
Zinc poly-carboxylate	Can be used under amalgam restoration	Very biocompatible, hence no varnish required prior to its placement. Varnish applied after base placement
Glass ionomer	Under amalgam and composites	When placing very close to the pulp, a liner of $Ca(OH)_2$ may be applied

Cements when used as bases are applied in thick layer (0.75 mm) under restoration to protect the pulp against the thermal injury, galvanic shock and chemical irritation depending on the restorative material used.

It should also be strong enough to withstand condensation forces during placement of restoration and to resist fracture under any masticatory stress induced on the restoration.

128. Metal Modified Glass Ionomer Cements/Ketac-Silver/ Miracle Mix.

This is a modified glass ionomer cement with the incorporation of metal particles to improve mechanical properties.

Methods of Reinforcement of Metal Particles

- Glass ionomer cements can be reinforced by physically incorporating silver alloy powder with glass powder usually referred to as 'silver alloy admix'
- By sintering silver particles to glass powder at a high temperature. These are called 'cermets'.

Available as

Powder and liquid composition in two bottles which have to be mixed by hand.

Powder

- It is a simple mixture of glass and silver incorporated in the glass powder
- It is produced from a mixture of glass, gold and silver of equal volumes (17.5/82.5 wt%)
- Particle size of silver is 3–4 µm
- The mixture is formed into pellets and then sintered at 800°C until the glass and silver fuse together and form a mass
- The sintered solid substance is then ground to produce right particle size for mixing and manipulation
- The particles are rounded by grinding process and each particle consists of a mixture of glass and silver tightly bonded to each other by sintering.

Liquid

Liquid consists of an aqueous solution of copolymer of acrylic or maleic acid 37% and tartaric acid 9%.

Properties

Hardness

- Has good strength and wear resistance due to incorporation of silver in glass
- They set rapidly.

Compressive Strength

Almost similar to conventional glass ionomer cement. Cermets also have a compressive strength of 150 MPa.

Tensile Strength

Metal modified glass ionomer cements have a diametral tensile strength of 6.7 MPa while conventional glass ionomer is 6.6 MPa.

Anticariogenic Property

Metal reinforced system releases fluoride but decreases in magnitude over time.

Esthetics

- These materials are slightly grey in color due to the presence of metallic phases within them and are not suitable as anterior restorative material
- Some of them contain whitening agent to improve appearance of the cement.

Clinical Considerations

- They are used as an alternative to amalgam or composite for posterior restorations
- They can be used for class II restoration
- They are used as core build up for teeth to be restored with cast crowns.

Advantages

- The dispersed phase of a tough, ductile metal within the material improves the mechanical properties as brittleness and abrasion resistance whilst maintaining adhesion to enamel and dentin
- The metal usually used is silver but other metals like tin, gold, titanium and palladium have been tried
- Improved compressive strength and fracture resistance
- They are fast-setting cement; can be used for core build up.

Disadvantages

- Difficult to mix to correct consistency
- Not esthetic
- Cannot be used as anterior restorative material.

129. Mechanical Bonding.

DEFINITION

Mechanical adhesion associated with bonding of an adhesive to a roughened adhered surface is termed as mechanical bonding.

Factors in Mechanical Bonding

- Mechanical bonding can be due to mechanical retention or by molecular attraction
- Mechanical bonding can be due to the penetration of the adhesive into microscopic or submicroscopic irregularities. (As in acid etching and bonding of composite)
- A bonding agent can increase the mechanical retention by penetrating into the surface defects formed by etching
- On hardening the numerous adhesive projections embedded in the adhered surface provide the anchorage for mechanical retention
- Mechanical bonding is also used to retain a cast gold alloy crown or a base metal endodontic post by mechanical attachment of the cementing agent into irregularities that exist on the internal surface of the casting
- In micromechanical bonding, the enamel is exposed to phosphoric acid for a short period. This is referred to as the acid-etching technique. The acid produces minute pores onto which the resin subsequently flows, thereby reducing the possibility of interfacial leakage.

Bond Formation to Tooth Structure

Enamel

- Enamel can be etched with phosphoric acid, increasing the surface area for the resin matrix or bonding agent
- Bonds that are formed between a low-viscosity polymer bonding agent and an enamel surface are primarily mechanical and depend on the penetration of the resin into irregularities on the enamel surface.

Dentin

The bonding of composite to dentin is not recommended as the dentinal tubules contain tissue fluid.

130. Cavity Liners used in Dentistry.

DEFINITION

Certain filling materials are not suitable for direct placement into the cavity. So a cavity lining material is placed on the base of the cavity and on the axial dentinal wall for class II cavities prior to placement of the filling.

Requirements of Cavity Lining Materials

- Depends on:
  - Depth of cavity
  - Type of filling material which is being used to restore the tooth
- A lining material may provide thermal, chemical and electrical barriers
- It must also have sufficient mechanical strength to resist disruption during placement of filling and to provide a firm rigid base which will support the filling above.

Materials Developed for Pulp Protection include the following:
- Varnishes
- Calcium hydroxide cement
- Zinc oxide-based cement
- Glass ionomer cement
- Visible light-cured resins
- Glass ionomer cement resin hybrids.

Functions of Cavity Liner

Thermal Barrier

- Liners act as a thermal insulating barrier to protect the pulp from sudden changes in temperature
- A thermal insulating cavity liner is required when a metallic filling such as amalgam is used. The thermal diffusivity of amalgam is about 40 times greater than that of dentin
- Thermal injury can also occur during the setting of light-activated composites when the temperature increases from 20° to 40°C, causing injury to pulp.

Chemical Barrier

Lining material acts as a protective barrier against chemical irritants presents in some filling materials.

For example, phosphoric acid in silicate materials.

Lining cements may themselves contain irritants so that they are only suitable for shallow to medium depth cavities.

Electrical Barrier

- When an amalgam restoration is placed adjacent or opposing a gold restoration, a galvanic cell results which may accelerate corrosion and also cause pain
- Hence, varnishes consisting of less polar resin, such as polystyrene can be painted onto the surface of metallic restorations giving temporary relief to symptom of galvanic pain
- Varnish is a natural gum (such as copal resin or a synthetic resin dissolved in an organic solvent) which evaporates to leave a thin layer of resin which helps to seal the ends of the dentinal tubules
- Varnish does not give adequate thermal protection in deep cavities since they form only a thin layer.

Against Bacteria and Endotoxins

- Bacteria and endotoxins can cause thermal shock of the pulp when the patient takes hot/ cold food. In shallow cavity, lining is less important
- Liner cements set by an exothermic reaction can cause pulp irritation
- The advantage of using a liner is to prevent bacterial microleakage (by use of adhesive techniques so that no gap exists between tooth and restoration)
- This antibacterial barrier protects pulp from infiltrating bacteria and their toxins.

Strength and Flow

- Liners are supplied as two components which are mixed together initiating a setting reaction
- The liner should remain intact during placement of the filling material.

Integrity of lining depends on

- The degree of set achieved at the time when the filling material is placed
- Strength of the set material and its thickness
- Type of cavity
- Pressure exerted during placement of the filling material
- Degree of support from surrounding structures
- Choice of correct operative techniques.

Radiopacity and Compatibility

- If the material is radiopaque it aids in the diagnosis of caries around the filling
- The lining should be compatible with the filling
- Its components should not have any effect on setting characteristics or properties of filling.

131. Cavity Varnishes.

COMPOSITION

Natural gums such as copals, resins or synthetic resins dissolved in an organic solvent such as acetone, chloroforms or ether.

Mode of Application

- Applied in two or three coatings on the cavity walls
- Applied using a thin brush
- A single layer application can result in evaporation of the solvent, leading to formation of voids.

Mode of Action

They form a coating on the tooth by evaporation of the solvent.

Function

- They reduce microleakage
- They prevent penetration of corrosion products of amalgams into the dentinal tubules
- They do not provide insulation.

Contraindications

- They are not indicated under adhesive material like glass ionomer and composites
- Under glass ionomer, they prevent the carboxylic groups from coming in contact with calcium of enamel and dentin
- Under composites, they interfere with the polymerization reaction and may cause softening of the resin.

132. Resin-bonded Cement (Kalzinol).

COMPOSITION

Powder	Liquid
ZnO—60%	Eugenol—85%
White resin—5–10%	Olive oil—15%
Natural or synthetic resin—10–40%	Acetic acid—1%
Zinc acetate—0.5%	

Properties

- Strength is more
- Compressive strength of Resin-bonded—40–60 MPa
- Solubility is less
- Low film thickness used for permanent cementation
- Setting time—Resin-bonded—5–9 minutes
- P/L ratio—Resin-bonded—4:1.

133. Dimensional changes occurring in amalgam and its control.

FACTORS CAUSING DIMENSIONAL CHANGES

During Manipulation

- After trituration, there is an initial contraction after first 20 minutes. This is due to the solution of mercury in the alloy particles
- After this period, expansion occurs, which is due to the reaction of mercury with silver and tin and the formation of inter-metallic compounds
- This expansion continues until the crystal reaches the grain boundaries, after which no further crystal growth takes place into the spaces between the crystals. This results in a slight contraction
- The maximum dimensional change permissible is ($^+$/-) 20 m/cm
- The dimension becomes nearly constant after 6–8 hours.

Other Factors in Manipulation

Manipulation factors that result in excess mercury leading to a net final expansion	Factors that cause net shrinkage
High mercury : alloy ratio	Low mercury : alloy ratio
Improper trituration	Trituration in sufficient force
Not squeezing out excess Hg	Squeezing out excess Hg
Not applying sufficient pressure during condensation	Applying condensation pressure

The newer high copper unicompositional amalgams show a net contraction due to a low mercury : alloy ratio.

Choice of Alloy

Expansion resulting from manipulation of Zn containing alloys

- Moisture contamination during trituration or condensation of Zn containing amalgam leads to the production of ZnO and H_2 gas
- This H_2 gas neither reacts with any other ingredients in the restoration nor is it able to escape from the restoration
- Thus, it applies force on the restoration which results in expansion after 48–72 hours. This is known as delayed expansion
- This can be controlled by proper isolation techniques during the manipulation steps.

Expansion resulting from formation of corrosion products in low copper amalgam

- Over a period of time, the tin-mercury phase (γ_2) in low copper amalgam reacts with atmospheric O_2 to form tin oxide and tin oxychloride releasing mercury

- This free mercury reacts with the unreacted alloy particles (γ phase) to form silver-mercury (γ_1) and tin-mercury (γ_2) phase which results in expansion.

$$\underset{(\gamma)}{Ag_3Sn} + Hg \rightarrow \underset{(\gamma_1)}{AgHg} + \underset{(\gamma_2)}{SnHg} + \underset{(\gamma)}{AgSn}.$$

$$SnHg + O_2 + Cl \rightarrow SnO + SnOCl + Hg.$$

$$Hg + AgSn \rightarrow AgHg + SnHg + AgSn.$$

This expansion is called *mercuroscopic expansion or Jorgenson's expansion*.

Dimensional Change due to Creep

- Under a continued application of force in compression, amalgam shows a continued deformation, even after the mass has completely set
- Maximum creep is seen with low copper amalgam (proportional to the amount of γ_2 phase)
- High copper amalgam shows minimum creep.

Factors Affecting Creep

More mercury $\rightarrow$ More creep.
More $\gamma_2 \rightarrow$ More creep.

MEASURES TO MINIMIZE DIMENSIONAL CHANGE

- Choose spherical, high copper alloy powder, minimal Hg
- Use the optimum mercury : alloy ratio
- Sufficient trituration pressure
- Squeezing out excess mercury
- Adequate condensation pressure
- Avoid moisture contamination during manipulation to prevent delayed expansion
- Use high copper amalgam to minimize corrosion and creep.

134. Types of High Copper Amalgam and its Advantages Over Conventional Silver Amalgam.

TYPES OF HIGH COPPER ALLOY POWDERS

- Admixed alloy powder
- Single composition/unicompositional alloy powder.

Admixed Alloys

- In 1963, Innes DBK and Youdelis WV.[1]
- Added spherical silver-Cu eutectic alloy (71.9 wt% Ag and 28 wt% Cu) to lathe-cut low copper amalgam alloy particle. These alloys are often called admixed alloys
- Amalgam made from these powders is stronger than amalgam made from low copper powder because of the increase in residual alloy and resultant decrease in matrix
- Silver-copper as well as silver in particles act as fillers in amalgam, strengthening the amalgam matrix
- Admixed amalgams are superior to those made from low copper amalgam restoration for their resistance to marginal breakdown.

Chemical Reaction

- Admixed alloy powders usually contain 30 wt% to 55 wt% high copper powder
- When mercury reacts with an admixed powder, silver absorbs into the mercury and both silver and tin dissolve into the mercury from silver-tin alloy particules
- The tin in solution diffuses to the surfaces of silver-copper alloy particles and react with the copper to form a phase
- γ_1 phase forms simultaneously with the n-phase and surrounds both Silver-Cu spherical alloy particles and silver-tin lathe-cut particles.

$$\underset{(\gamma)}{Ag_3Sn} + \text{(Ag-Cu) eutectic} + Hg \rightarrow \underset{(\gamma_1)}{AgHg} + \underset{(\gamma_2)}{SnHg} + \text{unreacted alloy particles.}$$

This is followed by a second reaction.

$$\underset{(\gamma_2)}{SnHg} + Ag\text{-}Cu \rightarrow \underset{(n)}{Cu_6Sn_5} + \underset{(\gamma_1)}{AgHg}.$$

Thus, the final amalgam contains little or no γ_2.

The Advantages Over Conventional Amalgam

- Higher compressive strength
- A more rapid set to full strength
- A more reduction in creep
- A reduced susceptibility to corrosion.

Single Composition Alloys

- Unlike admixed alloy powders, each particle of these alloy powders has the same chemical composition. Therefore, they are called single composition alloys
- Major components of the alloy are silver, copper and tin
- A number of phases are found in each single composition alloy particle.

Reaction

- The copper content ranges between 13 and 30%. Thus, its setting reaction produces no γ_2 phase. Hence also called as non-γ_2 amalgam.
- $\underset{(\gamma)}{Ag\text{-}SnCu} + \underset{(\gamma_1)}{Cu_3Sn} + Hg \rightarrow AgHg + \underset{(n)}{Cu_6Sn_5} + \gamma.$
- This single composition can either be all spherical or all lathe-cut.

Advantages and Disadvantages of Admixed High Copper and Spherical

Admixed high copper ***Advantages***	**Spherical high copper** ***Disadvantages***
Longer working time	Less working time
Adapts better to cavity walls and adjacent teeth	Lesser adaptability

Admixed high copper ***Disadvantages***	**Spherical high copper** ***Advantages***
Slower set	Faster set
More mercury mix	Less mercury mix
Less early strength	Higher early strength
Higher creep during condense	Lower creep
Difficult to finish	Low condensation pressure

Comparison with Conventional

- High copper amalgam has better mechanical properties, good marginal integrity and performance in clinical trial, when compared with traditional low copper alloys
- Available since the 1970s
- High copper amalgam contains more copper, typically 10 to 30%, compared to less than 6% in the conventional alloys.

REFERENCE

1. Innes DBK, Youdelis WV. Dispersion strengthened amalgams. J Can Dent Assoc. 1963;29:587-93.

135. What are the Steps in the Manipulation of Amalgam?

STEPS IN THE MANIPULATION OF AMALGAM

- Selection of alloy
- Proportion of mercury and alloy powder
- Trituration
- Condensation
- Carving, polishing and finishing.

Selection of Alloy

Particle Size

- Smaller particles give better condensation, greater strength, easy carving, smooth finish, less marginal failures, faster setting time and are easy to adapt and condense
- Large particles form porosity, leading to their low strength.

Shape of Alloy

Spherical alloys are preferred because they give better finish, good marginal adaptation, better condensation, high strength, easier carving, less mercury needed.

Composition

High copper amalgams are preferred since they produce less γ_2, phase in the setting reaction.

Proportion of Alloy and Mercury

Alloy : Mercury Ratio

- Alloy/Mercury ratios vary between 5:8 and 10:8. Those mixes containing greater quantities of mercury are 'wetter' and are generally used with hand mixing
- Mechanical mixes contain smaller quantities of mercury and are 'drier'
- For optimum properties, the final set amalgam should contain less than 50% mercury.

Particle Size

Mercury consumption depends on the size and shape of the alloy particle.

Lathe cut — 50%
Spherical — 43%.

Trituration

Excess mercury in the mix following trituration is squeezed out using a squeeze cloth (Squeeze Cloth Technique).

Condensation

- Condensing the amalgam in increments reduces mercury content, as each time it is condensed, the excess mercury comes to the surface layer which may be scarped out
- Each time the environment is dried of excess mercury and only then subsequent increment is condensed. This technique is called the Incremental Dryness Technique/Increasing Dryness Technique
- The disadvantage with this technique is that the chance of a lack of bonding between two increments of too much of mercury is removed. This is known as lamination.

Carving, Polishing and Finishing

- The amalgam should neither be polished before its initial set nor after it has hardened completely.
- Only after the initial setting period, it should be polished after the carving procedure.

136. Germicidal Cements.

Germicidal cements are highly effective in the caries inhibition because of their *fluoride releasing* property.

Action of Fluoride on Caries Inhibition

- Fluoride accumulates in the dental plaque from saliva, gingival fluid, diet, topically applied fluoride gel and demineralizing enamel
- Fluoride inhibits the carbohydrate metabolism by acidogenic plaque
- Fluoride enters cementation gradient and accumulates as the extracellular pH decreases
- The transport of hydrogen fluoride into the cells leads to dissociation into H^+ and F^- ions
- Ionic fluoride then induces enzyme inhibition leading to a lower caries rate
- Fluoride increases cell permeability and can rapidly diffuse out of bacterium, contributing again to the fluoride content within the plaque matrix.

TYPES OF GERMICIDAL CEMENTS

- Glass ionomer cements
- Silicate cements.

Glass Ionomer Cements

Composition

Powder

The powder is an acid soluble calcium fluoroaluminosilicate glass.

The alumina-silica reaction is high and increases its reactivity with liquid.

- Silica — 41.9%.
- Alumina — 28.0%.
- Aluminum fluoride — 1.6%.
- Calcium fluoride — 15.7%.
- Sodium fluoride — 9.3%.
- Aluminum Phosphate — 3.8%.

The fluoride component acts as a ceramic flux.

Lanthanum, strontium, barium or zinc oxide provide radiopacity.

Liquid

- Earlier the liquid was 50% aqueous solution of polyacrylic acid. It was very *viscous* and has a tendency to gel
- Hence, polyacrylic acid was copolymerized with other acids such as itaconic, maleic and tricarboxylic acid.

Anticariogenic Properties

- Type-II GIC used for restoration releases fluoride in amounts comparable to silicate cements initially and continues to do so over an extended period of time
- In addition due to its adhesive effect, it has the potential for reducing infiltration of oral fluids at the cement tooth interface, preventing secondary caries.

Silicate Cements

Composition

Powder

- Silica — 40%
- Alumina — 30%
- Sodium fluoride — 19%
- Cryolite, calcium fluoride, calcium phosphate or lime.

Liquid

- Phosphoric acid — 52%
- Aluminum phosphate — 2%
- Zinc phosphate — 6%
  (or)
- Magnesium phosphate
- Water — 40%.

Anticariogenic Properties

- The incidence of secondary caries is markedly less around silicate restorations
- Also the incidence of contact caries is less when compared to amalgam restorations
- The anticariogenic property is due to the presence of 15% fluoride
- Fluoride release is slow and occurs throughout the life of the restoration
- It makes the adjacent tooth structure more resistant to acid decalcification
- It acts as an antibacterial agent
- It acts as an enzyme inhibitor and thus prevents the carbohydrate metabolism.

137. Adhesive Cements/Any one in detail.

TYPES

- Zinc polycarboxylate cement
- Glass ionomer cement.

Zinc Polycarboxylate

- Cements are pulp friendly and form an adhesive bond to tooth structure by the formation of the carboxylate groups in the polymer molecule to chelate with calcium
- Are used primarily for luting permanent restorations and as bases
- Can also be used in orthodontics for cementation of bands, earlier were used for direct bonding of bands and direct bonding of brackets.

GLASS IONOMER CEMENT

Composition

The glass ionomer cements are supplied as powder that is mixed with liquid.

Powder

Powder is calcium fluoroaluminosilicate glass—(SiO_2-Al_2O_3-CaF_2-Na_3AlF_6-$AlPO_4$).

Chemical	Percentage by weight
Silica (SiO_2)	29.0
Alumina (Al_2O_3)	16.6
Aluminum fluoride (AlF_3)	5.3
Calcium fluoride (CaF_2)	34.3
Aluminum phosphate ($AlPO_4$)	9.9
Cryolite	5.0

Liquid

- 47.5% solution of 2:1 polyacrylic acid/itaconic acid copolymer (average molecular weight 10,000) in water
- The itaconic acid reduces the viscosity of the liquid and inhibits gelation by intermolecular hydrogen bonding
- Tartaric acid (5%)—serves as an accelerator
- Polyacids attack the glass to release cations and fluoride ions
- These metal fluoride complexes react with the polyanions to form salt gel matrix
- In the first 3 hours, calcium ions react with the polycarboxylate chains
- The trivalent aluminum ions react for at least 48 hours
- The polyacrylic acid chains are cross-linked by the calcium ions that are replaced by aluminum ions within the next 24 hours **(Fig. 53)**
- Sodium and fluorine ions do not participate in the cross-linking of the cement
- The cross-linked phase becomes hydrated over time with the same water used for mixing. This process is called maturation
- The unreacted portion of glass particles is sheathed by a silica gel

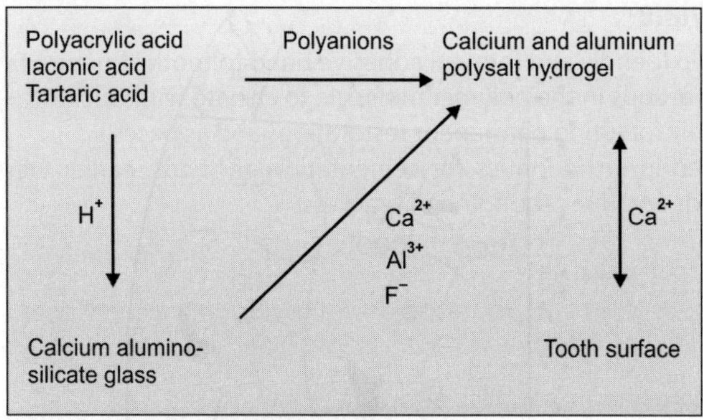

Fig. 53: Chemistry of setting

- Thus, the set cement consists of an agglomeration of unreacted powder particles surrounded by a silica gel in as amorphous matrix of hydrated calcium and aluminum polysalts.

The solid black particles represent unreacted glass particles surrounded by the gel (shaded) that form when Al^{+++} ions and Ca^{++} ions are leached from the glass as a result of attack by the polyacrylic acid.

The Ca^{++} and Al^{+++} ions form polysalts with the COO^- groups of the polyacrylic acid to form a cross-linked structure **(Fig. 54).**

The carboxyl groups react with calcium in enamel and dentin.

Mechanism of Adhesion

- The Ca^{2+} and Al^{3+} ions from the powder react with the carboxylate groups to cross-link the polymeric acid
- The same carboxylate groups interact strongly with surface Ca^{2+} ions in enamel or dentin to yield chemical adhesion to tooth structure
- The bond strength to enamel is always higher than that to dentin because of the greater inorganic content of the enamel.

Manipulation

- For mixing a wax paper and agate, spatula is used
- Mixing has three stages:
  1. The powder is divided into two equal halves
  2. The first half is folded into the liquid in 10 to 15 seconds
  3. The second increment is mixed into the resulting thin paste within the next 15 seconds.
- For luting cement, powder : liquid ratio is 1.5:1
- For restorative cement, powder : liquid ratio is 2.8:1.

Role of Water

- Serves as the reaction medium initially and it then slowly hydrates the cross-linked matrix, leading to an increase in strength

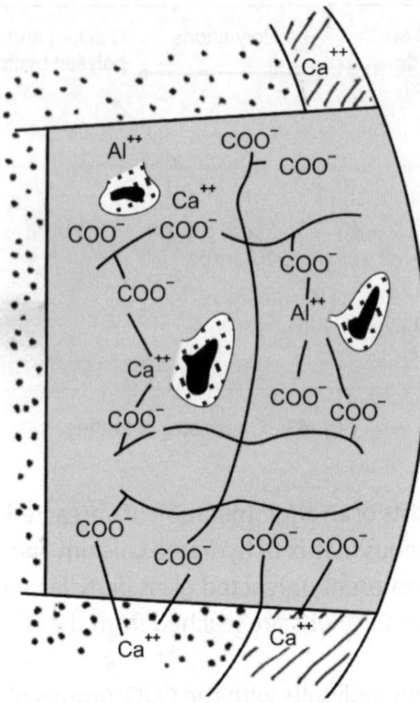

Fig. 54: Structure of glass ionomer cement

- Loosely bound water is readily removed by desiccation
- Tightly bound water hydrates the matrix
- Hydration yields a stable gel structure and builds the strength of the cement.

Bonding to Tooth Structure

- The adhesion to enamel and dentin is through carboxyl group calcium of the tooth
- Chelation takes place between the COO^- group of polyacids and calcium on the apatite of enamel and dentin.

TYPES

Wilson and McLean (1988)

Type I

- Luting

Type II

- Restorative material
- Esthetic filling material
- Bis-reinforced filling material.

Type III

- Liners/base and fissure sealing material.

PROPERTIES

- High compressive and low tensile strength
- Compressive strength type I—80–130 MPa, type II—150 MPa
- Diametrical tensile strength—type II—6.6 MPa
- It is a biocompatible material and is kind to pulp
- Anticariogenic, due to fluoride release
- Long working time, a rapid set at mouth temperature
- Strength—type I—6–8 minutes, type II—4–5 minutes
- Low viscosity and film thickness (film thickness—250–300 μm)
- Resistance to plastic deformation
- Modulus of elasticity—5.6–9.5 GPa
- Adhesion to tooth structure and restoration
- Translucent
- Radiopaque
- Good resistance to aqueous/acid attack
- Solubility—0.4%.

USES

- Restoration of erosion/abrasion lesions without cavity preparation
- Sealing and filling of occlusal pits and fissure
- Restoration of deciduous teeth
- Repair of defective margins in restoration
- As a base/lining material
- For core build up
- As a luting agent for indirect restorations.

138. Calcium Hydroxide.

Calcium hydroxide is a low strength base, supplied as a two-paste system, which, when mixed, sets to a hard mass. It is the chief ingredient in a cavity liner.

Applications

- Direct pulp capping
- Indirect pulp capping
- As low strength base beneath silicate and composite for pulp protection.

Availability

- Two-paste system containing base and catalyst paste in collapsible tubes
- Light-cured system.

Commercial Names

- Self-cured—Dycal
- Life
- Light-cured—Prisma VLC Dycal.

Composition

Base Paste

Component	Percentage	Function
Glycol salicylate	40%	Primary reactive ingredient.
Titanium dioxide		Filler, pigments
Calcium sulfate		
Calcium tungstate		Radiopacifier

Catalyst Paste

Component	Percentage	Function
Calcium hydroxide	50%	Principle reactive ingredient.
Zinc oxide	10%	
Zinc stearate	0.5%	Accelerator
Ethyl toluene		

Manipulation

Equal lengths of the two pastes are dispensed on a paper pad and mixed to a uniform color.

Setting Reaction

- The setting reaction occurs between calcium hydroxide and salicylate, yielding calcium disalicylate
- The zinc ions are responsible for chelation, with calcium present in reaction
- The setting reaction of light-activated calcium hydroxide cements involves light activated polymerization monomer

- Calcium hydroxide used as a cavity liner is suspended in a solvent carrier with a thickening agent. When it is placed on the pulpal floor, the solvent evaporates and leaves a thin film of calcium hydroxide.

Properties

The antibacterial action of calcium hydroxide makes these cements useful in indirect pulp capping procedures.

Mechanical Properties

- Compressive strength: 10–27 MPa
- Tensile strength: 1 MPa.
- Elastic modulus: 0.37 GPa/m^2.

Thermal Properties

In sufficiently thick layers, they provide some thermal insulation but thickness greater than 0.5 mm is not recommended.

Setting Time

It varies between 2.5 and 5.5 minutes.

Solubility

- Calcium hydroxide has the highest solubility
- It ranges from 0.4 wt% to 7.8 wt% in distilled water in 24 hours.

139. Pit and Fissure Sealants.

- The prevention of occlusal caries through the obturation of developmental pits and fissures in dental enamel
- Preventive resin restoration in minimal cavity preparation and placement of an enamel-dentin bonded composite restoration combined with a sealant application.

IDEAL PROPERTIES OF FISSURE SEALANT

- Inert in the mouth
- But should have a fluoride leach over time
- Should wet the surface of clean enamel

- Low viscosity on mixing so that surface spreading is rapid
- Should penetrate into the etched enamel pits
- Adequate mechanical properties on setting (strength, abrasion resistance, etc.)
- Physical properties of set material should match with those of enamel.

BOWEN'S RESIN-BASED FISSURE SEALANTS

Bowen's resin (BIS-GMA) is mixed with one part of methyl methacrylate to obtain a low viscosity. Several BIS-GMA sealants polymerize by an organic amine accelerator.

Available System

Two-component System

One contains BIS-GMA resin and benzoyl peroxide initiator, the other component contains 5% organic amine accelerator.

Composition

- Bowen's resin (BIS-GMA)—polymerizes to yield a highly cross-linked polymer
- Diluents (TEGDMA, BIS-DMA)—decrease the viscosity of BIS-GMA
- Opaquer (titanium dioxide, TiO_2)—allows placement of sealant to be monitored—optional
- Fluoride-releasing agent (ytterbium fluoride, or similar)—optional polymerization activation chemicals.

Materials used

Resin System

Cyanoacrylates, polyurethanes and BIS-GMA

Chemical activation, or by light activated.

- Filled resins
- Unfilled resins.

Polymerization of Fissure Sealants

Chemical Activation

- When mixed with the monomer, one of the electron pairs in the double bond unpairs
- These chemicals are *benzoyl peroxide* (white solid) and an *amine* (liquid).

Visible Light Activation

- This is called 'visible light curing' (VLC)
- Here the visible light, combined with a chemical called *camphoroquinone* together with an *Amine* will activate polymerization
- The percentage of conversion from monomer to polymer is significantly less for visible light-activation
- The residual monomer can act as a softening agent (plasticizer) in the set polymer and can be partly leached out in saliva.

BONDING RESIN-BASED FISSURE SEALANTS TO TOOTH MATERIAL

Procedure

- Prophylaxis (using a fluoride-free prophylactic paste)
- Rinsing
- Isolation and drying
- Acid-etch (37% phosphoric acid for ca 30 seconds)
- Rinsing and drying
- Application of sealant.

Enamel Surface Preparation

- 37% phosphoric acid, H_3PO_4 is used to etch enamel
- The etch system is available as a gel
- After it is rinsed and dried, sealant is applied.

Recent Advances

In recent advances, pit and fissure sealants containing fluoride as ytterbium fluoride are being tried which is supposed to be more resistant to caries attack.

140. Chemistry of Silicate Cement.

- Zinc silico-phosphate results from the mixing of zinc phosphate and silicate cements
- Type II Zinc silico-phosphate cement is used as a temporary filling material.

CHEMISTRY OF SETTING

It is basically an acid-base reaction in which metal ions in glass react with phosphoric acid to form a series of phosphate salts.

$$Al^{3+} + H_3PO_4 \rightarrow AlPO_4 + 3H^+$$
$$Ca^{2+} + H_3PO_4 \rightarrow CaHPO_4 + 2H^+$$
$$Na^+ + H_3PO_4 \rightarrow NaH_2PO_4 + H^+$$

Reaction is indicated as:

$H_3PO_4 \rightarrow H^+ + H_2PO_4^-$

$H^+ + nM^+$

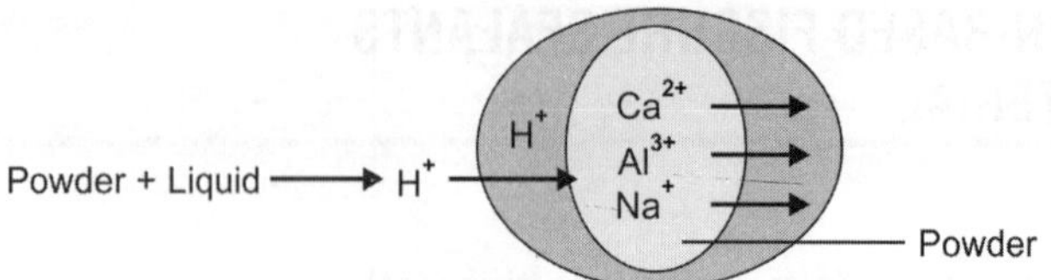

Fig. 55: Setting reaction of silicate cement

SETTING REACTION

When powder and liquid are mixed, the reaction is that of an acid and base. The surface of powder particle is attacked by acid liquid.

Alumino silicate glass + Phosphoric acid $\rightarrow H^+ + H_2PO_4^-$ (with release of Al^{3+}, Ca^{2+}, Na^+ and F^- ions)

- The liquid dissociates and the H^+ ions migrate into the surface layer of the glass particle. Al^{3+}, Ca^{2+}, Na^+ and F^- ions move from the glass into liquid **(Fig. 55)**
- The metal ions precipitate to form a gel matrix of phosphates and fluorides
- The matrix binds together the undissolved powder particles to form a composite material as set cement.

Stages in Setting Reaction

- The surface of the glass powder is decomposed by the liquid
- Hydrated protons from the liquid disrupt the aluminosilicate network by attacking the aluminum sites which are negatively charged
- Sodium and calcium are displaced by hydrated protons, resulting in degradation of the glass network to form a hydrated siliceous gel
- The powder is amphoteric, i.e. it can react chemically as an acid in the presence of strong bases. Hence, the reaction is an acid-base reaction in which the pH of the aqueous phase increases
- The ions liberated from the surface of the glass particles migrate to the liquid phase leaving a siliceous gel behind and later precipitated as phosphates and fluorides as the pH increases
- The material sets within 24 hours after the precipitation process is completed
- The binding agent is aluminophosphate gel which contains little crystalline basic phosphate $Al_2(OH)_3PO_4$
- Only the surface of the powder particle is attacked by phosphoric acid and 20% of powder is used
- The set material has a cored structure consisting of unreacted glass particles sheathed by a surface layer of siliceous gel and embedded in amorphous gel. The binding agent is aluminum phosphate **(Fig. 56)**
- The cations on the outer layers of glass particles are displaced by fluoride ions which are mobile and diffuse through the matrix (hence are fluoride releasing).

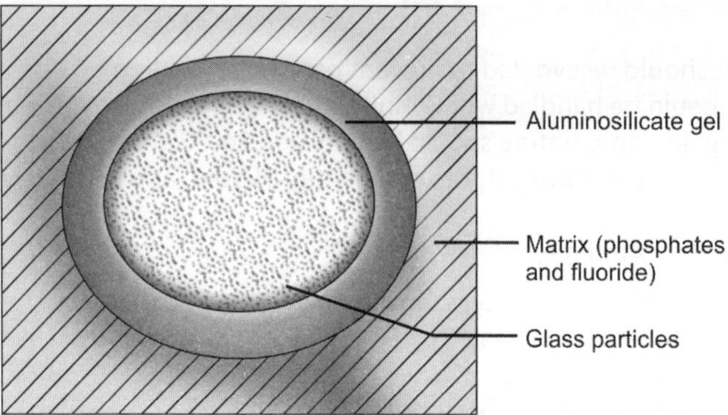

Fig. 56: Final set gel

141. Degassing.

Definition

- The direct filling golds except noncohesive golds are supplied in cohesive condition. But during storage and packaging, gas can adsorb on the surface of gold. So, the pellets need to be heated just before using it in oral cavity. This treatment is called *heat treatment, annealing or degassing*
- Noncohesive gold foil can be made to cohesive by heating noncohesive gold foil over a smokeless clean alcohol flame or electric heater over a preheated mica tray or table.

Significance

- Degassing aids in removing surface gases as oxygen, nitrogen, ammonia or sulfur dioxide due to improper storage
- Operator should wear chamois finger-tips to protect the gold from contamination
- Degassing is required to remove impurities from restorative material for total cohesion
- The cavity should be dried to ensure cohesion and maximize the physical properties in the restoration.

Methods of Heating

- Large quantities can be heated in a tray by gas flame or electricity
- Small pieces can be heated in a well adjusted alcohol flame
- Powdered gold must be heated in a flame till all the wax is eliminated, if heated in a tray, they get desorbed.

Rules to Follow

- Large quantities should be avoided to prevent prolonged heating
- The foil pieces should be handled with stainless steel wire points to prevent contamination
- The electric annealer temperature should be between 340°C and 370°C
- The time depends on the temperature and quantity of gold (approximately 5–20 minutes).

Problems with Electric Annealer

- Pellets may stick together, if the tray is moved
- Air currents affect uniformity in heating
- Greater exposure to contamination
- Size selection among the pieces of desorbed gold is limited
- Alcohol flame is preferred as chances of contamination are less (Methanol or Ethanol).

Advantages of Flame Desorption

- Ability to select a piece of gold of the desired size
- Desorption of only the pieces used
- Less exposure to contamination between time of degassing and use
- Less danger of oversintering
- Underheating causes incomplete cohesion
- Overheating leads to oversintering, incomplete cohesion and poor compaction characteristics.

142. What is Abrasive and Erosive Wear? Name the Methods of Bonding in the Bonded Abrasives. Explain the Truing and Dressing Procedures.

DEFINITIONS

Abrasion: Abrasion or abrasive wear is a material removal process that can occur whenever surfaces slide against each other.

Example: The process of finishing a restoration by using hard particles.

Abrasive: The surface material of an abrading instrument is referred to as an abrasive.

Substrate: It is the material being finished. This finishing depends on the rotational direction of a rotary abrasive.

Hard particle erosion: It is when the erosive wear is caused by hard particles impacting a substrate surface, carried by either a stream of liquid or a stream of air.

Chemical erosion: When acids and alkalis are used instead of hard particles to remove substrate material as in acid etching.

Abrasion

Classification

- Two-body abrasion
- Three-body abrasion.

Two-body Abrasion

Occurs when the abrasive particles are firmly bonded to the surface of the abrasive instrument and no other abrasive particles are used, e.g. a diamond bur abrading a tooth.

Three-body Abrasion

- Three-body abrasion occurs when abrasive particles are free to translate and rotate between two surfaces, e.g. as in the use of a dental prophylaxis paste.
- Lubricants are used to minimize the risk for unintentional shifts from two-body to three-body wear and vice-versa, to increase the efficiency of cutting and grinding.

Methods of Bonding in Bonded Abrasives

- Sintering
- Vitreous bonding (glass or ceramic)
- Resinoid bonding (phenolic resin)
- Rubber-bonding (Latex-based or silicone-based rubber).

Sintered Abrasives

Sintered abrasives are the strongest type with the abrasive particles fused together.

Vitreous-bonded Abrasives

Vitreous bonded abrasives are mixed with a glassy or ceramic matrix material, cold pressed to the instrument shape and fired to fuse the binder.

Resin-bonded Abrasives

Resin-bonded abrasives are cold pressed or hot pressed and then heated to cure the resin.

Rubber-bonded Abrasives

Rubber-bonded abrasives are made similar to resin-bonded abrasives.

TRUING AND DRESSING

- A bonded abrasive instrument should always be trued and dressed before its use
- Truing is a procedure through which the abrasive instrument is run against a harder abrasive block until the abrasive instrument rotates in the handpiece without eccentricity or run-out when placed on the substrate
- The dressing procedure is done basically to shape the instrument
- Dressing reduces the instrument to its correct working size and shape
- Dressing removes clogged debris from the abrasive instrument to restore grinding efficiency during the finishing operation
- The clogging of the abrasive instruments with the debris is called abrasive blinding
- Abrasive binding occurs when debris generated from grinding or polishing occludes the small spaces between abrasive particles on the tool and reduces the depth that particles can penetrate into the substance. This reduces abrasive's efficacy and greater heat is generated.

143. Cast Metal Bases/Metal Denture Bases.

REQUIREMENTS FOR CAST METAL BASES

- Metal bases should be thin but rigid
- Should be dense
- Accurate, having a positive fit on the master cast without rocking
- Biologically acceptable alloy.

Advantages of Metal Bases over Resin Bases (by Faber)

- Prevention of acrylic warpage
- Lack of bulk with more strength
- Increased accuracy
- Less tissue change under the base
- Less porosity and, therefore, easier to clean and keep clean
- Thermal conductivity
- Less deformation in function.

Disadvantages

- High cost
- Greater weight
- Inability to be easily rebased

- Poor esthetic qualities
- Time-consuming construction.

Materials for Cast Metal Bases

- Gold alloys—types III and IV
- Chrome-base alloys
- Aluminum alloys
- Anodized aluminum.

Gold Alloys—Types III and IV

They contain copper, silver, palladium, platinum and some trace elements.

Chrome-base Alloys

- All the cast chrome alloys for RPD can be used
- Examples: Ticonium, vitalium, nobelium, etc.

Aluminum Alloys

- Pure aluminum with 4% magnesium and slight amounts of silicon is more common
- The casting temperature of aluminum is between 704.5° and 815.5°C.

Design Principles

A design is drawn with pencil indicating the amount of coverage, placement of finishing lines and type of resin retention on the master cast.

Maxillary Bases

The design covers the complete palate and ridge crest, but leaves the denture borders in resin. Covering the posterior palatal seal area in the metal is also permitted and the resin periphery begins at the pterygomaxillary notch area.

Mandibular Bases

The mandibular cast base covers crest of the ridge with resin peripheries as this is easier to adjust and polish, though complete coverage of metal base can also be done.

Resin Retention

- Retention mesh
- Non-relieved retention of beads
- Nail heads and loops.

Blockout and Relief

- Blockout relief is provided under the soft-tissue undercuts
- This blockout reduces the number of sharp metal projections on the tissue surface to be removed during finishing.

Casting Procedure

- Vitalium and Nobelium need 982° to 1093°C temperature burnout
- Casting is done in automatic induction casting machines
- For aluminum at 343.5°C, the aluminum ingots are placed in the induction crucible of the casting machine. This crucible should be used only for aluminum
- Turn on the melt switch and probe the ingots with a quartz rod as they melt. When it is possible to push the top ingots into the mass, turn off the melt switch and allow the metal to cool
- Remove the mold from the furnace and place it in the cradle. Turn on the melt switch and watch the metal until it takes on the orange color of a harvest moon. At that point, throw the automatic cast switch and complete the casting. Keep the arm rotating for full 3 minutes
- Remove the cast and allow it to bench cool for 10 minutes before quenching it in running water
- Remove the bulk of the refractory material with a wax spatula or a similar hand instrument under running water
- The final cleansing of the refractory cast is done by blasting it with walnut-shell abrasives. Sand blaster will pit and dull the aluminum alloy.

BIBLIOGRAPHY

1. Anusavice Kenneth J. Philips Science of Dental Materials, Harcourt Asia PTE Ltd, 10th edn,1998.
2. Anusavice Kenneth J. Philips Science of Dental Materials, Saunders, 11th edn, 2004.
3. Combe EC. Notes on Dental Materials, Churchill Livingstone, 6th edn, 1992.
4. Graig Robert G, Powers John M, Wataha John C. Dental Materials Properties and Manipulation, Mosby, 9th edn, 2004.
5. McCabe John F. Applied Dental Materials, Blackwell Scientific Publications, 7th edn, 1990.
6. Powers John M, Wataha John C. Dental Materials Properties and Manipulation, Mosby, 9th edn, 2008.
7. Richard Van Noort. Introduction to Dental Materials, Mosby, 1994.

Multiple Choice Questions

Prosthodontics

Physical and Mechanical Properties

1. **Rockwell test is used:**
   a. To test resiliency of material
   b. To test color index
   c. To test hardness of material
   d. To test malleability.
2. **Change of length per unit when a dental material is subjected to load is known as:**
   a. Stress
   b. Creep
   c. Strain
   d. Diffusion.
3. **A metal which may be drawn readily into sheets is:**
   a. Ductile
   b. Malleable
   c. Plastic
   d. Elastic
4. **Green strength with reference to plaster means:**
   a. Dry strength
   b. Compressive strength
   c. Wet strength
   d. Strength due to green color.
5. **A stress that tends to resist a twisting motion or sliding of one portion of body over another is called:**
   a. Compressive strength
   b. Tensile strength
   c. Shearing strength
   d. All the above.
6. **The time-dependent plastic deformation is referred to as:**
   a. Creep
   b. Flow
   c. Static
   d. All the above.
7. **The greatest stress which may be produced in a material such that the stress is directly proportional to strain is known as:**
   a. Elastic limit
   b. Yield strength
   c. Modulus of elasticity
   d. Proportional limit.
8. **Bezold-Brücke effect is related to:**
   a. Galvanism
   b. Polymerization
   c. Color perception
   d. Welding.
9. **Time-dependent deformation produced by a stress is called:**
   a. Modulus
   b. Shear thinning
   c. Creep
   d. Sag.
10. **Surfactant is a material that:**
    a. Increases surface tension
    b. Decreases surface tension
    c. Does not affect surface tension
    d. Reacts chemically.
11. **The property by which a metal can be drawn into sheets is called:**
    a. Ductility
    b. Rigidity
    c. Wettability
    d. Malleability.
12. **KHN is a unit used for the measurement of:**
    a. Elasticity
    b. Resiliency
    c. Hardness
    d. Adhesiveness.
13. **An example of a material that behaves with Newtonian viscosity is:**
    a. Zinc-phosphate cement
    b. Zinc oxide eugenol cement

c. Composite resin
d. Cold cure resin.

14. The law which states that stress by strain is a constant is termed as:
a. Crook's law
b. Newton's law
c. Boyle's law
d. Hooke's law.

15. The greater the surface energy, the greater is the:
a. Adhesion
b. Toughness
c. Hardness
d. Brittleness.

16. Time-dependent plastic deformation is referred to as:
a. Adhesion
b. Viscosity
c. Creep
d. Cohesion.

17. To have a good wettability, the contact angle between adhesive and adherent should be:
a. 90
b. 60
c. 45
d. 0.

18. Unit of viscosity is:
a. MPa per second
b. mg/cm^2
c. cc
d. mms/Hg.

19. A refractory material is the one which is:
a. Resistant to acids
b. Obtained from factory
c. Chemically unstable
d. Resistant to heat.

20. Contact angle helps to know:
a. Wettability
b. Strength
c. Malleability
d. Resistance.

21. Maximum stress, which can act in a body without resulting in a permanent deformation, is:
a. Ultimate tensile stress
b. Flexure stress
c. Elastic limit
d. Endurance limit.

22. Modulus of elasticity:
a. Is the stress required to produce unit strain
b. Means toughness
c. Is the energy required to fracture
d. Is the same as proportional limit.

23. Coefficient of thermal expansion of tooth enamel (in ppm) is:
a. 81
b. 38.4
c. 11.4
d. 7.6.

24. The property of flow is important in:
a. Investments
b. Waxes
c. Gold alloys
d. Silicate cements.

25. Set elastic impression material has high:
a. Flexibility
b. Elastic recovery
c. Tear strength
d. All the above.

26. The ability of the alloy to withstand permanent deformation in the form of an indentation is:
a. Abrasion resistance
b. Modulus of elasticity
c. Hardness
d. Tensile strength.

Casting, Investments and Procedures

1. Thermal expansion of silica-bonded investment can be controlled by:
a. Rapid heating of investment mold
b. Increasing W/P ratio of investment materials
c. Vacuum investment technique
d. The amount of particle size and type of silica filler used.

2. Extra vent sprues are used to minimize:
a. Back pressure porosity
b. Microporosity
c. Surface porosity
d. Corrosion.

3. Satisfactory casting can be obtained if sprue former is attached at:
a. 90% angle to wax pattern
b. 20% angle to wax pattern

c. 65% angle to wax pattern
d. 45% angle to wax pattern.

4. It is preferred to attach sprue when:
a. The wax pattern is on the die
b. After the pattern is removed from the die
c. After washing in soap
d. After soaking in water.

5. The sprue former is attached to the:
a. Casting ring
b. Crucible former
c. Investment
d. Ring liner.

6. Before investing, the casting ring liner:
a. Is used along with separating media
b. Is coated with investment
c. Is immersed in water
d. Is heated in an oven.

7. For hygroscopic expansion, the casting ring is immersed in water at:
a. 27 to 28°C
b. 28 to 29°C
c. 37 to 38°C
d. 30 to 36°C.

8. Casting ring is heated for the sake of:
a. Elimination of wax
b. Thermal expansion
c. Both
d. None of the above.

9. Vacuum mixing of investment material results in:
a. Better visualization
b. Less power consumption
c. Porosity
d. Quick setting time.

10. Heating a discolored casting in an acid is called:
a. Acidifying
b. Pickling
c. Annealing
d. Cleaning.

11. The type of investment material used for casting cobalt-chromium alloy is:
a. Gypsum-bonded investment
b. Silica-bonded investment
c. Phosphate-bonded investment
d. All the above.

12. Dislocation is:
a. Fracture of a casting
b. Separation of metal from ceramic
c. Defect in the crystal
d. Breakage of the sprue.

Dental Ceramics

1. Zirconium and titanium are added in dental porcelain:
a. As sintering agents
b. To provide opacity
c. To provide lower fusion temperature
d. As a flux.

2. Metal ceramic crown consists of:
a. Cast metal coping into which porcelain is fired
b. Porcelain is fixed and fused on wrought metal
c. Body of core porcelain contains 40 to 50% of alumina crystals
d. Metal backing and porcelain facing.

3. The action of fluxes:
a. Is as a solvent
b. Presents oxide formation
c. Is reducing
d. All of these.

4. Cermet cement is:
a. Ceramic particle with composite
b. Glass ionomer with silver amalgam
c. Amalgam with composite
d. Glass ionomer with fluoride.

5. The glossy surface obtained by heating dental porcelain is:
a. Glaze
b. Overglaze
c. Frit
d. Body

6. Porcelain-fired article is toughened by:
a. Repeated firing
b. Vacuum firing
c. Interruption of crack propagation
d. Glazing.

7. Ceramming heat treatment causes:
a. Devitrification
b. Degassing
c. Tempering
d. Order hardening.

8. Ceramming causes:
a. More cracks
b. Vitrification
c. Decreased strength
d. Crystallization.

9. **High-fusing porcelain is used:**
   a. To fabricate metal-free crowns
   b. Inlays
   c. Denture teeth
   d. Bridges.
10. **Zirconium in ceramics is used as:**
   a. Incisal layer
   b. Dentin layer
   c. Opaquer
   d. Binder.

Dental Waxes

1. **Distortion of inlay wax is due to:**
   a. Relaxation of internal stresses
   b. Crazing
   c. Hygroscopic expansion
   d. Imbibition.
2. **Which property is not desirable in inlay wax:**
   a. It must flake
   b. Must be dimensionally stable
   c. Must not leave residue on burnout
   d. Must be carvable to a thin edge.
3. **Waxes used in dentistry solidify as:**
   a. Gel structure
   b. Amorphous material
   c. Crystalline material
   d. Formation of polymers.
4. **Distortion of inlay wax is due to:**
   a. Relaxation of internal stresses
   b. Presence of foreign particles
   c. Hygroscopic expansion
   d. Imbibition.

Wrought Metal Alloys

1. **Percentage of chromium in stainless steel is:**
   a. 1 to 4%
   b. 4 to 10%
   c. 11 to 30%
   d. Above 50%.
2. **Corrosion resistance is more in:**
   a. Austenitic steel
   b. Martensitic
   c. Ferritic
   d. b and c.
3. **Carbon is added to steel for:**
   a. Increasing the hardness
   b. Light weight
   c. As a filler
   d. Increasing young's modulus.
4. **18–8 stainless steel will lose its resistance to corrosion:**
   a. When carbon content is reduced
   b. When heated to a temperature of 400°C –900°C
   c. a and c
   d. When heated to a temperature of 200°C –365°C.
5. **Chrome-Cobalt-Nickel alloys have fusion temperature around:**
   a. 940°C
   b. 1150°C
   c. 1300°C
   d. 1575°C.
6. **Nickel-Titanium alloys have high.**
   a. Density
   b. Weldability
   c. Rigidity
   d. Flexibility.

Dental Casting and Soldering of Alloys

1. **In hygroscopic technique during burnout, the mold casting is heated:**
   a. Up to 468°C
   b. Up to 468°C and held in that temperature for 60 to 90°C
   c. Heated up to 700°C
   d. Temperature not critical.
2. **Role of copper in gold alloys is:**
   a. To increase strength
   b. To decrease strength
   c. To increase malleability
   d. To decrease ductility.
3. **Type of gold alloy used for removable partial denture casting is:**
   a. Type III
   b. Type IV
   c. Type II
   d. Type I.
4. **Gold-Copper alloy is a:**
   a. Solid solution
   b. Eutectic alloy
   c. Intermetalic compound
   d. Hypoeutectic.

5. **One of the characteristics of an alloy is that it is:**
   a. Only the parent metal
   b. Naturally found
   c. Has a melting range
   d. None.
6. **Which of the following is not used to melt base metals:**
   a. Oxygen and acetylene
   b. Compressed air and LPG
   c. LPG and oxygen
   d. Induction.
7. **Casting shrinkage of base metal alloys is:**
   a. 2 to 2.3%
   b. 1 to 1.3%
   c. 2.5 to 3%
   d. 0.5 to 1.2%.
8. **The modulus of elasticity of base metal in relation to gold is:**
   a. Same
   b. Twice
   c. Less
   d. Three times.
9. **The density of base metal alloys is:**
   a. 8.0 g/cm^3
   b. 18.39 g/cm^3
   c. 1.80 g/cm^3
   d. 0.80 g/cm^3.
10. **Palladium in gold alloys:**
    a. Increases whiteness and decreases strength
    b. Decreases yellowness and increases strength
    c. Decreases whiteness and decreases strength
    d. Increases malleability and decreases yield strength.
11. **Role of beryllium in dental casting alloys is to improve:**
    a. Strength
    b. Castability
    c. Malleability
    d. Ductility.
12. **Casting temperature of a molten alloy is:**
    a. 90°C to 98°C above its liquidus temperature
    b. 38°C to 66°C above its liquidus temperature
    c. 100°C–above its liquidus temperature
    d. 20°C less than its liquidus temperature.
13. **Discoloration of gold alloy casting is removed by:**
    a. Acid etching
    b. Pickling
    c. Conditioner solution
    d. Surfactant.
14. **Antiflux used in bracing is suspension of:**
    a. Potassium fluoride
    b. Borax
    c. Silica
    d. Rouge.
15. **Cold welding refers to:**
    a. Joining of two metals in cold climate
    b. Condensation of gold foils with condenser
    c. Repair of cast partial denture
    d. Repair of metal ceramic components.
16. **Lost wax technique for cast restorations was first reported by:**
    a. William Wordsworth
    b. William Taggart
    c. GV Black
    d. Buonocore.

Denture-base Resins

1. **The excess material which comes out of flask during packing of resin into mold is:**
   a. Dough
   b. Flash
   c. Bakelite
   d. Thrush.
2. **The fundamental difference between heat and self-cure resins is:**
   a. Method of activation of benzoyl peroxide
   b. Composition of powder
   c. Powder-liquid ratio
   d. Color of resin.
3. **During packing, polymer-monomer mixture should be packed into mold at the:**
   a. Sticky stage
   b. Fluid stage
   c. Dough stage
   d. Rubbery stage.
4. **The most popular separating agent is**
   a. Water soluble alginate
   b. Tin foil
   c. Soap
   d. Starch.
5. **Thermal conductivity of denture base should be:**
   a. Very low
   b. Same as enamel

c. High
d. Same as dentin.

6. **Activator in heat-cure acrylic is:**
a. Dimethyl-p-toluidine
b. Benzoyl peroxide
c. Dibutyl phthalate
d. None of the above.

7. **Heat-cure acrylic repair of denture-base resin is not preferred due to:**
a. Difficulties in processing
b. Higher strength
c. Distortion during curing
d. Poor bonding.

8. **Localized shrinkage porosity is reduced by using:**
a. Porous investment
b. Ring liners
c. Thin lone sprue
d. Reservoir.

9. **Boiling point of methyl methacrylate is:**
a. 90°C
b. 104°C
c. 96.4°C
d. 100.8°C.

10. **The main advantage of microwave polymerization of denture-base resin is:**
a. High strength
b. Short time polymerization
c. Decreased porosity
d. Less crazing.

11. **Microscopic or visible cracks occurring on denture-base resin due to surface stresses is known as:**
a. Porosity
b. Crazing
c. Voids
d. Grains.

12. **The powder component of denture base resin consists of:**
a. BIS-GMA
b. Un-polymerized methyl methacrylate
c. Polymerized methyl methacrylate
d. Pre-polymerized poly (methyl methacrylate).

13. **Mechanism to avoid crazing in denture bases is:**
a. Fast curing
b. Cross-linking
c. Using high heat for polymerization
d. Using veined acrylic.

14. **The co-polymer included in composition of acrylic resin is:**
a. Methyl methacrylate
b. Ethyl acrylate
c. Butyl acrylate
d. Ethyl methacrylate.

15. **A rapid flow of molten metal into mold can lead to:**
a. Pinhole porosity
b. Gas inclusion porosity
c. Subsurface porosity
d. Localized shrinkage porosity.

16. **Back pressure porosity can be avoided by:**
a. Using asbestos liners
b. Keeping a long sprue former
c. Keeping air vents
d. Using a short and wide sprue former.

Impression Materials

1. **The W/P ratio for plaster for manipulation is:**
a. 60 mL of water with 100 g of plaster
b. 100 mL of water with 60 g of powder
c. 60 mL of water with 30 g of powder
d. 28 mL of water with 100 g of power.

2. **The size and weight of Vicat needle for measuring the setting time of plaster are:**
a. Weight 200 g; diameter 2 mm; length 3 cm
b. Weight 300 g; diameter 1 mm; length 5 cm
c. Weight 100 g; diameter 1 mm; length 5 cm
d. Weight 500 g; diameter 5 mm; length 5 cm.

3. **Retarder in gypsum products acts by:**
a. Increasing the number of crystal size
b. Increasing the temperature of mix
c. Dissolving hemihydrate and increasing the crystal growth
d. Formation of absorbed layer on hemihydrate and inhibiting crystal growth.

4. **The best way to alter setting time of impression paste is to:**
a. Alter temperature of glass slab
b. Alter ratio of base to catalyst
c. Increase the humidity
d. Alter the mixing time.

5. **Alginate impression material:**
   a. is hydrophilic
   b. is inelastic impression material
   c. can be autoclaved
   d. is dimensionally stable for a prolonged period.
6. **Impression compound can be used for:**
   a. Edentulous impressions
   b. Border molding
   c. Both
   d. None.
7. **Reversible hydrocolloids refer to:**
   a. Chemical set
   b. Hardness on heating
   c. Softness on heating
   d. Edentulous impressions.
8. **Type-IV gypsum product refers to:**
   a. Impression plaster
   b. Modeling plaster
   c. Dental stone
   d. High-strength densite.
9. **Perforated stock trays are used for:**
   a. Elastomers
   b. Zinc oxide eugenol
   c. Irreversible hydrocolloids
   d. Reversible hydrocolloids.
10. **When mixing base paste and catalyst paste:**
    a. Both are incorporated into each other
    b. Catalyst is incorporated into base
    c. Base is incorporated into catalyst
    d. It makes no difference.
11. **Addition silicon impressions can be poured:**
    a. Immediately
    b. After 20 minutes
    c. After 6 hours
    d. After 8 hours.
12. **Impression compound should be kept in a patient's mouth at:**
    a. 40°C
    b. 45°C
    c. 50°C
    d. 55°C.
13. **Which of these elastomers has high viscosity:**
    a. Heavy body
    b. Medium body
    c. Light body
    d. Putty.
14. **The best and common method of controlling setting time of gypsum without altering its properties is to:**
    a. Add excess water in the mix
    b. Increase the spatulation
    c. Alter the temperature of water
    d. Add retarders.
15. **A material that changes chemically and hardens when subjected to heat is:**
    a. Thermoplastic
    b. Thermoform
    c. Thermoset
    d. None.
16. **Which is an amorphous material:**
    a. Investments
    b. Waxes
    c. Gold alloys
    d. Silicate cements.
17. **Organic glycols in alginate act to:**
    a. Increase setting time
    b. Decrease setting time
    c. Produce a pleasant taste
    d. Make the powder dustless.
18. **Average linear contractions of impression compound are:**
    a. 2 to 4%
    b. 0.7 to 0.9%
    c. 0.3 to 0.4%
    d. 4 to 7%.
19. **Stone castes can be heated/stored in a maximum temperature of:**
    a. 440°C
    b. 220°C
    c. 110°C
    d. 55°C.
20. **From which impression can electroformed dies not be prepared:**
    a. Polysulfide
    b. Polyether
    c. Alginate
    d. Impression compound.
21. **First synthetic elastomeric impression material introduced in dentistry was:**
    a. Addition silicone
    b. Condensation silicone
    c. Polyether
    d. Polysulfide.

22. The following impression material is set by chemical reaction except:
a. Impression compound
b. Dental plaster
c. Alginate hydrocolloid
d. Zinc oxide eugenol paste.

23. The temperature lag between gelation and liquefaction temperature of gel is known as:
a. Liquidus temperature
b. Solidus temperature
c. Syneresis temperature
d. Hysteresis.

24. The catalyst used in addition silicone impression material is:
a. Water
b. Dibutyl phthalate
c. Lead dioxide
d. Platinum salt.

25. Gelation of alginate occurs by:
a. Chemical reaction
b. Exothermic reaction
c. Physical reaction
d. None of the above.

26. One of the following is a reversible impression material:
a. Alginate
b. Zinc oxide eugenol paste
c. Agar-Agar
d. Polyether.

27. The most important requisite of an impression material is:
a. Retardation of setting time
b. Rigidity
c. Dimensional stability
d. Creep.

28. An ideal impression material for partially edentulous mouth is:
a. Impression plaster
b. Alginate
c. Impression compound
d. Zinc oxide eugenol impression paste.

29. Stiffest impression material is:
a. Condensation silicone
b. Polysulfide
c. Addition silicone
d. Polyether.

30. During manipulation of impression compound, water acts as a:
a. Reactor
b. Retarder
c. Catalyst
d. Plasticizer.

31. High-strength dental stone has setting expansion of:
a. 5%
b. 8%
c. 0.8%
d. 0.08%.

32. The most effective method for controlling setting expansion of plaster is:
a. Changing W:P ratio
b. Addition of chemicals
c. Changing mixing time
d. Intermittent mixing.

33. Water : powder ratio of type IV die stone is:
a. 46%
b. 23%
c. 19%
d. 11.4%.

34. Gillmore needles are used to find:
a. Wet strength
b. Dry strength
c. Setting expansion
d. Setting time.

35. Set impression material should have adequate:
a. Flexibility
b. Elastic recovery
c. Tear strength
d. All the above.

36. Accelerator for zinc oxide eugenol impression material is:
a. Calcium chloride
b. Inert oils
c. Potassium sulfate
d. Borax.

37. The best method to increase setting time of alginate impression material in clinics is by adding:
a. Trisodium phosphate
b. $CaSO_4$
c. More water
d. Cold water.

38. An useful property of elastomeric impression material is:
a. Incomplete elastic recovery
b. Thermal contraction
c. Flexibility
d. Polymerization shrinkage.

Properties

1. **A fluctuating dipole is a feature of:**
   a. Hydrogen bond
   b. van der Waals attraction
   c. Metallic bond
   d. All of these.
2. **Crystalline structure was described by:**
   a. Robert Hooke
   b. Carl Boucher
   c. Craig
   d. McLean.
3. **Interstitial impurity is an example of which crystal defect:**
   a. Point defect
   b. Line defect
   c. Planar defect
   d. None of these.
4. **Temperature at which the thermal expansion coefficient increases abruptly is called:**
   a. Heat capacity
   b. Latent heat of fusion
   c. Glass transition temperature
   d. Heat of vaporization.
5. **The minimum spacing between two adhering solid surfaces is:**
   a. 1.5 nm
   b. 1.7 nm
   c. 0.5 nm
   d. 0.7 nm.
6. **Contact angle is formed between:**
   a. Molecules of adhesive
   b. Molecules of adherent
   c. Adhesive and adherent
   d. Adhesive and the surrounding medium.
7. **For complete wetting, the contact angle should be:**
   a. 90
   b. 0
   c. 45
   d. 89.
8. **Smear layer:**
   a. Promotes marginal leakage
   b. Has a protective coating
   c. Causes delayed expansion
   d. Is formed by acid etching.
9. **Degree of saturation of a color is:**
   a. Value
   b. Hue
   c. Chroma
   d. None of these.
10. **Time-dependent plastic deformation of a set solid substance is:**
    a. Creep
    b. Flow
    c. Necking
    d. Flexibility.
11. **Irreversible deformation of metal framework at the firing temperature of ceramic is called:**
    a. Sag
    b. Creep
    c. Flow
    d. Necking.
12. **Thixotropic behavior is due to:**
    a. Breaking of chemical bond
    b. Structural break down and reformation
    c. Boiling and cooling of liquid
    d. All of these
13. **The ability of the material to withstand abrasion or wear is called:**
    a. Hardness
    b. Malleability
    c. Ductility
    d. Impact strength.
14. **Most malleable and ductile metal is:**
    a. Silver
    b. Copper
    c. Gold
    d. Iron.
15. **A fluid showing proportional shear stress and strain rate is termed as:**
    a. Dilatant
    b. Newtonian
    c. Pseudoplastic
    d. Plastic.
16. **Fluid denture-base resins are:**
    a. Newtonian
    b. Pseudoplastic
    c. Dilatant
    d. Plastic.
17. **Surface discoloration of a metal is called:**
    a. Corrosion
    b. Rusting
    c. Reduction
    d. Tarnish.
18. **Cathode exhibits:**
    a. Reduction
    b. Oxidization

c. Metal dissolution
d. None of these.

19. If dissimilar metals come to direct physical contact in the oral cavity, the effect produced is called:
a. Galvanic shock
b. Warpage
c. Tarnish
d. Erosion.

20. Fatigue is due to:
a. Impact load
b. Continuous load
c. Cyclic load
d. All of these.

21. Three-point loading is associated with:
a. Tensile stress
b. Compressive stress
c. Complex stress
d. Shear stress.

22. Necking is associated with:
a. Compressive load
b. Shear load
c. Tensile load
d. None of these.

23. Temperature affects malleability and ductility such that it:
a. Decreases malleability and increases ductility
b. Increases malleability and ductility both
c. Decreases malleability and ductility both
d. Increases malleability and decreases ductility.

24. The oldest hardness test is:
a. Rockwell test
b. Vickers test
c. Brinell test
d. Knoop test.

25. Hardness test applicable for brittle materials is:
a. Shore test
b. Barcol test
c. Knoop test
d. All of these.

Metallurgy

1. Supercooling is associated with:
a. Expansion of alloy
b. Purification of metal
c. Electroplating
d. Initial cooling of molten metal.

2. Small cluster of atoms, having long range atomic order found in solidified metal, is called:
a. Focus
b. Nucleus
c. Embryo
d. Center.

3. Rapid cooling of molten metal causes:
a. Heterogenous nucleation
b. Supercooling
c. Homogenous nucleation
d. None of the above.

4. The process of dendritic growth during solidification of pure metals is called:
a. Homogenous supercooling
b. Thermal supercooling
c. Heterogenous supercooling
d. Coring.

5. Interdendritic region serves as a site for:
a. Facile crack propagation
b. Interrupting crack propagation
c. No effect on crack propagation
d. Effect may vary.

6. Noble metal alloy casting shows:
a. Equiaxed polycrystalline microstructure
b. Monocrystalline microstructure
c. Equiaxed monocrystalline structure
d. Composite form.

7. If the atoms of solute metal occupy the positions in the crystal structure that are normally occupied by the solvent atoms in the pure metal, then the solution is called:
a. Substitutional solid solution
b. Interstitial solid solution
c. Disordered solid solution
d. Variable solid solution.

8. Solid solubility is influenced by all except
a. Atom size
b. Valence
c. Temperature
d. Chemical affinity.

9. Tie line helps to determine the composition of solid that is formed in a system. It is constructed by drawing a line:
a. From the solidus curve
b. From the liquidus curve parallel to the base line

c. From the liquidus curve perpendicular to the base line
d. From the solidus.

10. Microsegregation is:
a. Uniform composition and distinct boundaries
b. Uniform composition and indistinct boundaries
c. Grains have nonuniform composition and indistinct boundaries
d. None of these.

11. Eutectic system shows:
a. Unpredictable solid solubility
b. Limited solid solubility
c. Complete solid solubility
d. Absence of solid solubility.

12. Silver-copper binary eutectic composition is:
a. 28% Ag; 72% Cu
b. 34% Ag; 66% Cu
c. 66% Ag; 34% Cu
d. 72% Ag; 28% Cu.

13. Eutectic reaction is an invariant transformation because:
a. It occurs at single temperature and composition
b. It occurs at single temperature but different composition
c. It occurs at different temperatures but same composition
d. It occurs at different temperatures and compositions.

14. Peritectic systems can be represented as:
a. Liquid + beta solution → Alpha solid solution
b. Liquid → Alpha + Beta
c. Liquid+ Beta + Alpha → Liquid+ Beta
d. Liquid + Beta + Alpha → Liquid + Alpha.

15. Quenching produces alloys which are:
a. Hard and brittle
b. Soft and ductile
c. Soft and brittle
d. Hard.

16. When eutectic system solidifies, the structure formed is:
a. Dendritic
b. Equiaxial
c. Lamellar
d. Zigzag.

Polymers and Denture-base Resins

1. The main chain of a polymer is called:
a. Monomer
b. Master-chain
c. Back-bone
d. Copolymer

2. Ability of a polymer to behave as an elastic solid and viscous liquid is called:
a. Viscoelasticity
b. Thixotropy
c. Viscosity
d. None of these.

3. Identical monomer units occurring in relatively long sequences along the main polymer are called:
a. Random copolymers
b. Branched copolymers
c. Block copolymers
d. Homopolymers.

4. Agents added to resins to reduce their softening temperature are called:
a. Plasticizers
b. Cross-linking agents
c. Fillers
d. None of these.

5. Butyl methacrylate added to methyl methacrylate before polymerization acts as:
a. Internal plasticizer
b. External plasticizer
c. Cross-linking agent
d. Activator.

6. Induction, Propagation, Chain Transfer and Termination are the stages of:
a. Condensation polymerization
b. Step growth polymerization
c. Copolymerization
d. Cross-linking.

7. Free radicals are produced in which stage of polymerization:
a. Propagation
b. Termination
c. Induction
d. Chain transfer.

8. The initiator in cured dental resin is:
a. Benzoyl peroxide
b. Tertiary amine
c. Camphoroquinone
d. MMA.

9. **Derivatives of ethylene containing a vinyl group called:**
   a. Phenolic resins
   b. Urethane
   c. Acrylic resins
   d. Bakelite.
10. **Boiling point of MMA:**
   a. 108°C
   b. 10.8°C
   c. –48°C
   d. 100.8°C
11. **Density of MMA:**
   a. 9405 g/cc
   b. 0.945 g/cc
   c. 945 g/cc
   d. 9.45 g/cc
12. **Cross-linking agent in MMA is:**
   a. Glycol dimethacrylate
   b. Benzoyl peroxide
   c. Campharoquinone
   d. Tertiary amine.
13. **Inhibitor of polymerization in heat cure MMA is:**
   a. Hydroquinone
   b. Benzoyl peroxide
   c. Camphoroquinone
   d. Amine.
14. **Cold mold seal is:**
   a. Soap solution
   b. Starch
   c. Soluble alginate
   d. None of these.
15. **Volumetric shrinkage of MMA is:**
   a. 7%
   b. 21%
   c. 14%
   d. 2.1%.
16. **In what stage of polymer-monomer interaction, denture-base resin is packed in the mold cavity:**
   a. Stringy stage
   b. Sandy stage
   c. Rubbery stage
   d. Dough stage.
17. **Excess resin coming out of denture flask during packing is called:**
   a. Dough
   b. Micelle
   c. Flash
   d. None of these.
18. **Free monomer content in the chemically activated acrylic resin after polymerization is:**
   a. 0.2 to 0.5%
   b. 5 to 10%
   c. 0.5 to 1%
   d. 3 to 5%.
19. **Residual monomer content in heat-activated resin is:**
   a. 0.2 to 5%
   b. 3 to 5%
   c. 5 to 10%
   d. 0.5 to 1%.
20. **Stress relaxation which imparts a 'hazy' or 'foggy' appearance in the processed resin, is called:**
   a. Warpage
   b. Water sorption
   c. Crazing
   d. None of these.
21. **Soft denture liners are:**
   a. Plasticized acrylic resin
   b. Cross-linked acrylic resin
   c. Copolymerized resin
   d. Auto polymerized resin.
22. **The disadvantage of polyurethane MFP polymer is:**
   a. No natural feel
   b. Poor appearance
   c. Rapid deterioration
   d. High temperature for polymerization.

Implant Materials

1. **Reinsertion of a tooth back into its jaw socket, after accidental or intentional removal, is called:**
   a. Implantation
   b. Transplantation
   c. Reimplantation
   d. Transposition.
2. **Blade-vent implants were introduced by:**
   a. Branemark
   b. Linkow
   c. Goldberg
   d. Formiggini.

3. **An implant, that is placed into the mandible or maxilla and transects only one cortical plate, is called:**
   a. Subperiosteal implant
   b. Transosteal implant
   c. Endosteal implant
   d. Epithelial implant.
4. **Osseointegration requires:**
   a. No connective tissue between implant and bone
   b. Abundance of connective tissue
   c. Presence of epithelial cells
   d. None of these.
5. **Most common implant biomaterial is:**
   a. Pure titanium
   b. Ti6Al4V
   c. Ni Cr Mo Be
   d. Co Cr Mo.

Gypsum Products

1. **Gypsum is:**
   a. $CaSO_{4\frac{1}{2}}H_2O$
   b. $CaSO_4\,2H_2O$
   c. $CuSO_{4\frac{1}{2}}H_2O$
   d. $CuSO_4\,2H_2O$.
2. **Positive likeness of an object is called:**
   a. Cast
   b. Die
   c. Model
   d. None of these.
3. **Preconverted gypsum added to plaster as an accelerator is called:**
   a. Materia Alba
   b. Terra Alba
   c. Gum Arabic
   d. Surface active agent.
4. **Dead burnt plaster is:**
   a. Orthorhombic anhydrite
   b. Hexagonal anhydrite
   c. Stone
   d. Gypsum.
5. **Which gypsum product is irregular and spongy:**
   a. β Hemihydrate
   b. α Hemihydrate
   c. Stone
   d. Improved stone.
6. **W/P ratio of plaster is:**
   a. 0.6
   b. 0.28
   c. 0.34
   d. 0.53.
7. **Surface area per unit weight of stone (cm^2/g) is:**
   a. 4000 to 6000
   b. 6000 to 8000
   c. 8000
   d. 10,000.
8. **Calcination of gypsum in an autoclave (17 lbs/inch^2) at about 130–140°C in the presence of organic acids gives:**
   a. Crystacal base
   b. Hydrocal
   c. Densite
   d. Plaster.
9. **Antiexpansion (AE) solution contains:**
   a. K_2SO_4, Borax and Alizarin red
   b. K_2SO_4 and Borax
   c. Borax and Alizarin red
   d. K_2SO_4 and Alizarin red.
10. **Soluble plaster contains:**
    a. Potato starch
    b. Gum
    c. Alizarin red
    d. Stone plaster.
11. **Solubilities of $CaSO_4$ hemihydrate and dihydrate at 20°C are:**
    a. 0.8% and 0.2%
    b. 0.2% and 0.8%
    c. 0.6% and 0.4%
    d. 0.4% and 0.6%.
12. **Maximum concentration of $CaSO_4$ is present in:**
    a. Dissolution center
    b. Precipitation center
    c. Same in both centers
    d. None of the above.
13. **Size of spherulite**
    a. 5 to 20 μ
    b. 20 to 25 μ
    c. 30 to 35 μ
    d. 0 to 50 μ.
14. **Dimensions of Vicat needle are:**
    a. 500 g wt/3 cm long/2 mm^2 tip
    b. 100 g wt/6 mm long/4 mm^2 tip

c. 300 g wt/5 cm long/1 mm^2 tip
d. 400 g wt/1 cm long/8 mm^2 tip.

15. Weight of final Gillmore needle is:
a. 113.4 g
b. 453.6 g
c. 907.2 g
d. 1 kg.

16. Universal accelerator of gypsum is:
a. NaCl
b. Na_2SO_4
c. Borax
d. K_2SO_4.

17. Volumetric shrinkage of plaster during setting is:
a. 7.5%
b. 2.5%
c. 5%
d. 10%.

18. Synthetic gypsum is made from the byproducts of the manufacture of:
a. Sulfuric acid
b. Hydrochloric acid
c. Phosphoric acid
d. Nitric acid.

19. Crystals with low density, high surface area and poor packing ability can be formed by:
a. Wet calcination
b. Dry calcination
c. Any type of calcination
d. None.

20. Which gypsum product is formed by calcination of gypsum at 125°C and 17 lbs/inch in the presence of calcium chloride—30% or sodium succinate—0.5%:
a. Hydrocal
b. Improved stone
c. Crystacal base
d. Plaster.

21. The presence of residual water in set gypsum is seen as:
a. Angular spaces
b. Round spaces
c. Rough spaces
d. Pinhole spaces.

Impression Materials

1. Which of the following is a rigid impression material:
a. Alginate
b. Agar
c. Waxes
d. ZnO eugenol.

2. Which ingredient smoothens impression paste:
a. Silica
b. Lanolin
c. Balsam
d. Vegetable oil.

3. Plasticizer in impression paste is:
a. Lanolin
b. Vegetable oil
c. Balsam
d. Calcium chloride.

4. Mixing time of impression paste is:
a. 2 minutes
b. 15–30 seconds
c. 45 seconds–1 minute
d. 5 minutes.

5. Example of chelate is:
a. Zinc eugenolate
b. Eugenol
c. Lanolin
d. Balsam.

6. 24-hour shrinkage of impression paste is:
a. 0.1%
b. 0.2%
c. 0.3%
d. 0.4%.

7. 2-hour compression strength of impression paste is:
a. 2 MPa
b. 10 MPa
c. 8 MPa
d. 7 MPa.

8. Noneugenol pastes contains:
a. Phosphoric acid
b. Acetic acid
c. Carboxylic acid
d. Oil of cloves.

9. Modeling plastic is:
a. Putty elastomer
b. Impression compound
c. Light-body elastomer
d. Alginate.

10. Fusion temperature of green stick compound is:

a. 55°C
c. 75°C
b. 60°C
d. 43.5°C.

11. ADA specification of impression compound is:
a. 11
b. 7
c. 13
d. 3.

12. Synthetic wax added to impression compound is:
a. Copal resin
b. French chalk
c. Pumice
d. Diatomaceous earth.

13. Softening temperature of impression compound Is:
a. 80°C
b. 50 to 60°C
c. 60 to 70°C
d. 75°C.

14. Glass transition temperature of impression compound is:
a. 45°C
b. 39°C
c. 43.5°C
d. 55°C.

15. Coefficient of thermal expansion of impression compound is:
a. 0.2%
b. 0.3%
c. 0%
d. 0.05%.

16. Dispersed medium in hydrocolloid is:
a. Oil
b. Alginate
c. Agar
d. Water.

17. Absorption of water by hydrocolloid is called:
a. Syneresis
b. Hysteresis
c. Imbibition
d. Gelation.

18. Temperature lag between gelation and liquefaction temperature of agar is called:
a. Imbibition
b. Hysteresis
c. Syneresis
d. Gelation.

19. 'Micelles' are:
a. Fibrils in sol
b. Fibrils in gel
c. Fibrils in impression paste
d. None of these.

20. Gelation temperature of agar is:
a. 37°C
b. 107°C
c. 70°C
d. 80°C.

21. The ingredient(s) that provide(s) the brush heap structure in Agar is/are
a. Borates
b. Sulfates
c. Agar
d. Waxes.

22. Laminate technique involves:
a. Agar and alginate
b. Compound and plaster
c. Greenstick and impression paste
d. Elastomer and alginate.

23. Rim lock trays are necessary for making impression with:
a. Alginate
b. Elastomer
c. Agar
d. Compound.

24. Reactor in alginate is:
a. Zinc oxide
b. Potassium titanium fluoride
c. Sodium phosphate
d. Calcium sulfate.

25. Potassium titanium fluoride in alginate is:
a. Retarder
b. Accelerator of gypsum
c. Reactor
d. Filler.

26. Dust-free alginate contains:
a. Phosphoric acid
b. Glycol
c. K_2SO_4
d. Borax.

27. Chromic alginate is:
a. Tear-free alginate
b. Highly flexible alginate
c. Color-changing alginate
d. Normal setting alginate.

28. **Single component material with such shearing potential that it can be used as the syringe material and tray material is called:**
    a. Light body
    b. Medium body
    c. Monophase
    d. Heavy body.
29. **The process of heating natural rubber with sulfur to produce cross-linking is called:**
    a. Co-polymerization
    b. Cross-linking
    c. Vulcanization
    d. Calcination.
30. **ADA specification of nonaqueous elastomeric dental impression material is:**
    a. 8
    b. 3
    c. 19
    d. 21.
31. **Polymerization of polysulfide impression material:**
    a. Is exothermic
    b. Is endothermic
    c. Refers to where heat is neither produced nor absorbed
    d. Refers to where heat production\absorption may vary.
32. **Thiokol is a type of**
    a. Condensation silicon
    b. Polysulfide
    c. Addition silicon
    d. Polyether.
33. **Which of the following is a disadvantage of polyether:**
    a. Messy and stains clothes
    b. Short working time
    c. Poor tear resistance
    d. Highly hydrophobic.
34. **The byproduct in RTV silicones is:**
    a. Water
    b. Ethanol
    c. Acetic acid
    d. Phosphoric acid.
35. **Advantage of addition silicone is:**
    a. Not accurate
    b. Excellent shelf life
    c. Adequate tear strength
    d. Good dimensional stability.
36. **Vinyl polysiloxane impression material is:**
    a. Condensation silicone
    b. Polyether
    c. Polysulfide
    d. Addition silicone.
37. **Role of platinum salt in addition silicone material is:**
    a. Accelerator
    b. Retarder
    c. Filler
    d. Activator.
38. **Conventional addition silicones:**
    a. Are hydrophobic
    b. Are hydrophilic
    c. Show imbibition
    d. Show hysteresis.
39. **Too rapid polymerization of silicones causes:**
    a. Distortion
    b. Bubbles
    c. Rough surfaces
    d. Rough cast.

Casting Alloys, Waxes, Investment Procedures

1. **The first reported application of lost wax technique in dentistry is in:**
   a. Casting
   b. Acrylization
   c. a and b
   d. None of these.
2. **According to the National Bureau of Standards, Type III casting alloy is:**
   a. Hard
   b. Soft
   c. Medium
   d. Extra hard.
3. **Noble metal alloys contain:**
   a. <25 wt% of noble elements
   b. >25 wt% of noble elements
   c. > 40 wt% of noble elements
   d. 100 wt% of noble elements.
4. **Which one of the following is not noble in dentistry:**
   a. Gold-Silver
   b. Platinum-Silver
   c. Palladium-Gold
   d. Cobalt-Chromium.
5. **Number of parts of gold per 1,000 of gold is termed as:**
   a. Karat
   b. Fineness

c. Purity
d. Nobility.

6. Crown and bridge casting alloys are:
a. Type IV
b. Type III
c. Type II
d. Type I.

7. Heating alloy for 10 minutes at 700°C and then rapid quenching is referred to as:
a. Hardening treatment
b. Purifying
c. Softening treatment
d. None of these.

8. Solidification shrinkage of which alloy is more:
a. Type I Gold
b. Type II Gold
c. Type III Gold
d. Co-Cr-Mo.

9. Aging temperature of alloys generally is:
a. 700 to 750°C
b. 500 to 700°C
c. 1000°C
d. 200 to 450°C.

10. Which of the following is not a stage in alloy contraction:
a. Thermal contraction of the liquid metal between the temperature to which it is heated and the liquidus temperature
b. Inherent contraction of the alloy during liquid to solid stage conversion
c. Thermal contraction of the solid metal that occurs down to room temperature
d. None of these.

11. Which of the following statements is true:
a. Medium wax is used for direct technique
b. Medium wax is used for indirect technique
c. Synthetic waxes are used for direct technique
d. All are true.

12. Which wax is likely to flake when trimmed:
a. Paraffin wax
b. Gum dammar
c. Carnauba wax
d. Candella wax.

13. Ideal thickness of base plate wax is:
a. 2.3 mm
b. 0.5 to 1 mm
c. 4.5 mm
d. 1.2 mm.

14. Waxes tend to return to their original shape after manipulation by a property known as:
a. Plastic memory
b. Elastic memory
c. Elastic strain
d. Plastic strain.

15. Disadvantage(s) of gas entrapment in wax pattern is/are:
a. Causes pronounced contraction
b. Causes excessive porosity
c. Has poor esthetics
d. Causes pronounced expansion.

16. ADA specification dealing with inlay wax is:
a. 6
b. 8
c. 4
d. 9.

17. In Type II Gypsum-bonded investment, the compensation for alloy contraction is by:
a. Less purity
b. Density
c. Contraction
d. Hygroscopic expansion.

18. Slight expansion of gypsum investments occurs at:
a. 400 to 700°C
b. 200 to 400°C
c. 700 to 1000°C
d. >1000°C.

19. The maximum temperature raise possible for gypsum investments is:
a. 700°C
b. 650°C
c. 750°C
d. 800°C.

20. Surface tension-reducing agent is used before investing:
a. To regulate hygroscopic expansion
b. To regulate thermal expansion
c. To increase wetting of wax pattern
d. To decrease porosity.

21. Quartz is converted to β quartz at:
a. 625°C
b. 200 to 270°C
c. 575°C
d. 350°C.

22. **Forms of silica commonly used in investments are:**
    a. Quartz and tridymite
    b. Quartz and cristobalite
    c. Cristobalite and tridymite
    d. Quartz, cristobalite and tridymite.
23. **The form of silica not used normally in investment is**
    a. Quartz
    b. Cristobalite
    c. Fused quartz
    d. Tridymite.
24. **Maximum setting expansion of type I Gypsum Investment is:**
    a. 0.8%
    b. 0.6%
    c. 1.5%
    d. 1.2%.
25. **Hygroscopic setting expansion of type II Gypsum Investment is:**
    a. 1.6 to 2.2%
    b. 0.4 to 0.6%
    c. 0.6 to 0.8%
    d. 1 to 1.6%.
26. **Thermal expansion of type I Gypsum Investment is:**
    a. 1.6 to 2.2%
    b. 0.4 to 0.6%
    c. 1.2 to 2.2%
    d. 1.0 to 1.6%.
27. **ANSI specification II states that the compressive strength for inlay investment should have a minimum value of:**
    a. 24 MPa
    b. 2.4 MPa
    c. 0.24 MPa
    d. 5 MPa.
28. **The ingredient added to the investment to produce clean casting and to facilitate divesting is:**
    a. Chromium
    b. Silica
    c. Magnesium phosphate
    d. Carbon.
29. **Palladium reacts with carbon above:**
    a. 1054°C
    b. 1504°C
    c. 1540°C
    d. 1450°C.
30. **Binder in phosphate investment is:**
    a. $Mg_2P_2O_7$
    b. MgO
    c. $Mg_3P_2O_{42}$
    d. Silica.
31. **Investment useful for high-fusing base metal partial denture alloy is:**
    a. Phosphate investment
    b. Ethyl silicate investment
    c. Type II Gypsum investment
    d. Type I Gypsum investment.
32. **Green shrinkage is associated with**
    a. Ceramic plaster
    b. Ethyl silicate investment
    c. Amalgam
    d. Gypsum.
33. **Greening is associated with:**
    a. Ethyl silicate investment
    b. Plaster
    c. Amalgam
    d. Ceramic.
34. **Green strength is associated with:**
    a. Ceramic
    b. Silicate investment
    c. Plaster
    d. Amalgam.
35. **Powercast system is an example of:**
    a. Centrifugal casting system
    b. Air pressure casting system
    c. Ringless casting system
    d. Air press casting system.
36. **Divestment is a:**
    a. Gypsum-bonded material
    b. Phosphate-bonded material
    c. Silica-bonded system
    d. Ringless casting system.
37. **Spruing angle of wax pattern is:**
    a. 0°
    b. 45°
    c. 90°
    d. 75°.
38. **'Controlled water-added technique' is utilized for:**
    a. Thermal expansion
    b. Setting expansion
    c. Hygroscopic expansion
    d. Contraction.

39. **Maximum burnout temperature of carbon containing investment should be:**
    a. 550°C
    b. 500°C
    c. 700°C
    d. 900°C.
40. **Dark casting can be corrected by:**
    a. Electroplating
    b. Sand blasting
    c. Pickling
    d. Vibration.
41. **Premature termination of the flow of molten metal during solidification causes:**
    a. Localized shrinkage porosity
    b. Pinhole porosity
    c. Subsurface porosity
    d. Gas inclusion porosity.
42. **Hot spot causes:**
    a. Pinhole porosity
    b. Subsurface porosity
    c. Back pressure porosity
    d. Suckback porosity.
43. **Rapid solidification of molten alloy causes:**
    a. Microporosity
    b. Suckback porosity
    c. Pinhole porosity
    d. Subsurface porosity.
44. **Incomplete burnout causes:**
    a. Suckback porosity
    b. Fins
    c. Incomplete casting
    d. Distorted casting.

Finishing and Polishing Materials

1. **The process of producing lustrous surface through abrading action of fine abrasives bound to a nonabrasive binder medium is called:**
    a. Buffing
    b. Abrasion
    c. Contouring
    d. Finishing.
2. **Diamond bur abrasion of a tooth is an example of:**
    a. Three-body abrasion
    b. Finishing
    c. Two-body abrasion
    d. Buffing.
3. **KHN value of enamel is:**
    a. 340
    b. 70
    c. 40
    d. 75.
4. **The procedure through which the abrasive instrument is run against a harder block until the abrasive instrument rotates in a hand piece without eccentricity is called:**
    a. Dressing
    b. Two-body wear
    c. Truing
    d. Binding.
5. **Mineral form of aluminum oxide is:**
    a. Corundum
    b. Tripoli
    c. Garnet
    d. Kieselguhr.
6. **Dentifrice contains all except:**
    a. Cuttle
    b. Detergent
    c. Humectant
    d. Fluoride.
7. **The material being finished and polished is called:**
    a. Abrasive
    b. Interface
    c. Substrate
    d. Binder.

Wrought Metal Alloys

1. **All are the stages of annealing except:**
    a. Recovery
    b. Re-crystallization
    c. Grain growth
    d. Cold working.
2. **Maximum percentage of carbon in plain carbon steel:**
    a. 0.21%
    b. 2.1%
    c. 21%
    d. 12 to 30%.
3. **Percentage of chromium added in stainless steel is:**
    a. 2.1%
    b. 1 to 2%
    c. 12 to 30%
    d. 21%.

4. **ANSI number of ferritic and martensitic stainless steel is:**
   a. 300
   b. 302
   c. 400
   d. 18–8.
5. **A form of stainless steel which has got little application in dentistry is:**
   a. Martensitic
   b. Austenitic
   c. Ferritic
   d. None of these.
6. **18-8 stainless steel contains:**
   a. 8% Cr and 18% Ni
   b. 18% Cr and 8% Ni
   c. 18% Cr and 8% C
   d. 18% C and 8% Cr.
7. **Property by which austenitic steel looses its corrosion resistance is called:**
   a. Stabilization
   b. Annealing
   c. Sensitization
   d. Quenching.

Conservative Dentistry

Biocompatibility

1. **Ability of a material to elicit an appropriate biological response in a given application in the body is called:**
   a. Biointegration
   b. Biocompatibility
   c. Biomechanics
   d. Osseointegration.
2. **The most biocompatible metal used for dental implants is:**
   a. Yttrium
   b. Platinum
   c. Titanium
   d. Palladium.
3. **Biocompatibility may vary with:**
   i. Age
   ii. Condition of test
   iii. Area in the oral cavity
   iv. Color of the material.
      a. (i) and (ii) are correct
      b. (i) and (iii) are correct
      c. (iii) and (iv) are correct
      d. All are correct.
4. **The process in which living bony tissue forms within 100 Å of the implant surface without any interfering fibrous connective tissue is:**
   a. Allergy
   b. Hypersensitivity
   c. Biointegration
   d. Osseointegration.
5. **Most biocompatible cement used is:**
   a. Glass ionomer cement
   b. Zinc phosphate cement
   c. Zinc oxide eugenol
   d. Composites.
6. **Which of the following affects biocompatibility test:**
   a. Tarnish and corrosion
   b. Esthetics
   c. Location in oral cavity
   d. Presence of other restorations.
7. **Which of the following forms the criteria for a biocompatible material:**
   i. It should not be harmful to the pulp and soft tissues
   ii. It should have no carcinogenic potential
   iii. It should be free of allergic response
   iv. It should not contain any toxic diffusible substances that can be released and absorbed into the circulatory system to cause a toxic systemic response.
      a. (i) and (ii) are correct
      b. (i), (ii) and (iii) are correct

c. (ii) and (iv) are correct
d. All of the above are correct.

8. Primary tests are done for the evaluation of the following:
a. Cytotoxicity and genotoxicity
b. Teratogenecity
c. Phototoxicity
d. Allergy and hypersensitivity.

9. The most allergenic metal known is:
a. Nickel
b. Beryllium
c. Titanium
d. Silicon.

10. Symptoms of acute mercury toxicity are:
a. Paresthesia
b. Ataxia
c. Joints pain
d. All of the above.

11. Which of the following is the most toxic:
a. Mercury vapors
b. Mercury liquid
c. Amalgam scrap
d. Alloy powder.

12. Partial removal of pulp is called:
a. Pulp capping
b. Pulpectomy
c. Root canal treatment
d. Pulpotomy.

13. The most toxic form of mercury is:
a. Metal mercury (Hg^+)
b. Ethyl mercury
c. Methyl mercury
d. Mercuric sulfate.

14. The criteria for good endodontic procedures are:
a. It should seal the canal laterally and apically only
b. It should not be impervious to moisture
c. It should not irritate periradicular tissue
d. All of the above.

15. Which of the following induces reparative dentin formation:
a. $Ca(OH)_2$
b. Zinc oxide eugenol
c. Zinc phosphate
d. Silicate cement.

16. Which of the following factors affects biocompatibility:
a. Age
b. Systemic disease
c. Immunity
d. All of the above.

17. The process by which latex is converted to hard rubber by heating with sulfur is called as:
a. Vulcanization
b. Polymerization
c. Oxidation
d. Reduction.

18. Which of the following tests is done for assessing xenoestrogenic activity:
a. Enzyme immunoassay
b. Cytotoxicity
c. Genotoxicity test
d. E-screen test.

19. The phenomenon, where resin material penetrates the collagen network of the dentin 'incompletely' resulting in collagen resin hybrid, is known as:
a. Microleakage
b. Nanoleakage
c. Both
d. None.

20. Which of the following is most appropriate for osseointegration:
a. Steel-Cobalt
b. Ti-Al-Vanadium alloy
c. Ceramic
d. All of the above.

21. Which of the following is the reason for the disadvantage of zinc phosphate cement despite being regarded as 'universal luting cement':
a. Ill-fitting restoration
b. Long setting time
c. Pulp irritation
d. Difficulty in manipulation.

Dental Amalgam

1. Amalgam alloy requirements follow
a. ADA Specification No. 1
b. ADA Specification No. 2
c. ADA Specification No. 13
d. ADA Specification No. 8.

2. Mercury melts at:
a. 100°C
b. –78.36°C
c. 98.65°C
d. –38.87°C.

3. The recommended mercury-alloy ratio for most modern lathe cut alloys is:
a. 2:1
b. 1:2
c. 3:1
d. 1:1.

4. Average mercury levels in patients with amalgam restorations:
a. 0.7 mg/mL
b. 0.5 mg/mL
c. 0.1 mg/mL
d. 0.3 mg/mL.

5. The following are phases of silver amalgam except:
a. β
b. γ
c. ΰ
d. η.

6. The strongest phase of amalgam is:
a. Ag_3-Sn phase
b. Ag-Hg phase
c. Sn-Hg phase
d. Cu-Sn phase

7. Delayed expansion usually accounts for:
a. 5 to 6%
b. 25%
c. 2 to 4%
d. 10 to 15%.

8. Recommended condensation pressure for amalgam is:
a. 10 to 15 pounds/square inch
b. 85 to 100 pounds/square inch
c. 25 to 30 pounds/square inch
d. < 10 pounds/square inch.

9. The weakest phase in amalgam is:
a. Gamma 1 (γ1)
b. Gamma 2 (γ2)
c. Gamma (γ)
d. Beta (β).

10. The chemical compositions of amalgam are the following except:
a. Copper
b. Tin
c. Silver
d. Lead.

11. Surface discoloration on a metal is known as
a. Corrosion
b. Tarnish
c. Trituration
d. Condensation.

12. Mercuroscopic expansion is shown by
a. Zinc containing amalgam
b. High copper unicompositional
c. Low copper
d. High copper admixed.

13. When silver amalgam is mixed and used, 70% of its strength is achieved after:
a. 8 hours
b. 8 days
c. 8 minutes
d. 8 weeks.

14. Final polishing of amalgam should be
a. Immediately
b. After 24 hours
c. After 12 hours
d. After 48 hours.

15. Action of zinc in amalgam is:
a. Scavenger
b. Filler
c. Accelerator
d. Oxidizer.

16. Which phase of amalgam promotes tarnish and corrosion:
a. Gamma 1 (γ1)
b. Gamma (γ)
c. Gamma 2 (γ2)
d. Eta (η).

17. Epsilon phase in dental amalgam is:
a. Ag-Sn
b. Cu_3 Sn
c. Ag_3 Sn
d. Cu_2 Sn.

18. Trituration is:
a. Mixing of amalgam alloy with mercury
b. Surface discoloration of alloy
c. Corrosion of metal
d. Weighing of the alloy.

19. Mulling is the continuation of:
a. Condensation
b. Trimming

c. Trituration
d. Burnishing.

20. Time-dependent plastic deformation is known as:
a. Sag
b. Creep
c. Porosity
d. Delayed expansion.

21. (Eta) η phase is:
a. Sn_3Hg
b. Cu_3Sn
c. Ag_2Hg_3
d. Cu_6Sn_5.

22. High-copper unicompositional amalgam shows creep rate of:
a. 2%
b. 1%
c. 0.2%
d. 0.05%.

23. Mercury in dental amalgam can be replaced by:
a. Gallium/Indium
b. Copper/Manganese
c. Gold/Silver
d. Tin/Lead.

24. β (Beta) phase in dental amalgam is
a. Ag-Sn
b. Cu_3Sn
c. Ag_3Sn
d. Cu_6Sn_5.

25. Silver amalgam was first introduced by:
a. Bales
b. Gilmore
c. GV Black
d. Vermont.

26. Zinc containing amalgam contains:
a. More than 0.01% Zn
b. Less than 0.01% Zn
c. 0.01% Zn
d. 0.001% Zn.

27. Procedure done to smoothen the restoration after carving is:
a. Trimming
b. Burnishing
c. Mulling
d. Condensation.

28. The following is a binary alloy:
a. Silver-tin
b. Silver-tin-copper
c. Silver-tin-copper-indium
d. Silver-tin-copper-gallium.

29. High copper alloys contain:
a. Less than 6% copper
b. More than 10% copper
c. More than 6% copper
d. Less than 5% copper.

30. Low copper alloys are also known as:
a. Conventional alloys
b. Spherical alloys
c. Zinc-free alloys
d. Admixed alloys.

31. Function of palladium is:
a. It reduces strength
b. It increases setting expansion
c. It reduces resistance to tarnish and corrosion
d. It hardens and whitens the alloy.

32. Mercury release occurs if temperature rises above:
a. 80°C
b. 37°C
c. 60°C
d. 100°C.

33. Ageing of alloy is done by heating at:
a. 95°C to 100°C
b. 100°C to 130°C
c. 60°C to 100°C
d. 115°C to 120°C.

34. Working time of amalgam:
a. 1 hour
b. 25 seconds
c. 30 minutes
d. 10 to 20 minutes.

35. The creep value of low copper amalgam is:
a. 0.8 to 8.0%
b. 10 to 25%
c. 0.1 to 0.5%
d. 1 to 5%.

36. The creep value of high copper amalgam is:
a. 0.4 to 0.8%
b. 0.1 to 0.4%
c. 95 to 100%
d. 16 to 20%.

37. Zinc-free alloys contain:
a. Less than 0.01% Zn
b. More than 0.01% Zn
c. Less than 6% Zn
d. More than 6% Zn.

38. Function of platinum is:
a. Hardens the alloy
b. Causes delayed expansion
c. Increases setting expansion
d. Whitens the alloy.

39. Function of copper is:
a. Increases setting expansion
b. Whitens the alloy and acts as scavenger
c. Hardens and whitens the alloy
d. Causes delayed expansion.

40. The composition of silver in low copper alloys is:
a. 63 to 70%
b. 2 to 5%
c. 26 to 28%
d. 80 to 90%.

41. The compressive strength of low copper in one hour is:
a. 145 MPa
b. 510 MPa
c. 262 MPa
d. 431 MPa.

42. Overtriturated mix shows the below features except:
a. Reduced working time
b. Contraction of amalgam
c. Increased tensile strength in high copper alloys
d. Warm mix.

43. Normal mix shows:
a. Shiny surface
b. Increased creep
c. Reduced working time
d. Higher contraction of amalgam.

44. Undertriturated mix shows:
a. Reduced compressive and tensile strength
b. Shiny surface
c. Reduced working time
d. Higher contraction of amalgam.

45. The composition of zinc in admixed alloy is:
a. 1%
b. 2 to 5%
c. 25 to 30%
d. 18%.

46. Based on shape, alloys are classified as follows, except:
a. Lathe-cut alloy
b. Spherical alloy
c. Admixed alloy
d. Ternary alloy.

47. Based on copper content, alloys are classified as follows, except:
a. Low copper
b. Admixed
c. Zinc containing
d. High copper.

48. Primary risk of mercury intoxication is from:
a. Skin
b. Ingestion
c. Inhalation
d. Blood.

Direct Filling Gold

1. A metal which may be drawn readily into sheets is:
a. Ductile
b. Malleable
c. Plastic
d. Elastic.

2. Rockwell test is used:
a. To test resiliency of material
b. To test color
c. To test hardness of a material
d. To test malleability.

3. The density of pure gold is:
a. 20 g/cm^3
b. 10.1 g/cm^3
c. 10.9 g/cm^3
d. 19.3 g/cm^3.

4. A unique and useful property of direct filling gold is:
a. Biocorrosion resistance
b. Biocompatibility
c. Cold-welding
d. High coefficient of thermal conduction.

5. The main disadvantage of gold is the following except:
a. Esthetics
b. High coefficient of thermal conduction
c. It is welded at room temperature
d. Difficulty in manipulation.

6. Which gold foil is used in the manufacture of mat foil?
a. No. 1
b. No. 2
c. No. 3
d. No. 4.

7. The gold, which is fully free of impurities, is:
a. Cohesive gold
b. Noncohesive gold
c. Adhesive gold
d. Neutral gold.

8. Placing the gold foil between the sheets of paper and igniting in a closed container, which type of gold is obtained:
a. Corrugated foil
b. Laminated foil
c. Platinized foil
d. Sintered foil.

9. Platinized foil is obtained by placing:
a. Two platinum foils and in between gold foil
b. Two gold foils and in between platinum foil
c. Gold foil and over that gold particles
d. Carbon particles over platinum and gold.

10. Platinized foil increases the.................of restoration:
a. Thickness
b. Hardness
c. Malleability
d. Density.

11. The latest from of electrolytic gold is an alloy of gold and:
a. Sodium
b. Calcium
c. Carbon
d. Copper.

12. The process which removes the adsorbed gases from the gold foil is known as:
a. Purification
b. Degassing
c. Welding
d. Compaction.

13. Compaction of gold can be done among the following except:
a. Hand mallet
b. Hand cutting
c. Pneumatic vibratory condensers
d. Electrically driven condensers.

14. Low hardness of the gold indicates the presence of:
a. Impurities
b. Gases
c. Porosity
d. Purity.

15. Melting point of gold is:
a. 1000°C
b. 900°C
c. 200°C
d. 1063°C.

16. The percentage of elongation seen in gold is:
a. 10%
b. 9.1%
c. 11.3%
d. 12.8%.

17. Brinell hardness number of pure gold is:
a. 15
b. 20
c. 25
d. 30.

18. The gold restoration is contraindicated except in:
a. Class V cavity
b. Tooth with large pulp chamber
c. Periodontally weakened patient
d. Large carious teeth.

19. Type of gold alloy used for removable partial denture casting is:
a. Type I
b. Type II
c. Type III
d. Type IV.

20. Unit of viscosity is:
a. MPA per second
b. Mg/cm^2
c. cp
d. MMS/Hg.

Dental Composites

1. One of the most widely used resin-matrix ingredients in dental composite is:
a. MMA
b. BIS-GMA
c. PMMA
d. DMAEMA.

2. The units in a polymer are connected by:
a. Ionic bond
b. Covalent bond
c. van der Waals forces
d. Coordinate bond.

3. TEGDMA is added to BIS-GMA to:
a. Decrease fluidity
b. Increase viscosity
c. Decrease viscosity
d. Increase opacity.

4. **The addition of filler particles into resin matrix:**
   a. Decreases viscosity
   b. Decreases radio-opacity
   c. Decreases shrinkage
   d. Decreases workability.
5. **The most commonly used coupling agents is:**
   a. Zirconates
   b. Organo silanes
   c. Titanates
   d. Peroxides.
6. **The initiator used in chemically activated resin is:**
   a. N, N-dimethyl-P-toluidine
   b. Organo silane
   c. Camphoroquinone
   d. Benzoyl peroxide.
7. **Light-activated resins are activated using:**
   a. Visible blue light
   b. UV light
   c. IR light
   d. Visible green light.
8. **The photosensitizer used in light-activated resin is:**
   a. Hydroquinone
   b. Camphoroquinone
   c. Benzoyl peroxide
   d. N, N dimethyl-P-toluidine.
9. **The wavelength of light used for curing is:**
   a. 368 nm
   b. 568 nm
   c. 468 nm
   d. 300 nm.
10. **Inhibitors (Butylated hydroxytoluene) are added to resin systems to:**
    a. Prevent polymerization
    b. Absorb light of N 468 nm wavelength
    c. Increase polymerization
    d. Initiate polymerization.
11. **Metal oxides added to dental composites act as:**
    a. Inhibitors
    b. Coloring agents
    c. Opacifiers
    d. Fillers.
12. **The lamp source that uses xenon gas for production of curing light is:**
    a. QTH lamp
    b. PAC lamp
    c. LED lamp
    d. Argon laser lamp.
13. **The advantage of chemically activated curing process is:**
    a. Good control on working time
    b. Insensitivity to oxygen inhibition
    c. Absence of pore formation
    d. Insensitivity to room illumination.
14. **The materials that can be used with reliable results as a luting agent under metallic restoration are:**
    a. Light-activated composites only
    b. Chemically cured composites only
    c. Both light-cured and chemically cured composites
    d. Composites are contraindicated as luting agents under metallic restorations.
15. **The average size of filler particles in traditional composites is:**
    a. 8 to 12 mm
    b. 0.8 to 1.2 mm
    c. 0.5 to 3 mm
    d. 0 .08 to 1.2 mm.
16. **The composite material that exhibits the best physical and mechanical properties is:**
    a. Hybrid composite
    b. Microfilled composite
    c. Small-particle-filled composite
    d. Traditional composite.
17. **The smoothest surface finish is provided by:**
    a. Traditional composite
    b. Small-particle-filled composite
    c. Hybrid composite
    d. Microfilled composite.
18. **The term 'organic filler' is given to:**
    a. Colloidal silica
    b. PMMA particles
    c. Cured composite particles
    d. Fibrous filler particles.
19. **Most modern hybrid composites consist of:**
    a. Colloidal silica and glass
    b. Quartz and glass
    c. Colloidal silica and amorphous silica
    d. Amorphous silica and quartz.
20. **The best possible finish of composites is obtained by:**
    a. Aluminum oxide discs
    b. Curing against smooth matrix strip

c. Tungsten carbide burs
d. Fine and extrafine polishing pastes.

21. 'Rebonding' technique refers to:
a. Application of bonding agent on contaminated prepared surface of tooth
b. Bonding between filler particles and resin matrix
c. Applying bonding agent over polished finished surface of composite
d. Technique of bonding fractured composite.

22. Coupling agent is used to bond:
a. Filler and resin matrix
b. Metal and ceramic
c. Restorative and enamel
d. Restorative and dentin.

23. Acid etching of enamel:
a. Removes surface debris
b. Produces micropores in enamel
c. Allows for free flow of composite
d. Increases the contact angle.

24. Particle size of microfilled composite is:
a. 1 to 4 mm
b. 0.04 to 0.4 mm
c. 0.6 to 1 mm
d. 4 to 7 mm.

25. Filler used in composite resins:
a. Glass
b. Silica
c. Quartz
d. All of the above.

26. Size of resin tags after etching is
a. 10 μm
b. 20 μm
c. 30 μm
d. 40 μm.

27. Polishable restorative resins are:
a. Microfilled
b. Macrofilled
c. None
d. Both.

28. Concentration of acid used for etching enamel is:
a. 10 to 20%
b. 30 to 50%
c. 20 to 29%
d. More than 50%.

29. Light-curable mixture of composite and glass ionomer is:
a. Compomer
b. Activator
c. Inhibitor
d. Coupling agent.

30. Amine acts as:
a. Initiator
b. Activator
c. Inhibitor
d. Coupling agent.

31. Composite bonds to enamel by:
a. Chemical bond
b. Mechanical bond
c. Ionic bond
d. Covalent bond.

32. The largest type of filler particle is:
a. Microfillers
b. Macrofillers
c. Inserts
d. Midifillers.

33. Microprotection is:
a. Protection of composite by a narrow cavity
b. Protection of the pulp using a base
c. Protection of pulp using varnish
d. Protection of the matrix by the fillers.

34. Macroprotection is:
a. Protection offered by narrow cavity to composite restoration
b. Protection of pulp by base
c. Protection of matrix by filler particle
d. Protection of tooth using crown.

35. Ideal distance of tip of coring light from the surface of composite is:
a. 10 mm
b. 3 to 5 mm
c. 1 to 2 mm
d. > 2 mm.

Calcium Hydroxide, Glass Ionomer Cement, Zinc Polycarboxylate Cement

1. Based on the formulations and their potential uses, GIC used for luting applications is:
a. Type I
b. Type II
c. Type III
d. Type IV.

2. The type of bonding between glass ionomer and tooth structure is:
a. Chemical
b. Mechanical
c. Micromechanical
d. Partly by chemical and partly by mechanical.

3. Calcium hydroxide cement has:
a. Anticariogenic property
b. Low acidity
c. Ability to form reparative dentine
d. Obtundent.

4. Cermet cement is an example of:
a. Resin modified GIC
b. Metal modified GIC
c. Cavity varnish
d. Resin cement.

5. The cement, that is most stimulant to pulp for its repair, is:
a. $ZnPO_4$
b. $Ca(OH)_2$
c. GIC
d. Zinc oxide eugenol.

6. Light curable mixture of composite and glass ionomer is known as:
a. Compomer
b. Conventional composite
c. Hybrid composite
d. Microfilled composite.

7. Fluoride is incorporated into cement:
a. To act as a filler
b. To act as a binder
c. To increase cement bond to calcium of teeth
d. Because it has anticariogenic property.

8. Glass ionomer cement is:
a. A posterior restorative material
b. A root canal sealant
c. An anterior esthetic restorative material
d. A thermal insulating base for silver amalgam.

9. Luting cements must have a film thickness of:
a. 25 to 45 μm
b. 200 to 220 μm
c. 100 to 50 μm
d. 75–95 μm.

10. Zinc polycarboxylate cement bonds better with castings when there is:
a. Pickled surface of casting
b. Electroplated surface with tin
c. Electroplated surface with silver
d. Electroplated surface with gold.

11. Cement that can be used as cavity liner is:
a. Zn oxide eugenol
b. $Ca(OH)_2$
c. Glass ionomer
d. Zn polycarboxylate.

12. Ideal film thickness for luting cement is:
a. 12 μ
b. 15 μ
c. 25 μ
d. 35 μ.

13. Which of the following has maximum solubility?
a. $ZnPO_4$
b. Zn polycarboxylate
c. Glass ionomer
d. Silicate.

14. Glass cermets are:
a. Glass ionomer and silver alloy
b. GIC and gold alloy
c. GIC sintered with silver
d. GIC sintered with tin.

15. Cement with maximum solubility in oral environment is:
a. $ZnPO_4$
b. Zn polycarboxylate
c. Silicate
d. Zn oxide eugenol.

16. Glass ionomer cement is otherwise called except:
a. Crown and bridge cement
b. Polyalkenoate cement
c. GIC
d. Aluminosilicate polyacrylic acid.

17. GIC recommended for liners is:
a. Type I
b. Type II
c. Type III
d. Type IV.

18. GIC recommended for restoration is:
a. Type I
b. Type II
c. Type III
d. Type IV.

19. The following are commercial names of GIC except:
a. Aquacem
b. Chem fil

c. Ketae bond
d. Acqua gel.

20. The powder of GIC contains the following except:
a. Silver
b. Alumina
c. Magnesium
d. Sodium fluoride.

21. The component of powder of glass ionomer cement which acts as ceramic flux is:
a. Sodium
b. Chlorine
c. Fluoride
d. Aluminum.

22. Radiopacity of GIC is provided by:
a. Fluoride
b. Calcium
c. Strontium
d. Aluminum.

23. The main component of liquid of GIC is:
a. Tartaric acid
b. Water
c. Polyacrylic acid
d. Methyl methacrylate.

24. Copolymerizing with the following acids will increase the reactivity and decrease the viscosity of GIC, except:
a. Itaconic acid
b. Maleic acid
c. Tricarboxylic acid
d. Formic acid.

25. Setting time of type I GIC is:
a. 2 to 3 minutes
b. 3 to 4 minutes
c. 4 to 5 minutes
d. 5 to 6 minutes.

26. Setting time of type II GIC is:
a. 5 minutes
b. 9 minutes
c. 8 minutes
d. 7 minutes.

27. Compressive strength of GIC is less than:
a. Silicate cement
b. Zinc phosphate cement
c. Zn polycarboxylate
d. Zinc oxide eugenol.

28. Which type of GIC is relatively biocompatible:
a. Type I
b. Type II
c. Type III
d. Type IV.

29. In mixing of GIC, the plasticity is maintained by:
a. A cool dry glass slab
b. Powder taken in increments
c. Correct powder/liquid ratio
d. Correct mixing time.

30. Mixing time of GIC is:
a. 15 seconds
b. 45 minutes
c. 15 minutes
d. 45 seconds.

31. Mechanical mixing has certain advantages, except:
a. Better properties due to controller P/L ratio
b. Less mixing time required
c. Convenient delivery system
d. More setting time.

32. The GIC after being applied on to the tooth surface is protected with the following, except:
a. Varnish
b. Polyacrylic acid
c. Unfilled light-cured resin bonding agent
d. Cocoa butter.

33. Finishing of glass ionomer restorations done:
a. Within 2 days
b. After 2 days
c. After 24 hours
d. Before 24 hours.

34. Silver alloy admixed GIC is a combination of silver amalgam alloy powder with:
a. Type I GIC powder
b. Type II GIC powder
c. Type III GIC powder
d. Type II GIC liquid.

35. Metal modified glass ionomer cement is not used as anterior restorative material because:
a. Of less fracture toughness
b. It is grey-colored
c. Its anticariogenic property is less
d. It has less tensile strength.

36. The P/L ratio for type II GIC is:
a. 2:1
b. 3:1
c. 4:1
d. 1:2.

37. GIC that is set solely by acid-base reaction is:
a. Light-cured GIC
b. Metal-modified GIC
c. Traditional GIC
d. Conventional GIC.

38. Uses of zinc polycarboxylate cement are all except:
a. As bases and liners
b. As varnish
c. As root canal fillings in endodontics
d. In orthodontics for cementation of bands.

39. Basic ingredient in powder of Zn polycarboxylate cement is:
a. Zinc oxide
b. Magnesium oxide
c. Stannous fluoride
d. Aluminum oxide.

40. The ingredient in powder of Zn polycarboxylate, which acts as a modifier and also aids in sintering, is:
a. Zinc oxide
b. Aluminum oxide
c. Bismuth oxide
d. Magnesium oxide.

41. The P/L ratio of type I GIC is
a. 2:1
b. 3:1
c. 1.5:1
d. 2.5:1.

42. Setting time of zinc polycarboxylate cements is:
a. 6 to 7 minutes
b. 7 to 8 minutes
c. 7 to 9 minutes
d. 6 to 9 minutes.

43. pH of zinc polycarboxylate cement is:
a. 1 to 1.7
b. 3 to 4
c. 4 to 5
d. 5 to 6.

44. Zinc polycarboxylate cement is opaque due to the presence of:
a. Fluoride
b. Strontium
c. Unreacted zinc oxide
d. Barium.

45. P/L ratio of zinc polycarboxylate cement is:
a. 1:1
b. 2:1.5
c. 2.5:1
d. 1.5:1.

46. Calcium hydroxide cement is used as following except:
a. As liners
b. As baser
c. As direct and indirect pulp cappers
d. As permanent restoration.

47. The component which provides radiopacity in calcium hydroxide base paste is:
a. Zinc oxide
b. Fluoride
c. Calcium tungstate
d. Aluminum.

48. Accelerator used in catalyst paste of calcium hydroxide cement is:
a. Sulfur
b. Zinc oxide
c. Calcium hydroxide
d. Zinc stearate.

49. Setting time of calcium hydroxide cement is:
a. 1 to 2 minutes
b. 1.5 to 2.5 minutes
c. 2.5 to 3.5 minutes
d. 2.5 to 5.5 minutes.

50. pH of calcium hydroxide cement is:
a. 4 to 5
b. 5.5 to 6
c. 9.2 to 11.7
d. 10.3 to 12.5.

Silicate Cement, Zinc Phosphate Cement, Zinc Oxide Eugenol Cement, Cavity Liners and Varnishes

1. Severe pulpal response is observed in:
a. Glass ionomer
b. Zinc phosphate
c. Zinc oxide eugenol
d. Silicate cement.

2. All are true about varnishes, except that:
a. They form a coating by evaporation of the solvent
b. They are set by chemical reaction
c. They should not be employed under composite restoration
d. They are not indicated when GIC is used.

3. **Following cements are used as cavity liners, except:**
   a. Calcium hydroxide
   b. Type IV ZOE
   c. GIC
   d. Zinc phosphate.
4. **The purpose of calcium hydroxide as a liner is to promote:**
   a. Primary dentin formation
   b. Secondary dentin formation
   c. Reparative dentin formation
   d. Pre-dentin formation.
5. **The main ingredients of powder in zinc phosphate cement are:**
   a. Zinc oxide: 30%; Aluminum oxide: 70%
   b. Magnesium oxide: 90%; Zinc oxide: 10%
   c. Zinc oxide: 90%; Magnesium oxide: 10%
   d. Aluminium oxide: 30%; Zinc oxide: 70%.
6. **Type of Zinc Oxide Eugenol used for sedative dressings:**
   a. Type I ZnOE
   b. Type II ZnOE
   c. Type III ZnOE
   d. Type IV ZnOE.
7. **In zinc phosphate cement, aluminum acts as a:**
   a. Opacifier
   b. Accelerator
   c. Buffer
   d. Retarder.
8. **Silicate cement is contraindicated in:**
   a. Mouth breathers
   b. Diabetic patient
   c. Thumb sucker
   d. Hypertensive patient.
9. **Type of ZOE used for temporary restoration:**
   a. Type I
   b. Type II
   c. Type III
   d. Type IV.
10. **Which of the following cements acts as a cavity liner:**
    a. Type III GIC
    b. Type IV ZNOE cement
    c. Suspension of calcium hydroxide
    d. Type I ZOE.
11. **Zinc oxide eugenol, zinc polycarboxylate cements are similar in respect to:**
    a. Strength
    b. pH
    c. Chelation
    d. Working time.
12. **pH of Zinc phosphate cement after 1 hour of mixing is:**
    a. 3
    b. 4
    c. 5
    d. 7.
13. **Varnishes protect pulp from:**
    a. Chemical insult
    b. Thermal insult
    c. Mechanical insult
    d. Electrical insult.
14. **Purpose of water used in liquid of zinc phosphate cement is to:**
    a. Control the ionization of acid
    b. Decrease the concentration of acid
    c. Increase the setting tlme
    d. Decrease the setting time.
15. **Cement that is least irritating to pulp:**
    a. ZOE
    b. Zinc phosphate
    c. Silicate cement
    d. Glass ionomer cement.
16. **The role of orthomethoxy benzoic acid in ZOE is to:**
    a. Increase the strength
    b. Increase the setting time
    c. Increase the working time
    d. Increase the mixing time.
17. **Role of fluoride salts in silicate cements**
    a. Increase the fusion temperature of glass
    b. Anticariogenic property
    c. Increase the strength
    d. Decrease the strength.
18. **Following cements are set by acid-base reaction except:**
    a. ZOE
    b. Zinc polycarboxylate
    c. Glass ionomer
    d. Compomer.
19. **Compressive strength of zinc phosphate cement is:**
    a. 104 MPa
    b. 410 MPa
    c. 140 MPa
    d. 145 MPa.

20. By reducing powder-liquid ratio of zinc phosphate cement:
a. Working time is decreased
b. Setting time is increased
c. Tensile strength is decreased
d. Compressive strength is increased.

21. Following cements have anticariogenic property except:
a. Silicate cement
b. Glass ionomer cement (Type II)
c. Cermet
d. ZOE.

22. Cement that is most stimulant to pulp for its repair is:
a. Zinc phosphate cement
b. Calcium hydroxide
c. Glass ionomer cement
d. ZOE.

23. Cavity varnishes are
a. Natural gums dissolved in organic solvent
b. Natural resins
c. Wooden extracts
d. Nothing but cement.

24. Varnishes are contraindicated in:
a. Amalgam
b. GIC
c. ZOE
d. Zinc phosphate.

25. Compressive strength of zinc phosphate (luting) cement is:
a. 93 to 135 MPa
b. 100 to 350 MPa
c. 90 to 328 MPa
d. 328 to 400 MPa.

26. Liners are applied mainly on:
a. Cavosurface
b. Pulpal floor
c. Buccal lingual walls
d. Gingival seat.

27. Film thickness of zinc phosphate cement should be:
a. 50 μm
b. 40 μm
c. 18 μm
d. 25 μm.

28. Setting time of zinc phosphate cement is:
a. 2.8 to 5 minutes
b. 2.5 to 8 seconds
c. 2.5 to 8 minutes
d. 2.8 to 5 seconds.

29. pH of zinc oxide eugenol cement is:
a. 8
b. 9
c. 7
d. 5.

30. Which of the following is permanent luting type of ZOE:
a. Type I
b. Type II
c. Type III
d. Type IV.

31. Compressive strength of ZOE:
a. 3 to 55 MPa
b. 55 to 60 MPa
c. 140 MPa
d. 401 MPa.

32. In zinc phosphate cements, reaction between powder and liquid is:
a. Endothermic
b. Mesothermic
c. Exothermic
d. Chelation.

33. Powder: liquid ratio of zinc phosphate cement is:
a. 1.4 g of powder, 0.5 mL of liquid
b. 1.5 m of powder, 0.9 mL of liquid
c. 1.9 g of powder, 0.5 mL of liquid
d. 1 g of powder, 0.5 mL of liquid.

34. Tensile strength of zinc phosphate cement is:
a. 5.5 MPa
b. 6.6 MPa
c. 7.7 MPa
d. 8.8 MPa.

35. For temporary luting, the type of ZOE used is:
a. Type I
b. Type II
c. Type III
d. Type IV.

36. Following methods are used to compensate the exothermic reaction in zinc phosphate cement, except:
a. Mixing in wider area
b. Using cool glass slab
c. By refrigerating the liquid
d. Mixing in increments.

37. Modulus of elasticity of zinc phosphate is:
a. 17.3 GPa
b. 13.7 GPa

c. 71.3 GPa
d. 3.71 GPa.

38. Cement that is used as root canal sealer and periodontal dressings is:
a. Zinc phosphate cement
b. Silicate cement
c. ZnOE
d. GIC.

39. In ZOE, acetic acid acts as a:
a. Retarder
b. Buffer
c. Opacifier
d. Catalyst.

Tarnish and Corrosion

1. The process, by which a vital surface gets dull in brightness or discolored through the formation of a chemical film, is called:
a. Erosion
b. Corrosion
c. Abrasion
d. Tarnish.

2. Discoloration of silver by sulfur is a:
a. Dry corrosion
b. Wet corrosion
c. Electrochemical corrosion
d. Tarnish.

3. Dissimilar metal contact is otherwise called:
a. Crevice corrosion
b. Stern corrosion
c. Galvanic corrosion
d. Pitting corrosion.

4. Noble metal will not corrode because:
a. EMF is neutral
b. EMF is +ve
c. EMF is –ve
d. All of the above.

5. Noble metals possess:
a. More +ve electrode potential
b. Less +ve electrode potential
c. More –ve electrode potential
d. Not related to electrode potential.

6. Corrosion rate of Ni is reduced by:
a. Coating Ni with paint
b. Coating Ni with Zn
c. Coating Ni with Al
d. Coating Ni with chromium oxide.

7. Gold has electrode potential of:
a. + 1.36 V
b. + 0.86 V
c. + 0.80 V
d. + 1.50 V.

8. Corrosion is actually:
a. Surface deposit
b. Deterioration of metal
c. Surface discoloration
d. Disintegration of metal.

9. Crevice corrosion occurs:
a. Between restoration and tooth
b. On restoration dentin
c. On surface of restoration
d. On margin of restoration.

10. The correct statement is:
a. Corrosion is a forerunner of tarnish
b. Tarnish is a forerunner of corrosion
c. Tarnish and corrosion are not related to each other
d. Tarnish causes pitting of restoration.

11. The most important factor causing surface tarnish on a metal is:
a. Sulfides
b. Phosphate
c. Fluorides
d. Iodides.

12. Dry corrosion occurs in:
a. Absence of fluid electrolyte
b. Presence of fluid electrolyte
c. Presence of water
d. Absence of water.

13. Presence of amalgam and gold restorations on opposing teeth causes:
a. Stress corrosion
b. Galvanic corrosion
c. Crevice corrosion
d. Pitting of surface.

14. Galvanic shock is reduced by:
a. Coating with varnish
b. Coating with base
c. Adding more amalgam
d. Reducing the amount of gold.

15. An example of good passive metal:
a. Si
b. Cr

c. Fe
d. Mg.

16. Corrosion is a .... process.
a. Electromechanical
b. Electrochemical
c. Physicochemical
d. Physicomechanical.

17. Iron is alloyed with chromium to provide:
a. Physical resistance to corrosion
b. Mechanical resistance to corrosion
c. Chemical resistance to corrosion
d. Biological resistance to corrosion.

18. Which of the following alloys has superior resistance to corrosion against chlorides:
a. Stainless steel
b. Nickel-Chromium
c. Cobalt-Chromium
d. Titanium alloys.

19. Variation in electrolyte level causes
a. Tarnish
b. Concentration cell corrosion
c. Crevice corrosion
d. Pitting.

20. The potential difference when gold and amalgam restoration is in contact is:
a. 500 mv
b. 540 mv
c. 530 mv
d. 580 mv.

Answers to Multiple Choice Questions

Prosthodontics

Physical and Mechanical Properties

1. c
2. c
3. b
4. c
5. c
6. a
7. d
8. c
9. c
10. b
11. d
12. c
13. a
14. d
15. a
16. c
17. d
18. a
19. d
20. a
21. c
22. a
23. c
24. b
25. d
26. c

Casting, Investments and Procedures

1. d
2. a
3. d
4. a
5. b
6. c
7. c
8. a
9. c
10. b
11. c
12. c

Dental Ceramics

1. b
2. a
3. d
4. b
5. a
6. c
7. a
8. d
9. c
10. c

Dental Waxes

1. a
2. a
3. b
4. a

Wrought Metal Alloys

1. c
2. a
3. a
4. b
5. b
6. d

Dental Casting and Soldering of Alloys

1. b
2. a
3. b
4. a
5. c
6. b
7. a
8. d
9. a
10. b
11. b
12. b
13. c
14. d
15. b
16. b

Denture-base Resins

1. b
2. a
3. c
4. a
5. a
6. d
7. c
8. d
9. d
10. b
11. b
12. d
13. b
14. d
15. d
16. c

Impression Materials

1. a
2. b
3. d
4. a
5. a
6. a
7. c
8. d
9. c
10. a
11. b
12. a
13. d
14. d
15. a
16. b
17. d
18. c
19. c
20. c
21. d
22. a
23. d
24. d
25. a
26. c
27. c
28. b
29. d
30. a
31. d
32. a
33. c
34. d
35. c
36. a
37. a
38. c

Properties

1. b
2. a
3. a
4. c
5. d
6. c
7. b
8. b
9. c
10. a
11. a
12. b
13. a
14. c
15. b
16. c
17. d
18. a
19. a
20. c
21. c
22. c
23. d
24. c
25. c

Metallurgy

1. d
2. c
3. c
4. b
5. a
6. a
7. a
8. c
9. b
10. c
11. b
12. d
13. a
14. a
15. b
16. c

Polymers and Denture-base Resins

1. c
2. a
3. c
4. a
5. a
6. b
7. c
8. a
9. c
10. d
11. b
12. a
13. a
14. c
15. b
16. d
17. d
18. d
19. a
20. c
21. a
22. c

Implant Materials

1. c
2. b
3. c
4. a
5. a

Gypsum Products

1. b
2. c
3. b
4. a
5. a
6. a
7. a
8. a
9. a
10. a
11. a
12. a
13. a
14. c
15. b
16. d
17. a
18. c
19. b
20. b
21. c

Impression Materials

1. d
2. b
3. b
4. c
5. a
6. a
7. d
8. c
9. b
10. d
11. d
12. a
13. c
14. b
15. b
16. d
17. c
18. b
19. b
20. a
21. c
22. a
23. c
24. d
25. b
26. b
27. c
28. c
29. c
30. c
31. a
32. b
33. a
34. b
35. c
36. d
37. a
38. a
39. b

Casting Alloys, Waxes, Investment Procedures

1. a
2. a
3. b
4. d
5. b
6. a
7. c
8. d
9. d
10. a
11. a
12. a
13. d
14. b
15. d
16. c
17. d
18. a
19. b
20. c
21. c
22. b
23. c
24. b
25. d
26. d
27. b
28. d
29. b
30. b
31. b
32. b
33. d
34. c
35. c
36. a
37. b
38. c
39. c
40. c
41. a
42. d
43. a
44. c

Finishing and Polishing Materials

1. a
2. c
3. a
4. c
5. a
6. a
7. c

Wrought Metal Alloys

1. d
2. b
3. c
4. c
5. c
6. b
7. c

Conservative Dentistry

Biocompatibility

1. b
2. c
3. b
4. d
5. c
6. a
7. d
8. a
9. a
10. d
11. a
12. d
13. c
14. d
15. a
16. d
17. a
18. d
19. b
20. b
21. c

Dental Amalgam

1. a
2. b
3. d
4. a
5. c
6. a
7. c
8. a
9. b
10. d
11. b
12. c
13. a
14. b
15. a
16. c
17. b
18. a
19. c
20. b
21. d
22. d
23. a
24. a
25. c
26. a
27. b
28. a
29. c
30. a
31. d
32. c
33. c
34. d
35. a
36. b
37. a
38. a
39. a
40. a
41. a
42. c
43. a
44. a
45. a
46. d
47. c
48. c

Direct Filling Gold

1. b
2. c
3. d
4. c
5. c
6. b
7. a
8. a
9. b
10. b
11. b
12. b
13. b
14. c
15. d
16. d
17. c
18. a
19. d
20. c

Dental Composites

1. b
2. b
3. c
4. c
5. b
6. d
7. a
8. b
9. c
10. a
11. c
12. b
13. d
14. b
15. a
16. c
17. d
18. c
19. a
20. b
21. c
22. a
23. b
24. b
25. d
26. a
27. a
28. b
29. a
30. b
31. b
32. c
33. d
34. a
35. c

Calcium Hydroxide, Glass Ionomer Cement, Zinc Polycarboxylate Cement

1. a
2. a
3. c
4. b
5. b
6. a
7. c
8. c
9. a
10. b
11. b
12. c
13. d
14. a
15. c
16. a
17. c
18. b
19. c
20. c
21. c
22. c
23. c
24. d
25. c
26. d
27. a
28. b
29. a
30. d
31. d
32. b
33. c
34. b
35. b
36. b
37. d
38. b
39. a
40. d
41. c
42. c
43. d
44. b
45. d
46. d
47. c
48. d
49. d
50. c

Silicate Cement, Zinc Phosphate Cement, Zinc Oxide Eugenol Cement, Cavity Liners and Varnishes

1. d
2. b
3. d
4. c
5. c
6. a
7. b
8. a
9. c
10. c
11. c
12. b
13. a
14. a
15. a
16. a
17. b
18. d
19. a
20. b
21. d
22. b
23. a
24. b
25. b
26. b
27. c
28. c
29. c
30. b
31. a
32. c
33. a
34. a
35. a
36. c
37. b
38. c
39. d

Tarnish and Corrosion

1. d
2. a
3. c
4. b
5. b
6. d
7. d
8. b
9. c
10. b
11. a
12. a
13. b
14. a
15. b
16. b
17. c
18. d
19. d
20. a

Invited Review Articles

1. Recent Advances in Restorative Dental Materials.

INTRODUCTION

Dental biomaterials science is a rapidly growing area, especially the fields of adhesive systems and tooth-colored restorative materials. With all the advances in dental restorative materials, clinicians these days are facing a paradigm shift in material selection. Often the advances in physicomechanical properties are the only aspect that are considered for improving the clinical efficacy of restorative materials. It should be recognized that the true clinical performance of a restorative material can be established only after appropriate clinical investigations. Therefore, it is vital to carry out more effective clinical investigations with restorative materials for adequate period of time, before they are applied clinically. However, most dental materials are introduced into the market even before adequate clinical investigation is carried out. Clinicians today have a plethora of new materials to choose from though most of these products are brought to the market without proper clinical or laboratory-based testing. This review focuses on the recent developments in indirect and direct restorative materials, mostly based on clinical investigations.

DIRECT RESTORATIVE MATERIALS

Dental Amalgam

Modern amalgam restoration is an alloy composed of mercury, silver, tin and copper along with other metallic elements added to improve the physical and mechanical properties of the final restoration.[1] Amalgam restorations have various advantages over other direct restorations. They demonstrate particularly high resistance to wear, ability to tolerate wide range of oral environments (especially wetness), and excellent load-bearing properties.[2-4] However, the recent drop in the clinical usage of amalgam is primarily due to its poor esthetics, potential for toxicity, and ease of manipulation of other available materials. Another argument against the usage of amalgam is that these restorations are responsible for cuspal fractures, while bonded or adhesive restorations are not. Interestingly, a recent study has concluded that the reason behind increased number of cuspal fractures in teeth restored with amalgam as compared to other materials is because of the sheer high numbers of teeth restored with amalgam and not because of the true fracture rate or the properties of amalgam as a restorative material.[5]

Research on amalgam in the recent times has been less on the material aspects of amalgam, and more on the toxicity and environmental hazards caused by amalgam. Although biocompatibility, toxicity and allergic potential of mercury have been subjects of great concern, it has been suggested that the quantity of elemental mercury vapor, released from amalgam restorations during chewing is less than one-half of the estimated natural daily exposure.[6] The possibility of localized allergic reactions to amalgam has also been highlighted[7], but one of the recent studies has suggested low prevalence of such allergies.[8] The Federal Health Agencies in the United States of America have investigated the biocompatibility of amalgam. Mercury level of urine was chosen as the biomarker in this study and it was concluded that individuals having more than 20 dental amalgam surfaces in the mouth present the possibility of having the mean urine mercury concentration higher than that of the general population.[9] Major health organizations such as the National Institute of Dental and Craniofacial Research (NIDCR), the Centers for Disease Control and Prevention (CDC) and the US Food and Drug Administration (FDA), World Health Organization (WHO) and Federation Dentaire International (FDI) have declared dental amalgam safe and effective.[1]

In 2003, American Dental Association (ADA) Council on Scientific Affairs proposed certain guidelines to minimize mercury vapor exposure to dental professionals and prevent environmental hazard risk.[10] These guidelines include: 1. training all personnel in handling products of mercury; 2. making staffs aware of potential sources of mercury vapor; 3. working in well-ventilated spaces; 4. periodically checking the levels of mercury vapors in the dental operatory; 5. using proper work area design to minimize spills; 6. using only precapsulated alloys; 7. using amalgamators with a completely enclosed triturating arm; 8. using care in handling amalgam and recap single-use capsules; 9. following disposal regulations; 10. using high-volume evacuation; 11. salvaging and storing all scrap amalgam; 12 recycling scrap amalgam where feasible; 13. disposing mercury contaminated items in sealed bags according to applicable regulations; 14. cleaning up spilled mercury properly using trap bottles, tapes, or freshly mixed amalgams; and 15. removing professional clothing before leaving the workplace. More information regarding the safety regulations by ADA can be found elsewhere.[10]

Glass Ionomer Cements

Glass ionomer cements (GICs) have unique advantages such as the ability to form a physicochemical bond to the tooth structure, release fluoride,[11] ability to recharge the fluoride from fluoride varnishes and gels,[12] and coefficient of thermal expansion closer to that of dental hard tissues. Conventional GIC is a water-based material which sets by an acid-base reaction between polyalkenoic acid and flouroaluminosilicate glass. They are available in the market as Ketac Fil, Chemfil (Espe, Seefeld, Germany) and Fuji II (GC, Tokyo, Japan). GICs are recommended for small restorations and in low load-bearing areas due to their early wear resistance. However, limitations such as low wear resistance, high technique sensitivity, moisture susceptibility, poor esthetics due to high opacity and inferior flexural strength have led to the development of several new modifications in conventional GICs.

Metal reinforced GICs incorporate: 1. metal powders (silver-tin alloy) (Miracle mix); or 2. metal that is sintered to the glass (glass cermet cements) in GICs. The addition of silver-tin alloy powder to conventional GIC material increases the wear resistance of the cement, at the expense of esthetics.[13] Cermet cement does not show improved wear resistance and the amount of fluoride released from this material has been found to be insufficient for clinical benefits.[13,14] Resin Modified Glass Ionomer Cements (RMGICs) contain a small quantity of resin, such as HEMA, which, along with the activators, make this material sensitive to light activation without overwhelming the acid-base reaction.[15] Immediate stabilization of the water balance followed by light activation is the most significant advantage of this material. RMGICs have displayed better esthetic properties, improved strength and fracture toughness. The drawbacks of this material include marginal instability,[16] along with reduced direct adhesion and polyelectric characteristics, the amount of fluoride release is also less. RMGICs are continually being modified and specific products are now available according to different applications. Examples of some of the RMGIC products for restoration are Vitremer, Photac-Fil and Fuji II LC, while RMGICs for luting purposes are Rely X and Fuji Plus.[17]

GICs with higher powder-to-liquid ratio, lower water content, and smaller glass particles known as High Viscosity GICs (HVGICs) were introduced to improve the load-bearing properties of GIC. According to the manufacturers, the HVGICs could be packable like amalgam and will exhibit enhanced flexural strength characteristics. Yet the initial wear measured in vitro and the observed clinical wear during the first year contraindicate their use. Examples of these materials are non-metal-reinforced: Fuji IX, Ketac Molar; metal-reinforced: Hi Dense. New improved HVGICs with fast setting properties, such as Fuji IX Fast and Ketac Molar Quick, have also been introduced. Compared to their 'regular-set' analogues (Fuji IX and Ketac Molar), the time needed prior to finishing was reduced from 6 minutes to 3 minutes in the improved HVGICs. Further, except for hardness, no differences in mechanical properties (compressive strength, diametric tensile strength, and two-body wear) were observed between the regular-set Fuji IX and fast-setting Fuji IX Fast during the first week.[18,19] With growing interest in Atraumatic Restorative Treatment (ART) and Minimally Invasive (MI) treatment procedures, HVGICs are being looked up as a better alternative to amalgam.[20] Currently, attempts are being made to develop GICs with antibacterial effects. This is achieved by the addition of bactericides such as chlorhexidine in GIC.[21,22] Nevertheless the effect of addition of bactericides on the physico-mechanical properties of GIC and their clinical implications needs further investigations.

Biocompatibility of GICs

Conventional GICs are said to be biocompatible with little potential for tissue irritation or other adverse responses.[1] Postoperative sensitivity with GICs has been reported but it may be a consequence of placement technique rather than due to the direct effect of the material.[23] Conventional GICs have been shown to possess better biocompatibility than resin-modified glass-ionomers.[24-26] The cytotoxicity of RMGICs is attributed to the leachable resin components such as 2-hydroxyethyl methacrylate (HEMA)[26,27] present in the cement. HEMA can diffuse through dentinal tubules[28] and cause cytotoxic effects. However, this issue needs further investigation, since no conclusive evidence of any systemic or localized cytotoxic effects was reported.[29,30] In vivo studies have demonstrated that RMGICs are biologically acceptable.[31]

Compomers

Compomers are one of the recently introduced restorative materials. They are composite resin/ glass ionomer hybrids that combine the desirable properties of both in one material. They resemble composite resins in their mechanical strength, while their setting reaction is closer to that of GIC.[32] Compomers are one-paste, light-cured material, containing a dimethacrylate forming matrix with an ion-leachable glass as filler. The initial setting of the material is achieved by light curing (free radicals activated by light) followed by a limited acid/base reaction initiated by water ingress.[33] To ensure bonding between the matrix and the glass particles, the glass particles are partially silanized.[34] The ingress of water is useful because the expansion of compomers can offset the shrinkage by polymerization. On the other hand, this expansion can also lead to fracture which is a disadvantage.[32] Compomers are able to release fluoride and offer excellent esthetics.[35]

They are easy to manipulate and do not require mixing. Compomers demonstrate lesser wear resistance than composites and inability to bond to dentine like GICs. Yet, because of their ease of use and fluoride-releasing function, they are recommended for restoration of primary teeth.[36,37] Improvements in the properties of compomers with different types of monomers are being reported but long-term studies are warranted to validate their clinical performance.[38]

Giomer

Giomer is yet another attempt to combine GICs and composite resins to produce a material which has desirable properties of both. Giomers are resin-based material containing pre-reacted glass ionomer (PRG) particles. These particles are made up of fluorosilicate glass that has been reacted with polyalkenoic acid in water prior to being incorporated into the resin.[39,40] The pre-reaction can be of two types: 1. involving the surface of the glass particles (called surface pre-reacted glass ionomer or S-PRG) only and 2. involving the entire particle (termed fully pre-reacted glass ionomer or F-PRG). Giomers are more of a composite resin than glass ionomer since they are light-activated and can make use of a bonding agent to adhere to the tooth.

Giomers are mainly indicated for Non-Carious Cervical Lesions (NCCLs), Class V cavities, deciduous teeth and root lesions. They are available in one-paste form, and the currently available giomers are Beautifil (Shofu Inc, Kyoto, Japan) and Reactmer (Shofu Inc, Kyoto, Japan). Although it is a promising new material, few studies are available to date on its clinical efficacy. Fluoride release is an important advantage of Giomers. Consequently, they have been found effective in preventing caries, especially when used with a fluoride-releasing adhesive.[41] In a more recent study, a giomer (Reactmer) has been found effective in giving rise to a caries inhibition zone around the restoration.[42] In another study, the demineralization inhibition effect of giomers at the margins of restorations has been reported.[43] Some evidence of ion movement within the hydrophilic portion of the resin matrix has been reported and this is said to play a role in their caries preventive effect.[44] In addition, giomers have been found to have a fluoride-recharging effect.[39,40] The esthetics offered by giomers is significantly better than conventional and RMGICs, and is comparable to composite resins and compomers.[39,40] They are biologically compatible with vital pulps.[45,46] However, giomers, when subjected to water sorption, exhibit rapid and extensive expansion and, therefore, should be avoided in tooth preparations that involve thin unsupported enamel.[47] Also, in case of recurrent caries, they are not as beneficial as GICs.[48]

Ormocers

Most of the changes in composite resins have been occurring in terms of filler content, while ormocers are modification of composite resin in the type of monomer used. They have an inorganic/organic copolymer system based on multifunctional urethane and thioether (meth)-acrylate alkoxysilanes (Definate, Degassua, Hanau, Germany).[49] An ormocer-based composite has been established by the name Admira, which has a consistency corresponding to that of conventional hybrid composite resin. Admira has been later modified to a chemically identical, but lower-filled and, thus, low-viscous, flowable version known as Admira Flow. Ormocers are synthesized through a solution and gelation process (sol-gel process) and consists of 3-dimensionally cross-linked copolymers. The increased level of polymerization in these materials results in no residual monomer after curing. Consequently, ormocers show greater biocompatibility with tissues. Further, they have been known to have good wear resistance.[50]

Ormocers are showing promising data in short-term clinical studies[51,52] and some laboratory studies,[53–55] but according to a recent cyclic load testing, which evaluated the marginal and internal cavity adaptation of ormocers, their performance was suggested to be inferior to that of hybrid composite resins.[56] However, because of their greater biocompatibility and lower wear rate, these have been recommended for bonding of orthodontic brackets.[57]

Composite Resins

Composite resin materials are used to restore cavities, reconstruct anterior teeth, function as a core preparation for crowns, correct stains, attritions and erosion, fabricate provisional restorations, secure orthodontic brackets, and as a luting cement. These are highly esthetic material and have been originally designed for anterior restorations, but with the increasing concern of esthetics in patients, these materials have been further improved, and are now used in nearly all classes and types of dental restorations. While they are generally not as strong or durable as metals and amalgams, they have shown some promising performances in clinical studies of Class I and Class II restorations[1]. Some of the composite resins showed early fluoride releasing properties, while failed to show any evidence of fluoride uptake.[58,59]

Modern composite resins have a highly filled resin matrix, with inorganic glass fillers based on improved cross-linking polymers formulated from biphenyl glycide methacrylate (bis-GMA) or urethane dimethacrylate (UDMA) resins. Other components have been included to improve the efficacy of the combination and initiate polymerization. The resin matrix consists of monomers, an initiator system, stabilizers and pigments. The inorganic filler consists of particles such as glass, quartz and colloidal silica. The matrix and filler are bonded together with a coupling agent. The final clinical performance of composite resins depends upon its basic composition.[60] The recent improvement in these materials has been mainly focusing on filler technology, but the resin monomers have remained largely unmodified. It should be recognized that the greater the amounts of filler, the better will be the mechanical properties, while reducing the filler particle size would enhance the polishability of the final restoration. The type of filler and resin, the nature of polymerization and water sorption influence the optical properties of the final restoration.[61]

The resins such as bis-GMA currently employed in composite resins are extremely viscous under ambient conditions due to hydrogen bonding by hydroxyl groups.[61] Therefore, chemicals such as TEGDMA are added in various concentrations to resin to dilute bis-GMA. TEGDMA has a low molecular weight and enables to lower the viscosity of bis-GMA. This enables the addition of fillers and allows greater amounts of cross-linking within the polymer chains. This greater conversion and cross-linking of polymer chains is both advantageous and disadvantageous. On the one hand, it increases the resistance of the resin matrix to solvents;[62] on the other hand, it increases the polymerization shrinkage.[63] Volumetric polymerization shrinkage in the range of 1.9 to 7.1 percent is observed during polymerization.[64] The stresses produced due to polymerization shrinkage can cause failure of the tooth restoration interface. The polymerization shrinkage can be reduced by increasing the amount of filler particles. The commonly used fillers are aluminum and lithium. Barium, zinc, boron and yttrium are added to increase the radiolucency, while ytterbium fluoride is added to impart fluoride-releasing property to composite resins.[65] In this review, packable, flowable and nanofilled composite resin types are discussed further, since these are relatively new classes of composite resins.

Packable Composite Resins

Packable composite resins have been introduced to replace amalgam as a posterior restoration. This material has been claimed to overcome the drawbacks usually associated with posterior composite restoration such as loss of marginal integrity, postoperative sensitivity, increased wear, and difficulties in obtaining ideal interproximal contacts, when compared to metallic restorations.[66] Packable composite resins have also been called condensable composite resins, which is a misnomer because they are only packed and do not undergo condensation during restoration.[65] Currently, there are several packable resin composites in the market: SureFil Alert (Jeneric/Pentron), Solitaire 2 (Heraeus (Dentsply/Caulk), Kulzer), Prodigy Condensable (SDS/ Kerr), Filtek P60 (3M ESPE), Tetric Ceram HB (Ivoclar Vivadent), and Pyramid (Bisco). They have a high viscosity and are similar to amalgam in handling properties. In an attempt to make them appear similar to amalgam, some of the resins (e.g., Alert, SureFil) are packaged in blister packs that differ by spill size. SureFil also comes with an amalgam carrier which can be used to place it into the preparation. These materials are packed with amalgam condensers and are used with traditional metal matrix bands and wooden wedges. Packable composite resins are more viscous and stiffer than conventional composite resins. The mechanical properties of composites vary due to different types and quantities of fillers and viscosity modifiers used.[50,67] Apart from the handling and manipulating properties, no considerable difference in the clinical performance of packable and hybrid composites has been reported.[68,69] In a recent study on the clinical performance of packable (Surefil, Dentsply) and conventional hybrid (SpectrumTPH, Dentsply) composite resins for posterior restorations after 3.5 years, it was concluded that the clinical performances of both the above composite resins are similar and satisfactory for the restoring Class 1 and moderate-sized Class 2 cavities.[71] However, because of the increased risk of bulk fracture, use of the either composite resin type should be avoided in large intracoronal Class 2 molar restorations.[70]

Additionally, some studies have reported no difference in the tightness or contours of proximal contacts created with a packable or hybrid composite.[72,73] Another drawback for this material is that manufacturers have recommended bulk placement (usually 5 mm thick). It is important to note that none of these products can be adequately polymerized to a 5 mm depth.[71,74,75] In a recent in vitro study, placement techniques for composite resin increments versus bulk loading were compared. This study highlighted significantly lower mean gap formation for incremental placement technique (6.1%) when compared to the bulk condensation technique (18.7%).[76] Bisco and 3M ESPE no longer recommend bulk placement.

Flowable Composites

In a flowable composite, the filler particles are similar but the filler volume is lower than conventional direct composite resins. Consequently, these materials have a decreased viscosity, which makes them a good choice as a pit and fissure restorative. The flowable composite resins has been reported to have more water sorption than conventional composites, and high modulus of resilience than conventional resins.[77] However, they have increased shrinkage.[78] and decreased strength, and are not recommended in high-stress areas. They have less fluoride release as compared to the other composite resin materials. They have been recommended as: (1) class V restorative as they have good marginal adaptation to dentine,[79] (2) pit and fissure sealant, repair of marginal defects or as liners in deep cavities. Their higher flexure strength may enable them to serve as stress absorbers during such applications.[64,80]

Nanofilled Composite Resin

Nanocomposites are unique from other composite resins in that they contain nano-sized fillers. They have been marketed under the brand name Filtek Supreme since 2003. This product has nonagglomerated discrete nanoparticles (20–75 nm in diameter) called nanomers that are homogenously distributed in nanoclusters which are loosely bound agglomerates of nanosized particles. Manufacturers claim to combine the strength of hybrid resins and the polishability of microfill resins in nanofilled composite resin. It comes in 30 different shades and 4 different opacities (dentin, body, enamel and translucent). Most shades contain a combination of nonagglomerated 20-nm-sized nanosilica filler and aggregated zirconia/silica nanocluster (primarily 5- to 20-nm in size) filler. The cluster particle size ranges from 0.6 to 1.4 microns. The combination of nanomer-sized particles and the nanocluster formulations reduces the interstitial spacing of the filler particles. Decrease in particle size results in less interparticle spacing, more protection of the softer resin matrix, and less filler plucking, which results in better wear resistance.[81] The increased surface area of the sub-micron filler particles is believed to improve the adhesion at the filler/matrix interface.[82] Due to smaller particle size, the restoration has a better finish, which is observed in its surface texture and the chances of the material's biodegrading over time is reduced.[83] Premise (Kerr/Sybron, Orange, CA) is another nanocomposite launched in the market very recently.[84]

Mitra and Holmes (2003) compared the properties of nanocomposites with the other existing composite resins such as hybrid, microhybrid and microfilled composite resins. It was suggested based on this study that nanocomposites exhibited high translucency, high polish and polish retention similar to those of microfilled, while maintaining the physical properties and wear resistance equivalent to those of hybrid composites.[85] Based on another study (2004), the wear resistance of nanofilled composite resins and ormocer composites was suggested to be comparable or superior to polyacid-modified, microfilled and minifilled composites.[86] Nevertheless, some recent investigation suggests that the performance of all nano-structured composite resins is equivalent to the conventional hybrid composites.[87] It was also suggested that the new nano-structured dental composites are not likely to provide improved wear and fatigue resistance, performances over conventional microfilled composite resins.[88] Recently, nano-silica-fused whiskers have been incorporated into the resin matrix and this modification has been found to provide better wear properties and strength. Xu et al (2004) evaluated the mechanical properties of nano-silica-fused whiskers containing composite resin, and recommended that this material possesses high toughness and wear resistance.[89] It should be kept in mind that the nanocomposites are expensive materials and more clinical studies are required to establish their superiority over other composite resin types.

Composite Toxicity

Composite resin components are sensitizing agents and can cause type IV allergic reactions. Allergic reactions among dental personnel have also been reported.[90,91] In a carefully controlled experiment, Frank and Santierre reported that degradation of composites is possible by the salivary enzymes, although it is still not clear whether this degradation effect involves the surface or the whole restoration.[92] TEGDMA has been known to have unwanted biological responses in solitary form and there has been concern on the effects of TEGDMA that leaches out of composite resin before or after polymerization.[93] The quantity of TEGDMA which can potentially cause cytotoxicity and apoptosis in primary human gingival fibroblasts has been studied. This study suggested that short duration exposure for less than 4 hours did not produce toxic effects, while long duration exposure for 24 hours and concentrations of 5–7.5 mmoL caused reduction in cell growth and induced apoptosis.[94]

Another study (2004) investigated the concentration of leached components from a hybrid composite resin and their effect on female mouse fertility. Although the test groups in this study demonstrated a decrease in pregnancy rate by 54.5% compared to 100% in the controls, it should be noted that the amounts of composite resins used were significantly higher than that can be found in clinical situations. This study also highlighted that the use of ethanol as a solvent can magnify the concentration of components leached from the composite resin.[95] Wada et al (2004) investigated the estrogenicity of 24 commercially available resin composites. Although the release of estrogenic compounds is undesirable, the amount leached was far below the levels required to cause estrogenicity in humans.[96] Nevertheless, this issue of composite resin toxicity requires further studies.

INDIRECT RESTORATIVE MATERIALS

Indirect Composite Resins

Indirect composite resin restorations such as inlays and onlays are preferable over direct composite restoration in large cavities because they offer various advantages over direct composite resin restorations. In indirect composite resins, polymerization of the restoration is carried out in vitro and only polymerization of the luting resin occurs in vivo. This leads to an improved degree of cure, reduced polymerization shrinkage and improved wear resistance in the restoration. Further, it is easier to establish interproximal contacts and occlusal anatomy in indirect composite resin restoration.[1,97,98] It has been suggested that indirect composite resin restorations such as inlays and onlays overcome most of the drawbacks of direct composite resin restorations, and can be considered as an alternative to direct restorations, especially while restoring proximal areas of posterior teeth.[99] Their use has been recommended in premolars since they are subjected to less stresses than in a molar.[100-102] The common causes of failures of indirect composite resin restorations are fracture, loss of marginal integrity, secondary caries and postoperative sensitivity.[100,102] Some studies highlighted better surface texture, anatomic form, marginal integrity and less postoperative sensitivity with indirect composite resin inlays when compared to direct composite resin restorations.[101-103] Kaytan et al conducted a clinical study for a period of 24 months, and concluded that both indirect composite resins and ceramic onlays were successful clinically.[104] Moreover, it has been suggested that the physical properties of indirect composite resins require additional improvement for long-lasting restorations. More long-term clinical investigations are required in this area.

Ceramics

Dental ceramic materials have excellent esthetics, wear resistance, chemical inertness, low thermal conductivity, and low thermal diffusivity.[105] Ceramic materials are brittle, with relatively high compressive strengths but low tensile and flexural strengths.[106] Ceramic restorations are used as anterior and posterior restorations, but being a brittle material, it can fracture when subjected to extreme forces or sharp impact. Traditionally, ceramic inlays are made of feldspathic ceramic material either by sintering or hot pressing or by a more recent technique in which a prefabricated block is milled into a desired restoration.[2] Reinforced ceramic onlays may provide better restorations for posterior teeth.

The Cerec system for restoring teeth by CAD-CAM has been in the market for a while now, and is currently manufactured by Sirona Dental Systems. Initially, CEREC 1 was introduced into the market. Improvements in both the software and hardware technologies led to the development of CEREC 2, CEREC 3 and eventually CEREC 3-D which is the latest version of this computer-assisted technology. CEREC 3-D can be used for the chairside fabrication of ceramic and composite inlays, onlays, crowns and veneers. This system makes use of an optical impression of the prepared tooth obtained with an infrared camera. CEREC 3-D is capable of acquiring a three-dimensional view of the preparation and proposed restoration.[107] The final restoration is designed using a system software and is machined from a block of optimized high performance ceramic or glass ceramic composite, using two separate diamond burs in a separate milling chamber. Martin and Jedynakiewicz conducted a systematic review in 1999 of 15 clinical studies and concluded that Cerec system provided restorations with a high intracoronal mean survival rate of 97.4% over a 4.2-year period.[108] In a 10-year prospective evaluation of CEREC inlays, an estimated survival rate of 89% of the restorations was reported and they found better results with chemically-cured resin cement rather than a dual-curing resin cement.[109] Several long-term studies are conducted to evaluate the long-term survival rate (up to 10 years) of ceramic inlays and onlays, and almost all of them showed a survival rate of more than 90%.[110-113] Premolars showed a better survival rate than molars, and vital teeth provided better results than nonvital teeth.[110] The causes of failures of these restorations are fracture of restoration, fracture of the tooth, wear at the interface, and postoperative thermal hypersensitivity.[108,111]

REFERENCES

1. ADA Council on Scientific Affairs. Direct and indirect restorative materials. JADA. 2003;134(4):463-72.
2. Manhart J, Chen HY, Hamm G, Hickel R. Review of the clinical survival of direct and indirect restorations in posterior teeth of the permanent dentition. Operative Dentistry 2004;29(5):481-508.
3. Yap AU, Teoh SH, Chew CL. Effects of cyclic loading on occlusal contact area wear of composite restoratives. Dent Mater effects of cyclic loading on occlusal contact area wear of composite restoratives; 18:149–58.
4. Leinfelder KF. Do restorations made of amalgam outlast those made of resin-based composite? JADA 2000;131:1186-7.
5. Wahl MJ, Schmitt MM, Overton DA, Gordon MK. Prevalence of cusp fractures in teeth restored with amalgam and with resin-based composite. JADA. 2004;135(8):1127-32.
6. Berglund A. Estimation by a 24-hour study of the daily dose of intra-oral mercury vapor inhaled after release from dental amalgam. J Dent Res 1990;69:1646-51.
7. US Food and Drug Administration Center for Devices and Radiological Health. Consumer update: dental amalgams. *www.fda.gov/cdrh/consumer/amalgams.html;* http://*www.fda.gov/cdrh/consumer/amalgams.html.*
8. McGivern B, Pemberton M, Theaker ED, Buchanan JA, Thornhill MH. Delayed and immediate hypersensitivity reactions associated with the use of amalgam. Br Dent J 2000;188:73-6.
9. Life Sciences Research Office. Review and analysis of the literature on the potential health effects of dental amalgam Bethesda: FASEB Special Publications on 2004.pp.1-165.
10. ADA Council on Scientific Affairs. Dental mercury hygiene recommendations. J Am Dent Assoc. 2003;134:1498-9.

11. Gao W, Smales RJ. Fluoride release/uptake of conventional and resin-modified glass ionomers, and compomers. J Dent Res 2001;29:301-6.
12. Delbem AC, Pedrini D, Franca JG, Machado TM. Fluoride release/recharge from restorative materials—effect of fluoride gels and time. Oper Dent. 2005;30(6):690-5.
13. Yap AU, Teo JC, Teoh SH. Comparative wear resistance of reinforced glass ionomer restorative materials. Oper Dent 2001;26(4).
14. Kunzelmann KH, Burkle V, Bauer C. Two-body and three-body wear of glass ionomer cements. Int J Paediatr Dent. 2003;13(6):434-40.
15. Mount GJ. Glass ionomers: A review of their current status. Operative Dentistry 1999;24(2):115–24.
16. Attin T, Buchalla W, Kielbassa AM, Hellwig E. Curing shrinkage and volumetric changes of resin- modified glass ionomer restorative materials. Dent Mater. 1995;11:359-62.
17. Tyas MJ. Milestones in adhesion: Glass-ionomer cements. Journal of Adhesive Dentistry 2003; 5(4):259-66.
18. Yap AU, Pek YS, Cheang P. Physico-mechanical properties of a fast-set highly viscous GIC restorative, J Oral Rehabil. Physico-mechanical properties of a fast-set highly viscous GIC restorative, J Oral Rehabil. 2003;30:1-8.
19. Duinen RN, Kleverlaan CJ, de Gee AJ, Werner A, Feilzer AJ. Early and long-term wear of 'fast-set' conventional glass-ionomer cements. Dent Mater. 21(8):716-20.
20. Frencken JE, Holmgren CJ. ART: a minimal intervention approach to manage dental caries. Dent Update. 2004;31(5):295-8, 301.
21. Botelho MG. Inhibitory effects on selected oral bacteria of antibacterial agents incorporated in a glass ionomer. Caries Res 2003;37:108-14.
22. Sanders BJ, Gregory RL, Moore K, Avery DR. Antibacterial and physical properties of resin modified glass-ionomers combined with chlorhexidine. J Oral Rehabil. 2002;29:553-8.
23. Bayne SC. Dental composites/glass ionomers: clinical reports. Adv Dent Res. 1992;6:65-77.
24. Wilson AD. Resin-modified glass ionomer cements. Int J Prosth 1990;3:425-9.
25. McCabe JF. Resin-modified glass-ionomers. Biomaterial.1998;19:521-7.
26. Costa CAS, Hebling J, Garcia-Godoy F, Hanks CT, Garcia-Godoy F, Hanks CT. In vitro cytotoxicity of five glass-ionomer cements. Biomaterials 2003;24:3853-8.
27. Geurtsen W Substances released from dental resin composites and glass ionomer cements. Eur J Oral Sci 1998;106:687-95.
28. Hashimoto M, Ito S, Tay FR, Svizero NR, Sano H, Kaga M, et al. Fluid movement across the resin dentin interface during and after bonding. J Dent Res. 2004;83:843-8.
29. Sidhu SK, Schmalz G. The biocompatibility of glass-ionomer cement materials. A status report for the American Journal of Dentistry. Am J Dent. 2001;14:387-96.
30. Tyas MJ, Burrow MF. Adhesive restorative materials: A review. Australian Dental Journal 2004;49(3):112-21.
31. Souza PP, Aranha AM, Hebling J, Giro EM, Costa CA. In vitro cytotoxicity and in vivo biocompatibility of contemporary resin-modified glass-ionomer cements. Dent Mater. 2005: Dec 29; [Epub ahead of print].
32. Xie D, Chung ID, Wang GG, Mays J. Synthesis and evaluation of novel bifunctional oligomer-based composites for dental applications. Journal of Biomaterial Applications 2006;20(3):221-36.
33. Young AM, Rafeeka, S.A. and Howlett, J.A. FTIR Investigation of Monomer Polymerization and Polyacid Neutralization Kinetics and Mechanisms in various Aesthetic Dental Restorative Materials. Biomaterials 2004;25:823-33.
34. Ruse ND. What is a Compomer? Journal of Canadian Dental Association 1999;65:500-4.
35. Gross LC GA, Casamassimo PS. Compomers as class II restorations in primary molars. Pediatric Dentistry 2001;23:24-7.
36. Pascon FM, Kantovitz KR, Caldo-Teixeira AS, Borges AF, Silva TN, Puppin-Rontani RM, et al. Clinical evaluation of composite and compomer restorations in primary teeth:24-month results. J Dent Res. 2005 Oct 17; [Epub ahead of print]

37. Gross LC, Griffen AL, Casamassimo PS. Compomers as Class II restorations in primary molars. Pediatr Dent. 2001;23(1):24-7.

38. Adusei GO, Deb S, Nicholson JW, A, Berglund. Preliminary study of experimental polyacid-modified composite resins (compomers) containing vinyl phosphonic acid. Dent Mater. 2005;21(6): 491-7.

39. Yap AU, Mok BY. Surface finish of a new hybrid aesthetic restorative material. Operative Dentistry 2002;27(2):161-6.

40. Yap AU, Wattanapayungkul P. Effects of in-office tooth whiteners on hardness of tooth-colored restoratives. Operative Dentistry 2002;27(2):137-41.

41. Itota T, Nakabo S, Iwai Y, Konishi N, Nagamine M, Torii Y. Inhibition of artificial secondary caries by fluoride-releasing adhesives on root dentin. J Oral Rehabil 2002;29(6):523-7.

42. Itthagarun A, Tay FR, Pashley DH, Wefel JS, Garcia-Godoy F, Wei SH. Single-step, self-etch adhesives behave as permeable membranes after polymerization. Part III. Evidence from fluid conductance and artificial caries inhibition. Am J Dent. 2004;17(6):394-400.

43. Gonzalez Ede H, Yap AU, Hsu SC. Demineralization inhibition of direct tooth-colored restorative materials. Oper Dent. 2004;29(5):578-85.

44. Tay FR, Pashley EL, Huang C, Hashimoto M, Sano H, Smales RJ. The glass-ionomer phase in resin-based restorative materials. Journal of Dental Research 2001;80(9):1808-12.

45. Sonoda H, Sasafuchl Y, Kitasako Y, Arakawa M, Otsuki M, Tagami J. Pulpal response to a fluoride-releasing all-in-one resin-bonding system. Oper Dent. 2002;27(3):271-7.

46. Shimada Y, Seki Y, Uzzaman MA, Foxton RM, Tagami J. Effect of a fluoride-releasing one-step adhesive system on monkey pulp tissue. J Adhes Dent. 2005:241-5;7(3):241-5.

47. Huang C, Kei LH, Wei SH, Cheung GS, Tay FR, Pashley DH. The influence of hygroscopic expansion of resin-based restorative materials on artificial gap reduction. J Adhes Dent. 2002;4(1):61-71.

48. Yap AU,Tham SY, Zhu LY, Lee HK. Short-term fluoride release from various aesthetic restorative materials. Oper Dent. 2002;27(3):259-65.

49. Hickel R, Dasch W, Janda R, Tyas M, Anusavice K. New direct restorative materials. International Dental Journal 1998;48(1):3-16.

50. Manhart JK, J Kunzelmann, Chen H, Hickel, R. Mechanical properties and wear behavior of light-cured packable composite resins. Dental Materials 2000;16(1):33-40.

51. Hennig AC, Helbig FR, Haufe E, Richter G, Klimm HW. Restoration of Class V cavities with the Ormocer-based filling system Admira. Schweiz Monatsschr Zahnmed 2004;114(2).

52. Rosin M, Steffen H, Konschake C, Greese U, Teichmann D, Hartmann A, et al. One-year evaluation of an ormocer restorative—a multipractice clinical trial. Clin Oral Investig 2003;4;7(1):20-6.

53. Janda R, Roulet JF, Latta M, Ruttermann S. The effects of thermocycling on the flexural strength and flexural modulus of modern resin-based filling materials. Dent Mater. 2006 Jan 5; [Epub ahead of print].

54. Yazici AR, Celik C, Ozgunaltay G. Microleakage of different resin composite types. Quintessence Int 2004;35(10).

55. Yap AU, Tan CH, Chung SM. Wear behavior of new composite restoratives. Oper Dent 2004;29(3):269-74.

56. Kournetas N, Chakmakchi M, Kakaboura A, Rahiotis C, Geis-Gerstorfer J. Marginal and internal adaptation of Class II ormocer and hybrid resin composite restorations before and after load cycling. Clin Oral Investig. 2004;8(3):123-9.

57. Ajlouni R, Bishara B, Soliman, MM Oonsombat, C Laffoon, JF Warren, J. The use of ormocer as an alternative material for bonding orthodontic brackets. Angle Orthodontist 2005;75(1):106-8.

58. Attar N, Turgut MD. Fluoride release and uptake capacities of fluoride-releasing restorative materials. Oper Dent. 2003;28(4):395-402.

59. Attar N, Onen A. Fluoride release and uptake characteristics of aesthetic restorative materials. J Oral Rehabil. 2002;29(8):791-8.

60. Phillips RW Phillips Science of Dental Materials. 1996; 10th edition: p274.

61. Johnston WM, Reisbick MH. Color and translucency changes during and after curing of esthetic restorative materials. Dent Mater 1997;13(2):89-97.
62. Asmussen E Peutzfeldt A. Influence of selected components on crosslink density in polymer structures. Eur J Oral Sci 2001;109(4):282-5.
63. Braga RR, Ballester RY, Ferracane JL. Factors involved in the development of polymerization shrinkage stress in resin-composites: a systematic review. Dent Mater 2005;21(10):962-70.
64. Labella R, Lambrechts P, Van Meerbeek B, Vanherle G. Polymerization shrinkage and elasticity of flowable composites and filled adhesives. Dent Mater. 1999;15(2):128-37.
65. Fortin D, Vargas MA. The spectrum of composites: new techniques and materials. J Am Dent Assoc. 2000;131.
66. Lohbauer U, Frankenberger R, Kramer N, Petschelt A. Strength and fatigue performance versus filler fraction of different types of direct dental restoratives. J Biomed Mater Res B Appl Biomater. 2006;76(1):114-20.
67. Abe Y, Braem MJ, Lambrechts P, Inoue S, Takeuchi M, Van Meerbeek B. Fatigue behavior of packable composites. Biomaterials 2005;26(17):3405-9.
68. de Souza FB, Guimaraes RP, Silva CH. A clinical evaluation of packable and microhybrid resin composite restorations: one-year report. Quintessence Int 2005;36(1):41-8.
69. Cobb DS, MacGregor KM, Vargas MA, Denehy GE. The physical properties of packable and conventional posterior resin-based composites: a comparison. J Am Dent Assoc. 2000;131(11): 1610-5.
70. Poon ECM, Smale RJ, Yip KHK. Clinical evaluation of packable and conventional hybrid posterior resin-based composites. Results at 3.5 years. J Amer Dent Assoc. 2005;136:1533–40.
71. Choi KK, Ferracane JL, Hilton TJ, Charlton D. Properties of packable composites. J Esthet Dent 2000;12:216-26.
72. Klein F, Keller AK, Staehle HJ, Dorfer CE. Proximal contact formation with different restorative materials and techniques. American Journal of Dentistry 2002;15(4):232-35.
73. Peumans M, Van Meerbeek B, Ascherickx K, Simon S, Abe Y, Lambrechts P, et al. Do condensable composites help to achieve better proximal contacts? Dent Mater. 2001;17:533-41.
74. Herrero AA, Yaman P, Dennison JB. Polymerization shrinkage and depth of cure of packable composites. Quintessence Int 2005;36(1):25-31.
75. Wang L, Garcia FC, Amarante de Araujo P, Franco EB, Mondelli RF. Wear resistance of packable resin composites after simulated tooth brushing test. J Esthet Restor Dent 2004;16(5):303-14;14-5.
76. Lopes GC, Baratieri LN, Monteiro S Jr, Vieira LC. Effect of posterior resin composite placement technique on the resin-dentin interface formed in vivo. Quintessence Int 2004;35:156-61.
77. Tjandrawinata R, Irie M, Suzuki K. Flexural properties of eight flowable light-cured restorative materials, in immediate vs 24-hour water storage. Operative Dentistry 2005;30(2):239-49.
78. Tiba A, Charlton DG, Vandewalle KS, Cohen ME. Volumetric polymerization shrinkage of resin composites under simulated intraoral temperature and humidity conditions. Operative Dentistry 2005;30(6):696-701.
79. Li Q, Jepsen S, Albers HK, Eberhard. Flowable materials as an intermediate layer could improve the marginal and internal adaptation of composite restorations in Class-V-cavities. Flowable materials as an intermediate layer could improve the marginal and internal adaptation of composite restorations in Class-V-cavities. Dent Mater. 2006;22(3):250-7.
80. Gomec Y, Dorter C, Dabanoglu A, Koray F. Effect of resin-based material combination on the compressive and the flexural strength. J Oral Rehabil 2005;32(2):122-7.
81. Xing XS, Li RKY. Wear behavior of epoxy matrix composites filled with uniform-sized sub-micron spherical silica particles. Wear 2004;256:21-6.
82. Sawyer WG, Freudenberg KD, Bhimaraj P, Schadler L. A study on the friction and wear behavior of PTFE filled with alumina nanoparticles. Wear 2003;254:573-80.

83. Hervas-Garcia A, Martinez-Lozano MA, Cabanes-Vila J, Barjau-Escribano A, Fos-Galve P. Composite resins. A review of the materials and clinical indications. Med Oral Patol Oral Cir Bucal. 2006;11(2):E215-20.
84. Terry DA. Restoring the incisal edge. NY State Dent J. 2005;71(5):30-5.
85. Mitra SB, Wu D, Holmes BN. An application of nanotechnology in advanced dental materials. J Am Dent Assoc. 2003;134(10):1382-90.
86. Yap AU, Tan CH, Chung SM. Wear behavior of new composite restoratives. Operative Dentistry 2004;29(3):269-74.
87. Ernst CP, Brandenbusch M, Meyer G, Canbek K, Gottschalk F, Willershausen B. Two-year clinical performance of a nanofiller vs a fine-particle hybrid resin composite. Clin Oral Investig 2006; [Epub ahead of print].
88. Turssi CP, Ferracane JL. Wear and fatigue behavior of nano-structured dental resin composite. J Biomed Mater Res B Appl Biomater. 2006, Jan 30; [Epub ahead of print].
89. Xu HHK, Quinn JB, Giuseppetti AA. Wear and mechanical properties of nano-silica-fused whisker composites. Journal of Dental Research 2004;83(12):930-5.
90. Kenarva L, Jolanki R, Estlander T. Occupational skin allergy in the dental profession. Dermatol Clinics 12 1994. pp. 517-32.
91. Munksgaard EC, Hansen EK, Engen T. Self-reported occupational dermatological reactions among Danish dentists. Eur J Oral Sci 1996;104:396-402.
92. Finer Y, Santerre JP. Salivary esterase activity and its association with the biodegradation of dental composites. J Dent Res. 2003;83:22-6.
93. Allen EP, Bayne SC, Cronin RJ, Donovan TE, Kois JC, Summitt JB. Annual review of selected dental literature: Report of the Committee on Scientific Investigation of the American Academy of Restorative Dentistry. Journal of Prosthetic Dentistry 2004;92(1):39-71.
94. Janke V, von Neuhoff H, Schlegelberger B, Leyhausen G, Geursten W. EGDMA causes apoptosis in primary human gingival fibroblasts. J Dent Res. 2003;82:814-8.
95. Al-Hiyasat AS, Darmani H, Elbetieha AM. Leached components from dental composites and their effects on fertility of female mice. Eur J Oral Sci 2004;112:267-72.
96. Wada H, Tarumi H, Imazato S, Narimatsu M, Ebisu SI. In vitro estrogenicity of resin composites. J Dent Res. 2004;83:222-6.
97. Peutzfelt A. Indirect resin and ceramic systems. Oper Dent. 2001;6:153-76.
98. Suzuki S, Nagai E, Taira Y, Minesaki Y. In vitro wear of indirect composite restoratives. J Prosthet Dent. 2002;88:431-36.
99. Leirskar J, Nordbo H, Thoresen NR, Henaug T, von der Fehr FR. A four to six years follow-up of indirect resin composite inlays/onlays. Acta Odontol Scand 2003;61:247-51.
100. Donly KJ, Jensen ME, Triolo P, Chan D. A clinical comparison of resin composite inlay and onlay posterior restorations and cast-gold restorations at 7 years. Quintessence Int 1999;30(3):163-8.
101. Scheibenbogen-Fuchsbrunner A, Manhart J Scheibenbogen-Fuchsbrunner A MJ, Kremers L, Kunzelmann KH, Hickel R. Two-year clinical evaluation of direct and indirect composite restorations in posterior teeth. J Prosthet Dent. 1999;82(4):391-7.
102. Pallesen U, Qvist V. Composite resin fillings and inlays. An 11-year evaluation. Clin Oral Investig. 2003;7(2):71-9.
103. Manhart J NP, Scheibenbogen-Fuchsbrunner A, Hickel R. Three-year clinical evaluation of direct and indirect composite restorations in posterior teeth. J Prosthet Dent. 2000;84:289-96.
104. Pallesen U, Qvist V, Pamir T, Tezel H. Clinical evaluation of indirect resin composite and ceramic onlays over a 24-month period. Gen Dent. 2005;53(5):329-34.
105. Anusavice KJ. Degradability of dental ceramics. Adv Dent Res. 1992;6:82-9.
106. Phillips RW, Editor. Phillips' science of dental materials. 2003;11:655-719.
107. Allen KL, Schenkel AB. An overview of the CEREC 3D CAD/CAM system. Gen Dent. 2004;52:234-5.
108. Martin N, Jedynakiewicz NM. Clinical performance of CEREC ceramic inlays: a systematic review. Dent Mater. 1999;15:54-61.

109. Sjogren G, Molin M, van Dijken JW, Sjogren G MM, van Dijken JW. A 10-year prospective evaluation of CAD/CAM-manufactured (CEREC). Ceramic inlays cemented with a chemically cured or dual-cured resin composite. Int J Prosthont 2004;17:241-6.
110. Reiss B, Walther W. Clinical long-term results and 10-year Kaplan-Meier analysis of CEREC restorations. Int J Computer Dent. 2000;3:9-23.
111. Otto T, De Nisco S. Computer-aided direct ceramic restorations: a 10-year prospective clinical study of CEREC CAD/CAM inlays and onlays. Int J Prosthodont 2002;15:122-8.
112. Posselt A, Kerschbaum T. Longevity of 2328 chairside CEREC inlays and onlays. Int J Computer Dent. 2003;6:231-48.
113. Reich SM, Wichmann M, Rinne H, Shortall A. Clinical performance of large, all-ceramic CAD/CAM-generated restorations after three years: a pilot study. J Am Dent. Assoc. 2004;135:605-12.

BIBLIOGRAPHY

1. Anusavice Kenneth J. Philips Science of Dental Materials. Harcourt Asia P Ltd. 10th edn., 1998.
2. Anusavice Kenneth J. Philips Science of Dental Materials. Saunders 11th edn., 2004.
3. Combe EC. Notes on Dental Materials, Churchill Livingstone. 6th edn., 1992.
4. Craig Robert G, Powers John M, Wataha John C. Dental Materials Properties and Manipulation Mosby. 9th edn., 2004.
5. John M Powers, John C Wataha. Dental Materials Properties and Manipulation. Mosby. 9th edn. 2008.
6. McCabe John F. Applied Dental Materials, Blackwell Scientific Publications. 7th edn., 1990.
7. van Noort Richard. Introduction to Dental Materials. Mosby, 1994.

2. Recent Advances in Dental Materials

RECENT ADVANCES IN IMPRESSION MATERIALS

Modifications of Zinc Oxide Eugenol Paste

Surgical Paste

Modified zinc oxide eugenol paste can be used as an intraoral bandage to protect cut surfaces and to prevent infection of tissues after surgical procedure such as gingivectomy.

It is available in paste, powder and liquid forms respectively.

Paste

- Paste contains more amount of eugenol
- Gives antiseptic and sedative effect
- More amount of filler
- Gives fracture resistance under masticatory load
- More amount of plasticizer
- Increases the flow and softness
- Tetracycline—used as antibiotic.

Powder

- Zinc oxide : 36%—reactive ingredient
- Rosin : 30%—plasticizer, to increase the flow
- Asbestos fiber : 5%—to increase setting
- Zinc acetate : 2%—accelerator.

Liquid

- Eugenol : 80 cc—reactive ingredient
- Vegetable oil : 20 cc—placticizer and acts as a retarder.

Bite Registration Paste

Composition: Similar to the conventional zinc oxide eugenol with additional plasticizer (petroleum jelly) to reduce the tackiness to the soft tissues.

This paste is used to record the occlusal relationship of maxillary and mandibular teeth or arches during the preparation of complete dentures partial denture and crown and bridge, etc.

Noneugenol Paste

Eugenol present in zinc oxide eugenol causes burning sensation, allergic reaction, and chronic gastric disturbances in some patients.

To overcome this problem, carboxylic acid can be used instead of eugenol.

$$ZnO + RCOH \rightarrow (RCOO)_2Zn + H_2O$$

Eugenol is replaced by an organic acid like orthoethoxybenzoic acid (EBA) to overcome its disadvantages.

Alginate

Dust-free Alginate

The silica particles in the dust of alginate lead to the possible health hazards if it is inhaled. Few manufacturers incorporated glycerine or glycol as dedusting agents to the alginate powder to agglomerate the powder particles which makes the powder denser than in the uncoated state.

Siliconized Alginate

The drawback of unmodified alginate is low tear strength. To overcome this, silicone polymer is being incorporated in alginate to develop stronger material.

It is available in tray and syringe consistency. This is considered as hybrid of alginate and silicone elastomers.

Chromatic or Color Indicator Alginate

To show the different stages during mixing the color indicators are added which helps the operator during recording of the impression.

For example:

- Violet—spatulation
- Pink—loading
- Light yellow—setting.

Alginate-containing Disinfecting Agent

Quaternary ammonium salts are chlorhexamine are added to alginate powder to destroy the microorganisms. The patients have to be strictly informed not to swallow the impression materials.

Alginot FS

- It is a type of alginate which is available in the form of cartridge which sets fast to increase the patient comfort without compromising the performance or working time
- The improved thixotrophic consistency decreases the slumping and displacement from the tray
- Better dimensional stability.

Elastomers

Hydrophilic Addition Polysilicone

One of the disadvantages of silicone impression material is its hydrophobic nature.

Nonionic surfactant is added to the paste to render the surface of the impression hydrophilic. This surfactant migrates towards the surface of the impression material and has its hydrophilic segment oriented towards the surface.

This allows the impression material to wet the soft tissues and maximum details will be obtained on the gypsum product cast.

Another method to solve the hydrophobic nature of impression material is by using the surface active spray which is used to coat the surface of the hard or soft tissues prior to recording an impression.

This helps to improve the affinity between the impression material and the oral tissues during recording of the impression and also increases the compatibility with the water-based gypsum model material.

Note: Latex gloves have been shown to adversely affect the setting of the addition silicone material because the sulfur of latex rubber glove can migrate to the surface of the gloves. These compounds can be transferred onto the prepared teeth. And adjacent of soft tissues during tooth preparation and other procedures.

This compound can poison the platinum containing catalyst which results in retarded or no polymerization in the contaminated area of the impression. To overcome this problem the new type of gloves like vinyl or nitrile gloves can be used.

RECENT ADVANCES IN WAXES

1. *Orthodontic tray waxes:* Soft white plastic wax sticks for orthodontic use in extension of periphery.
2. *Gum orthodontic waxes:* Adhere to orthodontic appliances to help to relieve the irritated tissues.
3. *Disclosing wax:* A creamy wax used to repair the defects in the wax patterns.

It is also used to identify the pressure points in the denture which need to be relieved. It is also known as pressure indicator wax.

RECENT ADVANCES IN INVESTMENT MATERIALS

Two types of investment material have been developed recently for producing all ceramic restorations:

- First type is used for the cast glass technique. Investment material for this type is provided by the manufacturer of the glass casting equipment. And is composed of phosphate bonded refractories.
- Second type is used for all ceramic restorations. The refractory die type of material which is used for all ceramic veneers, inlays and crowns.

Refractory dies are made by pouring the investment into the impression. When the investment sets, the die is removed and heated to remove the gases (degassing).

Refractory die spacer may be added to the surface. Porcelain or other ceramic powder are added to the die surface and fired. This material also contains phosphate bonded investment material with fine grained refractory fillers to allow the accurate reproduction.

Investment Materials for Titanium

Pure titanium and its alloys have very high melting point (1668°C) requires special investment material to withstand the casting temperature and its high oxygen sensitivity causes oxidation quickly.

Phosphate bonded or alumina cement bonded investment material with different refractory material recently developed in Japan.

Example: $Al_2O_3 + ZrO_2$, $Al_2O_3 + SiO_2$, $Al_2O_3 + LiAlSiO_2$, $MgO + Al_2O_3 + ZrO$, etc. combinations.

The refractory materials contains ethyl silicate bonding agents and mold casting temperature is lowered to room temperature to avoid oxidation and to increase the setting expansion.

RECENT ADVANCES IN DENTURE BASE RESINS

Rubber Reinforced Acrylics or High Impact Strength Acrylic Resins

- Impact strength of acrylic resins can be significantly improved by the incorporation of elastomers/rubber
- The elastomers absorbs the energy on impact and thus protects the acrylic resin from fracture
- *These materials are:* butadiene-styrene, rubber reinforced polymethyl methacrylate
- The rubber particles are grafted to methyl methacrylate so that they bond well to heat polymerized matrix
- It is available in powder and liquid form.

Merits

- Better impact strength (2.1J) and fatigue properties
- Greater resistance to crack propagation
- Because of the rubber decrease in the water sorption.

Demerits

Expensive.

Hydrophilic Polyacrylates

Poly (hydroxyethyl methacrylate) has been used as a denture base material and a soft denture liner. Hydroxy substituted acrylic increase the water sorption and wettability of the copolymer by saliva. It gives enhanced denture retention.

Light Activated Denture Base Resins

- Dispended in the form of single component system
- Supplied in sheet and rope form
- *Composition:* Consist of urethane (dimethacrylate) matrix
- High molecular weight acrylic resin monomer camphoroquinone (initiator)
- Microfine silica
- Organic fillers
- Acrylic beads
- Visible light (activator)
- The denture is polymerized in a light chamber with blue light of 400–500 nm
- Teeth are arranged and the denture base is molded on an accurate cast
- The denture is rotated on a table in chamber to provide uniform exposure to the light source
- After polymerization, the denture is removed from the cast finished and polished in a conventional manner.

Radiopaque Denture Base Resins

- Acrylic resin is radiolucent and it cannot be imaged using radiographic techniques if accidentally swallowed by the patient
- Additives like Triphenyl bismuth (TPP) is added to conventional autopolymerized resins to get the radiopaque effect
- Required level of TPP is 14.5% otherwise acrylic resin will undrgo brittle fracture.
- Other additives like powdered metals, inorganic salts such as barium sulfate, comonomer containing heay metals (e.g. barium acrylate) can be added.

High Microhardness Denture Base Resins

- Conventional denture base resins made up of PMMA is low in strength, soft and brittle on impact
- The mechanical properties improved by adding different reinforcing phases to the PMMA matrix
- Wet ground muscovite mica is added to PMMA which increases the microhardness (conc 20%) and decreases the flexural strength.

Ceramopolymer

- It is a new generation color stable resin. These materials exhibit only slight change in chroma and no change in value or brightness with usage
- Additional advantage of the material is decreased shrinkage and wears rates.

PMMA Reinforced with Nanoparticles

- PMMA is reinforced with zinc oxide, titanium, gentamicin and ceramic nanoparticles
- This reinforcement gives antiseptic effect which prevents the growth of *Candida albicans* and other bacterial colonies over the denture surface.

Valplast

- This is a flexible denture base material used for partial denture made up of nylon thermoplastic resin
- Highly biocompatible.

Sunflex

- Flexible denture base material made from a strong biocompatible nylon thermoplastic
- Virtually invisible, unbreakable, metal-free, light weight and extremely comfortable
- More stain-resistant than other flexible acrylics.

RECENT ADVANCES IN TISSUE CONDITIONERS

Tissue Conditioners with Silver Zeolite

Tissue conditioners containing silver zeolite (SZ) have been shown to have antimicrobial effect on *Candida albicans* and *Staphylococcus aureus.*

RECENT ADVANCES IN NOBLE METAL ALLOYS

Pd-Cu-Ga

- Pd—75%, Cu—10%, Ga—5–10%, and trace metals.
- Because of gallium the surface oxide layer formed, will prevent the tarnish and corrosion and also helps in the bonding between metal and ceramic.
- This particular has better mechanical properties.
- Drawback of this alloy is—copper causes discoloration.

Pd-Ga-Ag

- Pd—80–85%, Ga—5–10%, Ag—5–8%, and trace metals.
- Drawback of this alloy is—silver causes the discoloration.

RECENT ADVANCES IN BASE METAL ALLOYS

Cast Ti-6Al-4V

- Microstructure have been refined by temporary alloying with hydrogen
- The microstructure of the alloy can have a grain size less than 1 μm
- This results in increased yield strength (974–1119 MPa), ultimate tensile strength (1025–1152 MPa) and fatigue strength (643–669 MPa).

RECENT ADVANCES IN POLISHING AGENTS

- The mechanical polishing results in surface abrasion
- To overcome this, the new chemical polishing technique is introduced
- In this technique, the prostheses after finishing procedure is immersed in heated MMA monomer bar with temperature of 750°C for 10 seconds
- The advantage of this technique is that it eliminates the polishing sequence and the possibility of smoothening intaglio surface.

RECENT ADVANCES IN DENTURE TEETH

- The resin posterior denture teeth usually undergo abrasion over a period of time
- The complete denture prepared using zirconia teeth showed relatively low abrasion of the posterior denture teeth and provides a longer useful life span than other denture teeth material.

RECENT ADVANCES IN GYPSUM

- To improve the mechanical properties, especially the abrasion resistance, lignosulfonates are added to gypsum products which acts as wetting agent
- Improves the wettability of the gypsum products
- Such additives, increases the wetting by reducing the surface tension and produce harder, stronger and denser set gypsum.

Aqueous Solution of Chemical Disinfectants

Sodium hypochlorite (0.5–5%) and povidone-iodine (0.1%) with no significant effect on the dimensional accuracy and reproducibility of the resultant cast.

RECENT ADVANCES IN LUTING AGENTS

Hybrid Ionomer Cement with Radiopaques

Composition

- *Powder*: Fluoroaluminosilicate and borosilicate glasses
- *Liquid*: Complex monomer with carboxylic acid that undergo acid base reaction with glass and vinyl groups when chemically activated.

BIBLIOGRAPHY

1. Anusavice KJ, Phillips RW. Phillips' science of dental materials. 11th ed. St. Louis: WB Saunders; 2003.
2. Craig RG, Powers JM, Sakaguchi RL. Craig's restorative dental materials. 12th ed. St. Louis: Mosby Elsevier; 2006.
3. Gladwin, Marcia and Bagby, Michael. 2004. Clinical Aspect of Dental Materials 2nd Edition. USA: Lippincot Williams and Wilkins.
4. Jeffrey D Fleigel, Alan J Sutton. Reliable and Repeatable Centric Relation Adjustment of the Maxillary Occlusal Device. Journal of Prosthodontics pages 233-236, April 2013.
5. John. F Mc Cabe, Angus, WG Walls "Applied dental materials, 8th ed. Blackwell science Oxford.1998.

6. Mattie PA, Rawls. HR, Cabassol. I "Development of a radiopaque autopolymerzing dental acrylic resin". J Prosthodont. 1994;3(4):213-8.
7. Mohammed Q. Al-Rifaiy. The effect of mechanical and chemical polishing techniques on the surface roughness of denture base acrylic resins. The Saudi Dental Journal Volume 2010;22(1):13-7.
8. Ronald L. Sakaguchi. Craig's Restorative Dental Materials, 13th edn.
9. S. Mahalakshmi, "Materials used in dentistry" 1st ed.Wolters Kluwer health (India) 2013.
10. Ulf Ortengren, Fredrik Andersson, Ulrika Elgh, Björn Terselius, Stig Karlsson. Influence of pH and storage time on the sorption and solubility behavior of three composite resin materials. Journal of dentistry. 1997;25:373-5.
11. V. Shama Bhat, BT Nandhish, "Science of dental materials". 1st ed. Satish kumar Jain CBS publishers (India) 2006.
12. V. Shama Bhat, BT Nandhish, "Science of dental materials". 2nd ed. Satish kumar Jain CBS publishers (India) 2013.
13. William J. O'Brien, "Dental Materials and Their Selection" 2nd ed. Chicago: Quintessence Pub. Co.1997.
14. *www.kerrdental.eu/lab/kerrlabwaxes/productfamily/orthodontictraywax.*
15. *www.kerrdental.ice/media/6574/01_e.pdf. (impression materials).*

Index

Page numbers followed by *f* refer to figure